Praise for *Self-Care for New and Student Nurses*

"In Self-Care for New and Student Nurses, *Dorrie Fontaine and colleagues have compiled a compendium of resources relevant to all nurses engaged in clinical practice, education, and leadership. In elevating the necessity of self-care, the authors acknowledge the reality that while nursing is one of the most noble professions, it is also one of the most difficult. From working in a global pandemic to countering systemic racism, the book identifies anticipatory challenges and provides tools and resources for self-care and leadership. This is an astonishingly rich and relevant text that truly should be required in every nursing program. If widely adopted, this text has the potential to transform the profession."*

–Mary Jo Kreitzer, PhD, RN, FAAN
Director, Earl E. Bakken Center for Spirituality & Healing
Professor, University of Minnesota School of Nursing

"Our work as nurses brings gladness into our lives and, at the same time, meets some of the world's greatest needs. But because these needs are so great, the work's demands can threaten this gladness. Self-Care for New and Student Nurses *teaches us all, including seasoned nurses, practices that safeguard our gladness. It is a timely and exigent wellness handbook. I highly recommend it."*

–Mark Lazenby, PhD, APRN, FAAN
He, him, his
Professor of Nursing and Philosophy
Associate Dean for Faculty and Student Affairs
University of Connecticut School of Nursing

"A rare intersection of essential, practical, science-based, and aspirational wisdom! Readers will appreciate the genuine emphasis on whole-person self-care and a focus on organizational aspects of healthcare that still require advocacy and effort. The authors provide a 360-degree view of self-care for student nurses that is also highly relevant and engaging for nursing faculty and clinical preceptors. A guide that readers can turn to repeatedly for renewed insights and inspiration."

–Teri Pipe, PhD, RN
ASU Chief Well-Being Officer
Founding Director, ASU Center for Mindfulness, Compassion and Resilience
Dean Emerita and Professor
Edson College of Nursing and Health Innovation
Arizona State University

"This book blends current scientific evidence with practical strategies to empower not only students and new-to-practice nurses but also experienced nurses in building resilience and enduring life skills that are as important as any learned in the simulation lab. Introduce this book early in their program and integrate it throughout to guide discussions of professionalism, nursing identity, patient and self-advocacy, and team-based care. It is life changing!"

–Kathleen McCauley, PhD, RN, FAAN, FAHA
Professor of Cardiovascular Nursing
Former Associate Dean for Academic Programs
NewCourtland Center for Transitions and Health
University of Pennsylvania School of Nursing

"A rich and powerful book on the importance of self-care for nurses and practices that enhance resilience and well-being. This is a must-read for every nurse!"

–Rev. Joan Jiko Halifax
Abbot, Upaya Zen Center
Santa Fe, New Mexico

Self-Care

for New and Student

Nurses

Dorrie K. Fontaine, PhD, RN, FAAN

Tim Cunningham, DrPH, MSN, RN, FAAN

Natalie May, PhD

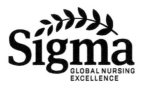

Sigma
GLOBAL NURSING
EXCELLENCE

Sigma Theta Tau International Honor Society of Nursing (Sigma) is a nonprofit organization whose mission is developing nurse leaders anywhere to improve healthcare everywhere. Founded in 1922, Sigma has more than 135,000 active members in over 100 countries and territories. Members include practicing nurses, instructors, researchers, policymakers, entrepreneurs, and others. Sigma's more than 540 chapters are located at more than 700 institutions of higher education throughout Armenia, Australia, Botswana, Brazil, Canada, Colombia, Croatia, England, Eswatini, Ghana, Hong Kong, Ireland, Israel, Italy, Jamaica, Japan, Jordan, Kenya, Lebanon, Malawi, Mexico, the Netherlands, Nigeria, Pakistan, Philippines, Portugal, Puerto Rico, Scotland, Singapore, South Africa, South Korea, Sweden, Taiwan, Tanzania, Thailand, the United States, and Wales. Learn more at www.sigmanursing.org.

Sigma Theta Tau International
550 West North Street
Indianapolis, IN, USA 46202

To request a review copy for course adoption, order additional books, buy in bulk, or purchase for corporate use, contact Sigma Marketplace at 888.654.4968 (US/Canada toll-free), +1.317.687.2256 (International), or solutions@sigmamarketplace.org.

To request author information, or for speaker or other media requests, contact Sigma Marketing at 888.634.7575 (US/Canada toll-free) or +1.317.634.8171 (International).

ISBN:	9781948057813
EPUB ISBN:	9781948057820
PDF ISBN:	9781948057837
MOBI ISBN:	9781948057844

Library of Congress Cataloging-in-Publication data

Names: Fontaine, Dorrie K., author. | Cunningham, Tim, 1978- author. | May, Natalie, author. | Sigma Theta Tau International, issuing body.
Title: Self-care for new and student nurses / Dorrie K. Fontaine, Tim Cunningham, Natalie May.
Description: Indianapolis, IN : Sigma, 2021. | Includes bibliographical references and index. | Summary: "Self-Care for New and Student Nurses presents self-care practices that must be learned and used consistently and in multiple settings to prepare new nurses for the clinical stressors to come. Filled with methods, tips, and exercises, this will book will guide new and student nurses to prioritize their own health needs in order to avoid burnout and premature exit from the nursing profession"-- Provided by publisher.
Identifiers: LCCN 2021007677 (print) | LCCN 2021007678 (ebook) | ISBN 9781646480807 (hardback) | ISBN 9781948057820 (epub) | ISBN 9781948057837 (adobe pdf) | ISBN 9781948057844 (mobi)
Subjects: MESH: Nurses--psychology | Self Care | Burnout, Professional--prevention & control
Classification: LCC RT86 (print) | LCC RT86 (ebook) | NLM WY 87 | DDC 610.73019--dc23
LC record available at https://lccn.loc.gov/2021007677
LC ebook record available at https://lccn.loc.gov/2021007678

First Printing, 2021

Publisher: Dustin Sullivan
Acquisitions Editor: Emily Hatch
Development Editor: Meaghan O'Keeffe
Cover Designer: Rebecca Batchelor
Interior Design/Page Layout: Rebecca Batchelor
Indexer: Larry Sweazy

Managing Editor: Carla Hall
Publications Specialist: Todd Lothery
Project Editor: Meaghan O'Keeffe
Copy Editor: Erin Geile
Proofreader: Gill Editorial Services

Dedication

We dedicate this book to nursing students and clinical nurses. We wish you the grit, grace, and wisdom to care for yourselves as well as you care for others.

Acknowledgments

We thank our students, fellow nurse clinicians, healthcare providers, and academic colleagues who inspired our collaboration, including Dorothe Bach, Danny Becker, Christina Beverage, Shelley Boyce, Joanne Braxton, Eboni Bugg, Forrest Calland, Marcia Day Childress, Joanne and Bill Conway, Zach Crowe, Joanne Davis, Gina DeGennaro, Becca Dillingham, David Germano, Sam Green, Roshi Joan Halifax, Rebecca Harmon, Amy Karr, Maria Tussi Kluge and the late John Kluge, Ramon Lavandero, Esther Lozano, Kelly McCaskill, Betty Mooney, Peggy Plews-Ogan, Cynda Rushton, Becky Ruegger, Hannah Schakat, John Schorling, Monica Sharma, Anita Thompson-Heisterman, Cheryl Thorpe, Juliet Trail, Richard Westphal, Diana Whitney, and the late Hannah Schakat. We also thank our encouraging, patient, and creative team who, with shared belief in the power of self-care, helped get this book across the finish line: Carla Hall, Emily Hatch, Meaghan O'Keeffe, Karen Davis, and designer and compositor Rebecca Batchelor.

Free Book Resources

PDF versions of the instructor's guide, student workbook, an extensive bibliography of additional readings, and a sample chapter can be found online from the Sigma Repository. Visit this book's page by following the link or the QR code below.

Print versions of both the instructor's guide and student workbook are available for purchase through online retailers.

http://hdl.handle.net/10755/21456

About the Authors

Dorrie K. Fontaine, PhD, RN, FAAN, is the Dean Emerita at the University of Virginia (UVA) School of Nursing, where she served as dean for 11 years until 2019. A champion of creating healthy work environments in clinical and academic settings, she is a past president of the American Association of Critical-Care Nurses (AACN). In 2009 she created the Compassionate Care Initiative at UVA, which has grown to be a guiding force in transforming the culture of the school with a focus on fostering human flourishing and resilience for students, faculty, and staff. A noted author of critical-care texts, a leadership book, and multiple papers and presentations on creating healthy work environments through compassionate care, Fontaine credits a retreat at Upaya Zen Center, Santa Fe in Spring 2009 with the Abbot Roshi Joan Halifax for setting her on the path of mindfulness, meditation, and a renewed focus on self-care. She attended Villanova University and the University of Maryland, and she received her PhD from The Catholic University of America. Her four-decade career of teaching and academic leadership includes the University of Maryland, Georgetown University, and the University of California, San Francisco (UCSF). Fontaine lives in Washington, D.C. and the Blue Ridge Mountains of Virginia with her husband Barry.

Tim Cunningham, DrPH, MSN, RN, FAAN, began his professional career as a performing artist and clown. As a clown, he worked for two organizations that changed his life. The first, The Big Apple Circus, employed him to perform as a clown doctor at Boston Children's Hospital, Yale New Haven Children's Hospital, and Hasbro Children's Hospital. Concurrently, he volunteered for Clowns Without Borders (CWB) performing in various refugee camps, war zones, and other global zones of crisis. He later served as Executive Director of CWB. It was in pediatric hospitals and refugee camps where he witnessed and began to learn about the true meaning of resilience and self-care. This performance work inspired him to pursue a career in nursing, and he completed a second-degree nursing program at the University of Virginia. Cunningham became an emergency trauma nurse and worked clinically in Charlottesville, Virginia, Washington, D.C., and New York City. It was during his time in New York City that he completed his doctoral degree in public health at the Mailman School of Public Health, Columbia University. Cunningham is the former Director of the Compassionate Care Initiative at the University of Virginia, where he had the opportunity to work closely with Drs. Fontaine and May as this book came to fruition. He currently lives in Atlanta, Georgia, and serves as the Vice President of Practice and Innovation at Emory Healthcare, where he also holds a joint appointment as an Adjunct Assistant Professor at the Nell Hodgson Woodruff School of Nursing at Emory University. Cunningham began his academic journey receiving his BA in English from the College of William and Mary in 2000. For self-care, he is an avid runner and wanna-be gardener. He also loves any chance he can get to swim in the ocean or meditate as the sun rises.

Natalie May, PhD, recently transitioned to the University of Virginia (UVA) School of Nursing after 30 years as Associate Professor of Research in the Division of General Medicine in the UVA School of Medicine. She is a founding member of the UVA Center for Appreciative Practice. Certified as an Appreciative Inquiry facilitator and lead author of *Appreciative Inquiry in Healthcare*, she enjoys developing appreciative inquiry projects and teaching appreciative practice workshops at her home institution and beyond. May is an experienced qualitative researcher, and she has extensive grant writing, program and curriculum development, and program evaluation experience. Her current research projects include the Mattering in Medicine study and the Medical Subspecialties HOME Team Program for high utilizer patients. She was also an investigator for the Wisdom in Medicine Project: Mapping the Path Through Adversity to Wisdom, a study funded by the John Templeton Foundation. She is coauthor of *Choosing Wisdom: The Path Through Adversity* and coproducer of a PBS film, *Choosing Wisdom*. She has codeveloped and implemented an innovative curriculum for medical students, The Phronesis Project, designed to foster wisdom in young physicians, and has implemented a similar program, Wisdom in Nursing, in the UVA School of Nursing. May earned a BA in economics and urban studies from Wellesley College, an MA in creative writing from Boston University, and her PhD in educational research from the University of Virginia Curry School of Education. She lives in Richmond, Virginia, with her husband Jim. Her most consistent and effective self-care practices are modern quilting and walking near water, especially the James River and the ocean at the Outer Banks, North Carolina.

Contributing Authors

Kim Acquaviva, PhD, MSW, CSE, is the Betty Norman Norris Endowed Professor at the University of Virginia School of Nursing. Prior to that, she spent 15 years as a faculty member at the George Washington University (GW) School of Nursing and the GW School of Medicine and Health Sciences. Her scholarly work focuses on LGBTQ aging and end-of-life issues, and her clinical work has been with patients and families facing life-limiting illnesses in both hospital and hospice settings. Her book *LGBTQ-Inclusive Hospice & Palliative Care: A Practical Guide to Transforming Professional Practice* was awarded first place in the AJN Book of the Year Awards in the Palliative Care and Hospice Category. She's the host of *em dash*, a podcast that explores the lived experiences of patients and healthcare professionals in the healthcare arena. Acquaviva has a PhD in human sexuality education from the University of Pennsylvania Graduate School of Education, an MSW from the University of Pennsylvania School of Social Policy and Practice, and a BA in sociology from the University of Pennsylvania College of Arts and Sciences. She is an AASECT-Certified Sexuality Educator.

Ryan Bannan, BSN, RN, CCRN, earned a BSN from Georgia Baptist College of Nursing of Mercer University and a BS in psychology from Michigan State University. Bannan's experiences caring for patients with COVID-19 have reinforced his interests in staff and patient safety, resiliency, and healthy work environments. He prioritizes self-care through exercise, meditation, nutrition, and relaxing with friends and family.

Jonathan Bartels, BSN, RN, has been a practicing nurse since 1998. He has worked in a variety of settings over the past 22 years, including emergency trauma, medical/surgical, and palliative care, and currently is the Palliative Care Liaison Nurse for the adult population at the University of Virginia Health System. Bartels has pursued several academic degrees, including bachelor of arts in psychology from Canisius College, Buffalo, New York (1990); comparative religion graduate program at Western Michigan University in Kalamazoo, Michigan (1991–1993); and bachelor of science in nursing from D'Youville College, Buffalo, New York

(1997). He has also been a member of the University of Virigina School of Nursing Compassionate Care Initiative since its inception in 2010. Since 2009, he has been a retreat and meditation/compassion facilitator. He is currently the Liaison to the Medical Center for the Compassionate Care Initiative. To support his role as retreat facilitator, he has received training from John Kabat Zinn (MBSR) and was an apprentice for the Being with Dying program at Upaya Institute and Zen Center in 2010. In 2009, Bartels started a practice to honor a patient who died called The Pause. The Pause is now practiced in hospitals around the United States and on seven continents around the world. Bartels was one of seven people nominated nationally for the Schwartz Center Compassionate care provider of the year in 2017. In 2018, he won the American Association of Critical Care Nurses Pioneering Spirit Award.

Susan Bauer-Wu, PhD, RN, FAAN, has held leadership, academic, and clinical roles in healthcare and higher education, with a focus on mind-body science and fostering resilience through mindfulness and other contemplative approaches. She began her career as an oncology, psychiatric, and hospice nurse, followed by doctoral training in psychoneuroimmunology and post-doc in psycho-oncology. From 2013–2016, Bauer-Wu was the Director of the Compassionate Care Initiative and Kluge Professor in Contemplative End-of-Life Care at the University of Virginia School of Nursing. Previously she held faculty appointments at Emory University, Dana-Farber Cancer Institute, Harvard Medical School, and the University of Massachusetts Medical School. She is a Fellow in the American Academy of Nursing, was a Robert Wood Johnson Executive Nurse Fellow, and has authored more than 80 scholarly articles and chapters plus a book for the lay public, *Leaves Falling Gently: Living Fully With Serious & Life-Limiting Illness Through Mindfulness, Compassion & Connectedness.*

Robin C. Brown-Haithco, MDiv, has served as the Director of Spiritual Health and Staff Support at Emory University Hospital for more than 14 years. An ordained minister with the American Baptist Churches, USA, she served as the President for the Association for Clinical Pastoral Education, Inc from 2012 to 2013. She is also an ACPE Certified Educator. She graduated from Mary Washington College with a BA in psychology and from Virginia Union University School of Theology with an MDiv.

Reynaldo "Ren" Capucao, Jr., MSN, RN, CNL, is a second-generation Filipino American nurse and alumnus of the University of Virginia. He specializes in the history of nursing and healthcare, Asian American studies, and digital humanities to address larger questions about the nursing labor supply, transnational exchange of people and knowledge, social history of nursing and immigration, and racial disparities and inequities. His current research examines the racialization of Filipino nurses across the Greater United States since the nascence of the twentieth century. He is the curator of the traveling exhibition *A Culture to Care: The History of Filipino Nurses in Virginia* and serves as a stakeholder for the Philippine Nurses Association of Virginia, APIDA Committee at the Library of Virginia, and Filipino Nursing Diaspora Network. Capucao is the 2020 Alice Fisher Society Fellow at the University of Pennsylvania Barbara Bates Center for the Study of the History of Nursing.

Ebru Çayir, MD, PhD, received her MD degree from the Istanbul University Cerrahpasa Medical Faculty in 2006. After graduation, she worked and was trained as a resident physician in the Department of Public Health at the Hacettepe University Medical Faculty. In 2011, she received a Fulbright Scholarship to study in the US, and in 2017, she earned her PhD from the Department of Health Promotion, Education and Behavior at the Arnold School of Public Health, University of South Carolina. Çayir is currently a postdoctoral research associate with the Compassionate Care Initiative at UVA's School of Nursing. Her research examines multilevel factors that influence self-care, resilience, and psychosocial well-being among caregiving professionals and how social identity categories such as race, ethnicity, gender, and nationality intersect to shape healthcare providers' work experiences and sense of professional belongingness.

Elgin Cleckley, Assoc. AIA, NOMA, is a designer, educator, and principal of _mpathic design, a Design Thinking initiative, pedagogy, and professional practice focusing on sociocultural interdisciplinary design projects. A graduate of the University of Virginia's School of Architecture and Princeton University, Elgin has collaborated with DLR Group (Seattle), MRSA Architects (Chicago), and Baird Sampson Neuert Architects (Toronto) on award-winning projects. Elgin currently facilitates Design Thinking Workshops and project development with national clients through _mpathic design. Before joining UVA's Design Thinking program in 2016, he was the 3D Group Leader and Design Coordinator at the Ontario Science Centre (Toronto), Visitor Experience / Science Content and Design, and Agents of Change Initiative, since 2001. This work produced award-winning exhibitions and public art with international artists David Rokeby, Michael Awad, Steve Mann, and Stacy Levy. Elgin teaches the university-wide Introduction to Design and Thinking course for undergraduates, and Design Thinking seminars on dynamic topics ranging from James Monroe's Highland to Dr. Carter G. Woodson's Birthplace in New Canton, Virginia. He also directs the School's Design Thinking program in Ghana, focused on community-supported innovations in the eastern region of the country.

Hannah R. Crosby, BA, RYT, is the Assistant Director of the Compassionate Care Initiative at the University of Virginia School of Nursing. A graduate of the College of Wooster, her passion for promoting holistic well-being was sparked in 2011 when she was an original member of the UVA School of Nursing's award-winning Healthy Work Environment team.

Anna DeLong, MSW, CEAP, a Mindfulness Teacher with more than 27 years' experience as a Licensed Clinical Social Worker, is a Certified Employee Assistance Professional who has been sanctioned to teach Mindfulness-Based Stress Reduction by the University of Massachusetts Medical School. Currently DeLong is employed as a Consultant for the University of Virginia's Faculty and Employee's Assistance program (FEAP), but she also has an Honorary Faculty Appointment in UVA School of Nursing. Prior to accepting a position with FEAP, DeLong spent 14 years working within UVA Medical Center, 8 of which were in leadership roles. She also has more than 10 years' experience in private practice.

Dallas Ducar, MSN, RN, PMHNP-BC, CNL, NREMT-B, NP, is the founding Chief Executive Officer of Transhealth Northampton. Inspired by others, she draws together psychology, philosophy, queer theory, and contemplative science in her daily work. Clinically, she works with gender-expansive patients providing holistic, gender-affirming, psychiatric care. Ducar's main research interests include moral psychology, trauma, and resilience. She seeks to harness the power of morality and prosociality, collaborating with vulnerable gender-expansive populations to direct community-based research. She continually works to create a more celebratory and open-hearted queer-friendly healthcare environment. With a BA in philosophy and cognitive science and an MSN in clinical nurse leadership, she is a board-certified registered nurse and psychiatric-mental health nurse practitioner.

Lerner L. Edison, MSN, MA, RN, CNL, is a proud United States Veteran with more than a decade of healthcare experience, holding both clinical and administrative positions. He continues to promote healthy environments through mentorship and non-profit organizations. His passion to serve humanity led to a career change as a graduate student at the University of Virginia School of Nursing Direct-Entry Clinical Nurse Leadership Program from 2017–2019. He joined Carilion Roanoke Memorial Hospital Cardiovascular Institute as a Cardiac Surgery Intensive Care Unit Registered Nurse in 2020 and recently became a member of the Cultural Competency Committee. The goal of this committee is to foster the core values of the organization through workshops, courses, and discussion forums to promote inclusivity. In 2020, Edison was the recipient of a DAISY Award as a Critical Care Registered Nurse for HCA Healthcare. He desires to be a change agent in healthcare with a focus on culture to elevate the nursing profession. In his free time, he enjoys reading, hiking, traveling, and socializing with close friends and family.

Danielle (Dani) Giaritelli, BSN, RN, has been a nurse for four years and currently works in the Acute Respiratory ICU at Emory University Hospital, Emory Healthcare. She graduated from the University of South Florida. She is currently completing a masters degree in Transformational Leadership and Nursing Administration. She aspires to bring positive influences to our nursing profession while helping to create a stronger and more resilient workforce.

Linda Grabbe, PhD, FNP-BC, PMHNP-BC, FAAN, is a board-certified Family Nurse Practitioner and Psychiatric/Mental Health Nurse Practitioner. As a Clinical Assistant Professor, she teaches psychiatric and population health nursing at Emory University's Nell Hodgson Woodruff School of Nursing and Community Advanced Practice Nurses, Inc. Her clinical expertise is in primary care and mental healthcare for homeless or incarcerated women and youth, providing Community Resiliency Model (CRM)® and Dialectical Behavior Therapy (DBT) skills trainings in group settings. Grabbe's current research includes measuring the impact of a brief Community Resiliency Model (CRM)® training on well-being of women in substance abuse treatment, as well as on well-being, resiliency, burnout, and effects of secondary traumatic stress in nurses, first responders, emergency department staff, and nursing students. She received her nurse training at the University of Hawaii and completed a master's degree in nursing education from Emory University. Her PhD was in family and community nursing from Georgia State University, and she has since trained as a Family Nurse Practitioner (Emory University) and Psychiatric/Mental Health Nurse Practitioner (Augusta University). Prior to becoming a nurse, Grabbe received a degree in Japanese language and civilization from the University of Paris.

Valérie Gruhn, BSN, RN, MPH, is an emergency trauma nurse, author, and humanitarian aid worker. Her public health work has taken her to the Philippines and Gaziantep, Turkey, where she worked on the Syrian Refugee Crisis. She has worked with Médecins Sans Frontières since 2016, assisting in Kenya, Chad, and Iraq. Gruhn recently worked on the Ebola epidemic in the Democratic Republic of Congo. Her piece "Ebola Patients Are Human Beings Not Biosecurity Threats" in Reuter's Foundation challenges the response of improving community engagement in Ebola care.

Julie Haizlip, MD, MAPP, is Clinical Professor at the University of Virginia School of Nursing and Faculty in the University of Virginia (UVA) Department of Pediatrics. She is board certified in pediatrics and pediatric critical care, having completed medical school and residency at the University of North Carolina and doing her pediatric critical care training at the University of Utah. Haizlip also earned a master's degree in applied positive psychology. She has published and presented internationally on using applications of positive psychology to create culture change in academic healthcare. Her article titled "The Negativity Bias, Medical Education, and the Culture of Academic Medicine: Why Culture Change Is Hard" earned her and her coauthors the ABIM Foundation Professionalism Article Prize. She has been a faculty member of the UVA Center for Appreciative Practice since its inception and became Director in 2016.

Susan Hassmiller, PhD, RN, FAAN, is the Robert Wood Johnson Foundation Senior Adviser for Nursing. She directs *The Future of Nursing: Campaign for Action,* a nationwide initiative led by RWJF and AARP that seeks to implement the recommendations of the Institute of Medicine report, *The Future of Nursing: Leading Change, Advancing Health,* and build a Culture of Health. Hassmiller has worked in public health and taught community health nursing at the University of Nebraska and George Mason University. A member of the National Academy of Sciences and a fellow in the American Academy of Nursing, she sits on several boards and committees.

Ashley R. Hurst, JD, MDiv, MA, is an Assistant Professor at the University of Virginia School of Nursing and affiliate faculty of the Center for Health Humanities and Ethics UVA School of Medicine. She is a member of the UVA Health System Ethics Committee and a consultant for its Ethics and Moral Distress Consultation Services. A licensed attorney, Hurst was previously a partner with the law firm Rogers & Hardin in Atlanta, Georgia, specializing in employment discrimination litigation. She writes and researches clinician moral distress, burnout, and preventive ethics. She has a JD from the University of Florida Levin College of Law, an MDiv from Yale Divinity School, and an MA in religious studies (with an ethics concentration) from the University of Virginia.

Nicole Jefferson, BSN, RN, began her professional caregiver career as a certified nursing assistant (CNA) while in high school but then went on to receive her BSN from the University of Virginia. While in college, she worked in the float pool at UVA Hospital as a patient companion and a patient care technician (PCT). As a patient companion and PCT, she floated to all floors of the hospital, where she was able to learn various skills. After graduating from college, she started her first nursing position as a Nurse Resident on a general medicine floor at Emory University Hospital. She worked on the general medicine unit for a year and a half before transferring to labor and delivery. She currently works as a labor and delivery nurse at Emory Decatur Hospital in Atlanta, Georgia.

Master Hiromi Hangai Johnson is the Founder and Director of Charlottesville T'ai Chi Center, an award-winning non-profit whose mission includes spreading the health benefits of T'ai Chi and related internal martial arts in the wider community. She is an International Cheng Ming Instructor certified in T'ai Chi, Ch'i Kung (Qigong), Hsing I, and Ba Gua. Her teacher, Grandmaster Wang Fu Lai, is the lineage holder of the International Cheng Ming Association in Taiwan.

Mick Krasner, MD, FACP, is a Professor of Clinical Medicine, University of Rochester School of Medicine and Dentistry, and practices full-time primary care internal medicine in Rochester, New York. Krasner has been teaching mindfulness-based programs to patients, medical students, and health professionals for more than 20 years and was the project director of *Mindful Communication: Bringing Intention, Attention, and Reflection to Clinical Practice.* This program led to the establishment of Mindful Practice Programs, which he codirects, at the University of Rochester. Krasner is engaged in a variety of research projects, including the effects of mindfulness practices on the immune system in the elderly, on chronic psoriasis, and on caregivers of Alzheimer's patients. A graduate of the University of California, Berkeley, in 1983, he received the doctor of medicine degree from the University of California, San Diego School of Medicine in 1987, completing residency in both internal medicine and pediatrics at the University of Rochester School of Medicine and Dentistry, where he is currently a full-time faculty member engaged in direct patient care, medical student and residency education, post-graduate medical education, and research in the University's Center for Mind-Body Research.

Irène P. Mathieu, MD, is an academic pediatrician, writer, and public health researcher. She holds a BA in international relations from the College of William & Mary and an MD from Vanderbilt University. Mathieu completed her residency in pediatrics at the Children's Hospital of Philadelphia, where she was selected as a Global Health Track resident. She has received fellowships from the Fulbright Program, Callaloo Creative Writing Workshop, and Virginia Center for the Creative Arts and is the author of three poetry collections: *Grand Marronage* (Switchback Books, 2019), *orogeny* (Trembling Pillow Press, 2017), and *the galaxy of origins* (dancing girl press, 2014). Currently a candidate for a master's degree in public health at the Johns Hopkins Bloomberg School of Public Health, Mathieu is an Assistant Professor of Pediatrics at the University of Virginia. There she serves as Director of Equity & Inclusion for the Department of Pediatrics and affiliate faculty of the UVA Center for Health Humanities & Ethics.

Michelle Maust, MD, FAPA, is a Clinical Psychiatrist at MindPath Care Centers in Raleigh, North Carolina, where she practices a holistic approach to psychiatric care. She earned her medical degree from the University of Virginia School of

Medicine and completed her psychiatry training as an Army officer at Tripler Army Medical Center. She has served in hospital and clinic settings on Oahu, deployed to Kuwait, at Fort Bragg, and currently is in the Triangle community. Working with service members has honed her focus on integrating lifestyle factors into treatment plans as a means of creating long-lasting wellness. Maust has presented at recent annual meetings of the American Psychiatric Association on lifestyle factors to foster health and sexual function.

Carrie McDermott, PhD, APRN, ACNS-BC, is the Corporate Director of Professional Nursing Practice for Emory Healthcare and is responsible for the leadership of Emory Healthcare's Nursing Residency Programs. She received her PhD from the University of Colorado Denver, College of Nursing, her MSN from the University of Missouri in Kansas City, and her BSN from the Rockhurst University/ Research College of Nursing in Kansas City, Missouri. McDermott's research interests are in the areas of workplace culture, incivility, leadership, competency development, and symptom management. She is also an adjunct faculty at Emory University Nell Hogson Woodson School of Nursing and at the University of Colorado Denver, College of Nursing.

Joy Miller, BS, MSN, RN, CPNP-PC, CPN, is a Pediatric Nurse Practitioner on the Pediatric Palliative Care team at the University of Virginia Children's Hospital. There, she coordinates the care of children with life-threatening/limiting illnesses and specializes in working through ethical issues in the care of vulnerable children and families. Miller earned her BS in health sciences from James Madison University and her BSN-RN from Seton Hall University in New Jersey. In 2007, she returned to UVA to work in Acute Care Pediatrics and earned her MSN/pediatric nurse practitioner degree. She joined the Pediatric Palliative Care service in 2011.

K. Jane Muir, BSN, RN, is an emergency department nurse and PhD student. Her research focuses on quantifying the cost of nurse burnout within healthcare organizations, as well as cultivating systems-level interventions that decrease nurse burnout-attributed turnover. She continues to practice in the emergency department setting and serves as a Compassionate Care Initiative clinical ambassador at University of Virginia Health. Within her ambassador role, Muir teaches self-care and resiliency practices to onboarding new nurse graduates as well as various clinician groups within UVA Health.

Sharon Pappas, PhD, RN, NEA-BC, FAAN, is the Chief Nurse Executive for Emory Healthcare (Atlanta). A member of Emory Healthcare and the Woodruff Health Science Center's senior leadership teams, she is responsible for nursing practice across Emory's eleven hospitals, ambulatory care, and post-acute agencies. With Emory University Hospital, Emory St. Joseph's Hospital, Emory Orthopedics & Spine Hospital, and Emory Johns Creek Hospital designated as Magnet® hospitals, she works to establish this same nursing excellence as a distinctive competency throughout Emory Healthcare. Prior to Emory, Pappas served in nurse executive roles in Centura Health (Englewood, Colorado). She completed her PhD at the University of Colorado, Denver College of Nursing with research focus on clinical and financial outcomes that are sensitive to nursing. She holds a master of science in nursing administration from Georgia College, School of Nursing and a bachelor of science in nursing from the School of Nursing, Medical College of Georgia.

Kate M. Pfeiffer, MS, PMHCNS-BC, PMHNP-BC, is a clinical instructor at the Nell Hodgson Woodruff School of Nursing. She is an Advanced Practice Nurse who is board certified as a Family Psychiatric Mental Health Nurse Practitioner and as a Psychiatric Mental Health Clinical Nurse Specialist. Pfeiffer graduated with a BS in nursing from Emory University in 2004, a master's in nursing from Georgia State University in 2009, and is currently enrolled in the doctor of nursing practice program at Emory University. Her specialty area is adult mental health nursing, with interest in enhancing nursing education in the areas of high-fidelity simulation, high-touch learning in an online environment, trauma-informed care and self-care for students, and integration of mental healthcare education into community and interprofessional settings. A member of Sigma Theta Tau International Honor Society of Nursing and the American Psychiatric Nurses Association, Pfeiffer is also a certified Community Resiliency Model trainer.

Elizabeth A. (Lili) Powell, PhD, is an Associate Professor at the Darden School of Business and the Kluge-Schakat Professor in Compassionate Care, School of Nursing, at the University of Virginia. During her time at Darden, Powell created an innovative experiential Executive MBA elective and a novel executive education program titled "Leading Mindfully." Powell brings her expertise to expand on the efforts of the Compassionate Care Initiative, which promotes resilient healthcare professionals and healthy work environments. Powell's general management teaching and consulting make her work applicable in industries ranging from banking to biotech. She is coauthor of *Women in Business: The Changing Face of Leadership* (Greenwood, 2007). She earned her PhD in rhetoric and performance studies from Northwestern University.

Millie Sattler, DNP, MSN, RN, CCRN, is the Corporate Director of Nurse Retention and Career Development for Emory Healthcare. She is part of the Emory Healthcare senior leadership team and the executive sponsor for the Professional Lattice Advancing Nurses (PLAN), Emory Nurse Peer Mentoring Program, and the Emory Nurse Extern and InEmory Program across the nine-hospital system and ambulatory care. Sattler has published several peer-reviewed articles and done several conference presentations throughout her nursing career focused on lifelong learning committed to patient care, patient safety, nurse engagement, team vitality, and nurse advocacy. She completed her DNP at Chamberlain University, Downers Grove, Illinois, in healthcare systems and executive leadership, focusing on interprofessional communication and collaboration. She holds a master of science in nursing administration and a bachelor of science in nursing from Chamberlain University. She received a diploma in nursing from St. Elizabeth's School of Nursing in Youngstown, Ohio.

Victoria Tucker, BSN, RN, has worked as a registered nurse for eight years. She joined the inpatient Thomas Palliative Care unit at Virginia Commonwealth University in 2014, where she currently resides. A nursing doctoral student at the University of Virginia, her dissertation focuses on Black nurses' and nursing students' experiences and contributions in Virginia, 1950s–1980s. Her research utilizes oral histories to address fragmented archives and enhance historical records.

Kath Weston, PhD, is an Indoor Student of Master Hiromi Hangai Johnson and Professor of Anthropology at the University of Virginia. She previously held positions at Cambridge University, University of Tokyo, Harvard University, and Arizona State University. She received her doctorate in anthropology from Stanford University and holds a master's degree in anthropology from the University of Chicago. Among her awards are a 2011 Guggenheim Fellowship and a 2019–2023 British Academy Global Professorship hosted by the University of Edinburgh. Her most recent book is *Animate Planet: Making Visceral Sense of Living in a High-Tech Ecologically Damaged World*. The study of T'ai Chi has deepened her understanding of embodiment, one of her research specialties.

Table of Contents

Foreword

You've decided to be a nurse. Perhaps you're pursuing your life's dream or an intentional career change. As you start your chosen career, you'll find there are some aspects of nursing that you won't fully appreciate until you have lived the experience. This begins as a student when you comprehend the immense responsibility you have for another human being's welfare and witness their cheerful moments as well as their pain, suffering, and grief. You accept the challenges as a learner who must build self-confidence, think critically, learn to trust instincts, act decisively, be able to work under pressure, and somehow power through long hours meeting multiple demands on your time.

Nurses are welcomed into a person's most intimate moments in life—when sick and vulnerable, when celebrating new life or restoration of quality of life, or when recovering from the brink of death. The work that nurses and other healthcare clinicians do across the continuum of joy to heartache is emotional labor, and it affects their well-being.

Nursing is stressful. Of the more than 10,000 nurses who responded to the American Nurses Association's Healthy Nurse, Healthy Nation Health Risk Appraisal in 2016, 82% said they are at a "significant level of risk for workplace stress," which is twice the average for the public (ANA, 2017). The survey also assesses work environment, physical activity, nutrition, quality of life, and safety—all important aspects of being a healthy nurse. Stress compels our body to respond to changes in its normal balanced state, leading to either manageable stress or negative and overwhelming distress. Stress activates our central nervous system to warn us in response to a threat. The body moves from an initial state of alarm to one of resistance, and then it tries to adapt to the stressor. If our bodies cannot adapt and our resources become depleted, we reach a state of collapse. Emotional exhaustion then gives way to emotional depletion, depersonalization, and depression—all drivers of burnout.

In 2019, the World Health Organization (Woo et al., 2020) elaborated on the occupational phenomenon of burnout, describing its three dimensions as "feelings of energy depletion or exhaustion; increased mental distance from one's job, or feelings of negativism or cynicism related to one's job; and reduced professional efficacy." Nurses gave voice to the term "burnout" decades ago. More recently, burnout has been associated with compassion fatigue, stress injury, moral distress and moral injury, perceptions of powerlessness, and dissatisfaction with the work environment, which transcend the excessive emotional and spiritual demands placed on nurses.

A systematic review of 113 studies with more than 45,000 nurse subjects across 49 countries revealed that burnout affects greater than 11% of the global nurse workforce, with the highest prevalence among critical care nurses (Woo et al., 2020). Numerous other country-level studies report burnout rates of 30% to 45%. Although many nurses may escape large doses of sustained periods of stress, one glaring exception is the intense situations of caring for COVID-19 patients and the deleterious effects on mental health for those clinicians who for weeks faced their own mortality, confronted unprecedented rates of death, served as surrogate family to dying patients, and endured daily moral adversity. The emotional and physical exhaustion rarely seen outside time-limited disasters or in conflict zones laid bare the consequences associated with intense human caring, social isolation, and inability to fulfill one's duty to care. Additionally, nurses and other clinicians were treated as pariahs and potential COVID spreaders rather than as self-sacrificing professionals who risked their own safety and that of their families to care for COVID patients. No amount of personal courage alone could resist the unprecedented stress and emotional turmoil felt across the front lines in such a crisis.

Nurses are not new to adversity in the workplace. Some comes with the territory—feeling vulnerable when there's a bad outcome despite all best efforts when someone dies, or when an ethical dilemma causes moral distress. Discrimination on the basis of gender, gender identity, race, religion, and ethnicity has, for years, presented challenges for nurses to be treated with respect. They have had to overcome harassment and stereotyping to be seen as well-educated and intelligent clinicians serving the public regardless of circumstances. These conditions call for self-care as survival.

The National Academy of Medicine (NAM) acknowledged the growing epidemic of burnout among health professionals, students, and trainees and took the lead to reverse the trends in clinician burnout through its Action Collaborative on Clinician Well-Being and Resilience. The Collaborative recognized that promoting clinician well-being is essential for safe, high-quality patient care and posited that the absence of well-being could lead to dire consequences such as increased medical errors and clinician suicide. NAM also conducted an influential consensus study that recommended systems approaches to improving clinical work and learning environments as well as imperatives for preventing burnout and promoting professional well-being.

You may be wondering how to deal with all this and create a personal force field that protects against burnout. Practice self-compassion and be kind to yourself? Boost your resilience? Be an activist for a supportive work environment? Sounds like a lot of work! First consider this advice I've given to many nurses throughout my career: No one else will ever look out for your personal welfare as well as you will look out for yourself. No matter the issue, we need to be good to ourselves. This derives from the ANA *Code of Ethics for Nurses with Interpretive Statements* (American Nurses Association, 2015) that states, "The nurse owes the same duties to self as others, including the responsibility to promote health and safety…" By nature, we care for others—family, friends, and strangers. We learn to care for patients and are just now learning the importance of caring for ourselves.

The good news is that you are not alone. Your organization's leaders have a shared responsibility to provide a supportive workplace with everything from appropriate staffing; a safe, satisfying, and inclusive environment; a sense of community; brave spaces that are free from discrimination, violence, harassment, and bullying; and a variety of opportunities to enhance resilience. It shouldn't be a solo journey.

This book's editors have decades of experience crafting positive environments that focus on the well-being of nurses as students and clinicians. With a commitment to excellent patient care and quality education, Dean Emeritus Dorrie Fontaine founded the Compassionate Care Initiative at the University of Virginia School of Nursing. She has decades of experience building healthy work environments in clinical and academic settings with a focus on human flourishing. Research professor Natalie May has helped countless clinicians and students develop resilience using appreciative practices. Her work has explored the role of adversity in fostering wisdom, particularly when clinicians experience a harmful error. Tim Cunningham is a clinical nurse leader with a doctorate in public health. Now a vice president for nursing professional practice and innovation, he uses his prior work with Clowns Without Borders to bring humanistic compassion into everyday clinical work. Their messages of self-care and resilience instill a focus on positive and restorative practices for daily living, one they believe is essential and achievable for all.

In the pages that follow, these and other experts will answer your questions, guide you, and help you prepare for the exciting work to come. The editors have created a scholarly yet practical guide that demonstrates the importance of self-care in addressing the current state of stress and burnout in nursing. In twenty-three chapters written by nurses, researchers, teachers, and other frontline healthcare workers, they have crafted a must-read book for every nursing student and early career clinician who aspires to not only provide excellent and compassionate patient care, but have a meaningful, purposeful life. The writers present both the realities of the workplace as well as concrete steps to develop your own personal resilience, or your "force field." Throughout the book, self-care and resilience research is enriched by compelling stories and vignettes, shared generously by working nurses. I cannot think of anything more valuable than reading the wisdom of these clinicians— nurses who have succeeded in establishing self-care practices amid busy clinical work, many during times of crisis and upheaval.

This book adds to the self-care literature in many ways, not in a superficial manner, but by delving deeply into both the art and the science of what works. The experts highlighted in this book explore self-care and resilience from many perspectives, often in fresh, new ways. Topics include appreciative practices, developing your resilience skills, narrative and contemplative practices such as T'ai Chi, and caring for your physical as well as mental health. There is particular attention given to nurses and student nurses who face an additional layer of stress and threat to their wellbeing: our LGBTQIA+, underrepresented, and international nurses. The authors address the challenges new graduates face as they transition to practice, and once in a clinical setting, the skills they will need to maintain their compassion and vitality. This book has unique value because it does not ignore the role that institutions, work environments, and the broader culture play in the well-being of our nurses.

Finally, this work goes further than many others, recognizing that new nurses can, and should, see themselves as advocates for their patients and as formal and informal leaders within their work environments. As I think about the future of healthcare, I appreciate that they have acknowledged the importance of empowering you, our future nurse leaders.

As you turn the pages of this book, you will see that the authors care deeply for you, the reader, and your well-being. Their compassion and wisdom are revealed throughout. Please take that to heart and know that there is an entire nursing profession in your cheering section, wishing you great success and happiness.

–Pamela F Cipriano
Dean and Sadie Heath Cabaniss Professor, University of Virginia School of Nursing
Past President, American Nurses Association
Steering Committee Member, NAM Collaborative on
Clinician Well-Being and Resilience

References

American Nurses Association. (2015). *Code of ethics for nurses with interpretive statements.* Retrieved from https://www.nursingworld.org/coe-view-only

American Nurses Association. (2017). Grand challenge: healthy nurse healthy nation. Retrieved from https://www.nursingworld.org/~4aeeeb/globalassets/practiceandpolicy/work-environment/health--safety/ana-healthriskappraisalsummary_2013-2016.pdf

Woo, T., Ho, R., Tang, A., & Tam, W. (2020). Global prevalence of burnout symptoms among nurses: A systematic review and meta-analysis. *Journal of Psychiatric Research, 123,* 9–20, 2020 04. doi:https://doi.org/10.1016/j.jpsychires.2019.12.015

World Health Organization. (2019). Burn-out an "occupational phenomenon": International Classification of Diseases. Retrieved from https://www.who.int/mental_health/evidence/burn-out/en/

Introduction

"I have met myself and I am going to care for her fiercely."
–Glennon Doyle

Self-care. Well-being. Resilience. Happiness. Self-compassion.

These are among today's self-help buzzwords. There are countless books, articles, and podcasts on these topics, and many of them are essential resources for anyone seeking solid footing in the world today. Self-care remains an imperative for nurses and other healthcare professionals as burnout, high attrition rates, emotional fatigue, and moral distress loom large over us. The people who so compassionately care for others are in dire need of care themselves.

This book, we hope, will be valuable specifically to the student nurse and early career nurse. No matter where you are in your nursing trajectory, we hope that keeping your mind and body safe and strong is a high priority for you. We hope that is why you picked up this book. You understand that the knowledge and skills you learn in school are important, but they are not all it takes to be an extraordinary nurse. You understand that your work will be challenging and that caring for yourself will help you care for others.

Self-care practices are important because we need you.

We need all the gifts that you bring to the nursing profession. Your future patients need you. Your future colleagues need you. We need you to become the best nurse you can possibly be so that you can support other young nurses as they, too, enter this profession. Nursing will afford you daily interactions that will change the lives of your patients, strengthen the resolve of your colleagues, and ripple beyond your immediate circle to surprising places. The gifts that you bring are beyond measure.

Imagine for a moment a patient who is a young mother. Perhaps she is facing her health challenges while trying to be strong for her children and partner. The kindness, wisdom, and support that you bring to your interactions with her will have a downstream impact on her children and family. Even her children's children. Think about yourself or your nursing school peers who, when asked why they wanted to become a nurse, tell a story about growing up and seeing a nurse who cared for them or a loved one during a health crisis. So many nurses are nurses because they experienced the compassion of someone like you when they were in need. These nurses' compassion may have started you on your own journey to nursing, even though they may never know the impact they had on you. That is one of the superpowers of nursing: the impact you have on others. *You will matter* in ways big and small, in ways that the universe may never even be able to reveal to you.

But here is the hard, honest truth: While you have chosen one of the most noble professions, you have also chosen one of the most difficult. In your career, you will face challenges big and small, whether it is a problematic coworker, the death of a favorite patient, or a global pandemic. You will have bad days or weeks when you ask yourself why you didn't choose a less demanding path in life. You will experience exhaustion, frustration, and grief. You will balance not only your nursing responsibilities, but your commitments to your family and community. But as you question your life choices and wonder how you can take one more step forward, that voice inside you will whisper, "You are a nurse."

Our goal in writing this book is that you never have to betray that voice. No matter what comes your way, you will have the strength, skills, and resilience to keep moving forward. But let us be clear: We do not want you to move forward at the expense of yourself or your well-being. We want you to move forward with wisdom and clarity of purpose by using every resource you can muster. We hope that what is contained in this book will become a valuable resource throughout the early years of your career, and even beyond.

We welcome you on this journey, and we hope you welcome the opportunity to explore the concept of self-care, what it means, what works best for you, and how it can help you flourish in good times and help you grow in difficult ones. We are especially grateful and humbled that we can do it with you.

Self-Care May Not Be What You Think

What comes to mind when you hear the words "self-care"? Does the idea of caring for yourself sound selfish? Do you think of a good night's sleep, a meal that includes a vegetable, or a workout at the gym? Is self-care something you'll do later, when you're in the throes of a stressful nursing job?

Let's examine these common assumptions about self-care.

The concept of self-care has all too often been considered selfish care. As a profession, nurses are recognized for their empathy, compassion, and—to a fault—giving so much of themselves to their patients that many suffer exhaustion, moral distress, and burnout. Some people even call this *pathological altruism*—caring so much for others that you, yourself become mentally or physically ill (Halifax, 2018; Oakley et al., 2011). These mental afflictions are all too real in the nursing profession. Early career nurses are especially vulnerable. Thirty-three percent of new registered nurses look for a new job within the first year of practice (Lucian Leape Institute, 2013), and they generally aren't leaving because the job wasn't satisfying or rewarding. Studies show that feeling burned out leads to concurrent feelings of depression and a desire to leave the profession (Rudman & Gustavsson, 2011). Not surprisingly, nurse burnout results in lower job performance and quality of patient care (Dall'Ora et al., 2020). In this same review study (Dall'Ora et al., 2020), the authors found that higher nurse burnout is linked to worse patient safety and increased errors and adverse events. A national study linked nurses' physical and mental health to medical errors; nurses who were mentally and physically healthy were less likely to make medical errors than nurses with worse health (Melnyk et al., 2018). Nurses are also more likely than the general population to die by suicide (Davidson et al., 2020). We believe it is an easy argument to make: Self-care is far from selfish. Healthy nurses, both physically and mentally, lead to healthier patients.

Let us underscore the importance of self-care as we move on to nurses' physical health. Ironically, nurses do a terrific job of teaching their patients about self-care, but they don't do as well regarding their own health (Ross et al., 2017). Registered nurses have poorer lifestyle behaviors, a higher prevalence of depression, and poorer health than physicians and the general population (Blake & Chambers,

2012; Priano et al., 2018). Further, nurses who work night and evening shifts have increased all-cause mortality as well as increased mortality from cardiovascular disease, diabetes, Alzheimer's disease, and dementia (Jørgensen et al., 2017; Vetter et al., 2016).

Your physical health is vitally important. Period. Your overall strength and resilience will depend on the strength and resilience of your body. We will explore some aspects of physical health in this book—namely, sleep, exercise, and nutrition—but our primary focus will be on your mind and your thinking. Our reasoning is this: Many excellent resources exist to keep you healthy and strong. There is little we can add to that body of work. However, there is no comprehensive resource specifically addressing the self-care needs of the student and early-career nurse. Your work as a nurse will be as challenging as it is important, and we hope that after reading this book, you will fully grasp the potential power of your mind to keep you safe, resilient, and well.

Another assumption about self-care is that it's something you can simply wait to do once you're a practicing nurse. This notion has arisen alongside the increase in well-being, stress management, and resilience programs that are offered in many health systems today. The 12-week Stress Management and Resilience Training (SMART) program is a well-studied worksite program to help healthcare workers make choices that foster well-being (Berkland et al., 2017). Many of the activities included in the SMART program (and others) reflect some that are included in this book because they have demonstrated effectiveness, and the activities are easily accessible to almost everyone. Some of these activities include gratitude, mindfulness, narrative reflection, spirituality, and more.

We hope to convince you that waiting until you're in the middle of a crisis is too late, that *there is no better time to begin a self-care practice than right now*. Begin to strengthen your resilience and well-being muscles now while you are a student. Start today to notice how your mind and body feel at any given moment. Notice how things change at the introduction of a stressor. Once you have noticed these shifts in your well-being, only then can you begin to intentionally explore the best practices that work *for you* to help you regain solid footing. It will take practice, but we are excited to imagine you with a well-honed self-care practice that will kick into high gear when you are facing the challenges of nursing. Think of this time as your runway, and imagine yourself soaring in flight, into your nursing career. A plane cannot take off without a runway, and a healthy nurse needs the time and reflection required to develop a self-care practice to prepare for liftoff.

There is one more assumption, or misconception, that we need to address. Unfortunately, the concept of self-care has been tainted by healthcare systems abuses themselves. Research consistently demonstrates that an unhealthy work environment is strongly linked to burnout and nurse dissatisfaction (Aiken et al., 2012; Casalicchio et al., 2017; Dall'Ora et al., 2020). Organizations that offer mindfulness classes but don't address staffing shortages or equipment failures cannot be let off the hook. Self-care as it has often been presented, as a workshop or a pamphlet, is not a panacea for the well-being of our nurses, physicians, and others who care for patients (Cunningham, 2020). We have been pleased to see calls for systemic approaches to clinician well-being in recent years (National Academies of Sciences, Engineering, and Medicine, 2019).

We hope, of course, that you will come to see yourself as part of the solution, and you will contribute to much-needed changes in our society and health systems. We hope that you will use your voice and your experience to advocate for yourself and others when you see systemic injustice at any level. But the burden is not all on you. Much of what you will read in this text stems from the work of psychologists and positive psychology researchers, and we caution you (and ourselves) "not to be complicit in the move to interiorize well-being" (Prilleltensky, 2020). As Davis (2015, pp. 5–6) wrote in his book *The Happiness Industry*, "The risk is that this science ends up blaming—and medicating—individuals for their own misery and ignores the context that has contributed to it." Davis's words can be applied to any organization or method that says, "You, not we, are responsible for your own well-being."

To begin, we would like to push back on these all too common assumptions. Instead, we propose that:

- Self-care is not selfish.
- Nurses don't flourish simply by fostering the well-being of others.

- Self-care is about the mind as much as it is about the body.

- Self-care is a lifelong *practice*, and it is best to practice on the safety of the runway, rather than in mid-air.

- Individual self-care practices do not let organizations off the hook.

What Is Self-Care?

A standard definition of self-care is elusive in part because of the breadth of the topic and the individual nature of self-care practices. As you will see in this book, one size definitely does not fit all. Practices that have been taught in nursing schools include but are not limited to feng shui; T'ai Chi and other martial arts; music, art and pet therapy; Reiki and healing touch; drum circles; aromatherapy; mindfulness and guided meditation; hypnotherapy; and yoga (Blum, 2014). Nursing researchers Pam Ashcraft and Susan Gatto (2018, p. 140) offer that self-care "can be described as deliberate decisions made and actions taken by individuals to address their own health and well-being." We appreciate their emphasis on "deliberate decisions" and the recognition that we are all empowered to manage our behaviors and resulting health and well-being. This is an excellent starting point.

The idea of our own empowerment resonates with us, as well as several other authors in this book. Self-care generates the energy and wisdom that you will draw upon when the going gets rough. Self-care is a collection of personally and culturally appropriate practices that provide nurses with skills to be with their stress, to experience growth during difficult times, and to provide compassionate care always. Self-care takes time, effort, and reflection. Self-care is a conscious decision to be aware of your thoughts and feelings and to be curious about them. Self-care is gentle and self-compassionate. It follows then that self-care is not judgmental or harsh. It's not a failed diet or New Year's resolution—we should never feel guilt or shame for struggling periodically or even frequently.

We have found that the diversity of self-care definitions mirrors the diversity of our nursing workforce—there are countless meaningful and critical self-care practices. We would be remiss to say there is only one definition that is "right," that there is only one correct way to do self-care. Use this book and every resource at your disposal to find the practices that resonate with you, that make your heart leap a bit and cause you to think, "Yes, that sounds like a good fit for me." Your self-care practice should complement—even enhance—who you are and what you're already doing. Your self-care practice will evolve as you grow and as your life circumstances change. With this book and workbook, we hope you'll find what fits for you now and that you will store away ideas for future use. Exploration and practice are the guiding principles of this text.

Self-care is *not* a magical elixir. It alone will not fix the problems that create stress in your life as a student or new nurse; however, a self-care practice can help you develop the necessary tools to find creative solutions to problems, to enjoy and rely on the camaraderie of your team, and ultimately to flourish in a meaningful and exciting career.

Your self-care journey will take effort on your part, and this book aspires to guide you along the way.

How to Use This Book: Explore, Practice, Reflect, and Journal

There is no better opportunity to explore and develop self-care practices than during your years as a student nurse. There is growing recognition that new graduate nurses will benefit from developing self-care practices and the ability to be resilient when facing new stressors (Ashcraft & Gatto, 2018). Nurse training programs are recognizing the value of teaching self-care skills to their students (Bartlett et al., 2016). This book shares many authors' wisdom about self-care and how it can be accessible to all nursing students, new graduates, and early career nurses. Together, we present complex ideas and illustrate them with practical exercises in the accompanying workbook. As a student nurse, you will have the opportunity to explore an array of self-care techniques and to choose those that fit you best. Our instructor's guide offers ideas, resources, and curriculum suggestions. We challenge you, as individuals and members of the most trusted professional community, to explore, practice, and imagine the power of a lifelong practice of self-care.

Throughout this book, we will underscore our belief that self-care practices are just that—*practices*—that must be learned and used consistently and in multiple settings to prepare the new nurse for the clinical stressors to come. Just as we wouldn't expect you to run a marathon with no training, we have seen tremendous value in "training" nurses for self-care before they even reach the starting line, or their first weeks or months of their nursing practice. When you read in this book about a practice that resonates with you, try it out. Do it consistently for a period of time. Reflect on its impact on your well-being. Make adjustments. Repeat. Our hope is that when you finish reading this book, you will have several tools in your self-care tool kit that will have become second nature to you. When your patient misses her fourth appointment, your manager schedules you on nights (even though you've been requesting days), or you simply feel like you are spinning 20 plates at a time, you will remember, "I am a nurse. I've got this."

We have organized the book into five sections. In Section I, "Fundamentals," we provide an overview of why self-care is so important in nursing, what we mean by resilience, and concrete practices to get you started. In Section II, "The Mind of a Nurse," we explore practices that address the needs of underrepresented nursing students, LGBTQIA+ students, international students, as well as narrative and mindfulness practices. Section II also includes an important chapter about the risks of "one-sided" resilience training; as we discussed earlier, a healthy work environment is critical to nurses' health and well-being.

In Section III, "The Body and Spirit of a Nurse," we explore the physical and spiritual needs of the resilient nurse. We talk more about strengths-based resilience, and we introduce our work bringing T'ai Chi practice to nurses and student nurses. We include a chapter on your physical well-being, with a focus on sleep, exercise, and nutrition.

Section IV, "The Transition to Nursing Practice," was designed to help you navigate that anxiety-provoking period between finishing your studies and beginning your practice. Will you be prepared? What is the role of a mentor? How do you choose a healthy work environment? We even include a chapter about humanitarian aid nursing as a possibility you might want to explore. We hope this section helps you navigate this exciting, if fraught, period.

The final section, "The Heart of a Nurse," focuses on your early years of nursing. No matter where you land professionally, you will not be working alone. Section V hopes to spark ideas about ways to navigate the interpersonal, interprofessional, and organizational issues you may face.

Each chapter includes sidebars, often including vignettes, that further illustrate the chapter topic. We have also included several stand-alone essays, written by nurses from many backgrounds at various points in their careers. We find these voices of practicing nurses compelling, shining light on self-care practices in the "real world."

This book has an accompanying workbook, providing the opportunity for you to explore the ideas within the book, to practice some of the ideas presented here, and to reflect upon the "fit" for you as a student and nurse.

We strived to present a wide array of self-care concepts, but you will probably notice that there are common threads that weave throughout the chapters, and we call this "synergy." But you may also notice some redundancy. If you see a topic or idea multiple times, please assume that it is something we think is very important. As Jon Kabat-Zinn (2010) said, "There are a million doors into the same room." We want you to try opening as many doors, or to try as many practices, as time will allow.

We hope that this book opens your mind to the value of self-care and its power to change the way you work, interact with others, and respond to adversity. This is such an exciting time. You are "meeting yourself" during these years of training and preparation for your nursing practice. You are a nurse. Our wish for you: Care for yourself fiercely.

Let's begin.

References

Aiken, L. H., Sermeus, W., Van den Heede, K., Sloane, D. M., Busse, R., McKee, M., Bruyneel, L., Rafferty, A. M., Griffiths, P., Moreno-Casbas, M. T., Tishelman, C., Scott, A., Brzostek, T., Kinnunen, J., Schwendimann, R., Heinen, M., Zikos, D., Strømseng Sjetne, I., Smith, H. L., & Kutney-Lee, A. (2012). Patient safety, satisfaction, and quality of hospital care: Cross sectional surveys of nurses and patients in 12 countries in Europe and the United States. *British Medical Journal (Clinical Research Ed.), 344,* e1717. https://doi.org/10.1136/bmj.e1717

Ashcraft, P. F., & Gatto, S. L. (2018). Curricular interventions to promote self-care in prelicensure nursing students. *Nurse Educator, 43*(3), 140–144. https://doi.org/10.1097/NNE.0000000000000450

Bartlett, M. L., Taylor, H., & Nelson, J. D. (2016). Comparison of mental health characteristics and stress between baccalaureate nursing students and non-nursing students. *Journal of Nursing Education, 55*(2), 87–90. https://doi.org/10.3928/01484834-20160114-05

Berkland, B. E., Werneburg, B. L., Jenkins, S. M., Friend, J. L., Clark, M. M., Rosedahl, J. K., Limburg, P. J., Riley, B. A., Lecy, D. R., & Sood, A. (2017). A worksite wellness intervention: Improving happiness, life satisfaction, and gratitude in health care workers. *Mayo Clinical Proceedings: Innovations, Quality, and Outcomes, 1*(3), 203–210. https://doi.org/10.1016/j.mayocpiqo.2017.09.002

Blake H., & Chambers, D. (2012). Supporting nurse health champions: Developing a 'new generation' of health improvement facilitators. *Health Education Journal, 71*(2), 205–210. doi:10.1177/0017896910396767

Blum, C. A. (2014). Practicing self-care for nurses: A nursing program initiative. *OJIN: The Online Journal of Issues in Nursing, 19*(3), 3. https://doi.org/10.3912/OJIN.Vol19No03Man03

Casalicchio, G., Lesaffre, E., Küchenhoff, H., & Bruyneel, L. (2017). Nonlinear analysis to detect if excellent nursing work environments have highest well being. *Journal of Nursing Scholarship, 49*(5), 537–547. https://doi.org/10.1111/jnu.12317

Cunningham, T. (2020). The burden of resilience should not fall solely on nurses: Healthcare organizations should manage resilience from the top down. *American Journal of Nursing, 120*(9), 11. https://doi.org/10.1097/01.NAJ.0000697544.96740.a6

Dall'Ora, C., Ball, J., Reinius, M., & Griffiths, P. (2020). Burnout in nursing: A theoretical review. *Human Resources for Health, 18,* 41. https://doi.org/10.1186/s12960-020-00469-9

Davidson, J. E., Proudfoot, J., Lee, K., Terterian, G., & Zisook, S. (2020). A longitudinal analysis of nurse suicide in the United States (2005–2016) with recommendations for action. *Worldviews on Evidence-Based Nursing, 17*(1), 6–15. https://doi.org/10.1111/wvn.12419

Davis, W. (2015). *The happiness industry: How the government and big business sold us well-being.* Verso.

Halifax, J. (2018). *Standing at the edge: Finding freedom where fear and courage meet.* Flatiron Books.

Jørgensen, J., Karlsen, S., Stayner, L., Hansen, J., & Andersen, Z. (2017). Shift work and overall and cause-specific mortality in the Danish nurse cohort. *Scandinavian Journal of Work, Environment & Health, 43*(2), 117–126. Retrieved December 12, 2020, from http://www.jstor.org/stable/26386129

Kabat-Zinn, J. (2010, March). *Mindfulness in medicine and psychology: Its transformative and healing potential in living and in dying.* Talk presented at the University of Virginia, Virginia, U.S.

Lucian Leape Institute. (2013). *Through the eyes of the workforce: Creating joy, meaning, and safer healthcare.* National Patient Safety Foundation.

Melnyk, B. M., Orsolini, L., Tan, A., Arslanian-Engoren, C., Melkus, G. D., Dunbar-Jacob, J., Rice, V. H., Millan, A., Dunbar, S. B., Braun, L. T., Wilbur, J., Chyun, D. A., Gawlik, K., Lewis, & L. M. (2018). A national study links nurses' physical and mental health to medical errors and perceived worksite wellness. *Journal of Occupational and Environmental Medicine, 60*(2), 126–131. doi:10.1097/JOM.0000000000001198

National Academies of Sciences, Engineering, and Medicine. (2019). *Taking action against clinician burnout: A systems approach to professional well-being.* The National Academies Press. https://doi.org/10.17226/25521

Oakley, B., Knafo, A., Madhavan, G., & Wilson, D. S. (Eds.). (2011). *Pathological altruism.* Oxford University Press.

Priano, S. M., Hong, O. S., & Chen, J. L. (2018). Lifestyles and related health consequences of US hospital nurses': a systematic review. *Nursing Outlook. Jan–Feb;66*(1), 66–76. doi:10.1016/j.outlook.2017.08.013

Prilleltensky, I. (2020). Mattering at the intersection of psychology, philosophy, and politics. *American Journal of Community Psychology, 65*(1–2), 16–34. https://doi.org/10.1002/ajcp.12368

Ross, A., Bevans, M., Brooks, A. T., Gibbons, S., & Wallen, G. R. (2017). Nurses and health-promoting behaviors: Knowledge may not translate into self-care. *AORN Journal, 105*(3), 267–275. https://doi.org/10.1016/j.aorn.2016.12.018

Rudman, A., & Gustavsson, J. P. (2011). Early-career burnout among new graduate nurses: A prospective observational study of intra-individual change trajectories, *International Journal of Nursing Studies, 48*(3), 292–306. https://doi.org/10.1016/j.ijnurstu.2010.07.012

Vetter, C., Devore, E. E., Wegrzyn, L. R., Massa, J., Speizer, F. E., Kawachi, I., Rosner, B., Stampfer, M. J., & Schernhammer, E. S. (2016). Association between rotating night shift work and risk of coronary heart disease among women. *JAMA. 315*(16), 1726–1734. doi:10.1001/jama.2016.4454

section I
Fundamentals

1
The Fundamentals of Stress, Burnout, and Self-Care

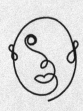

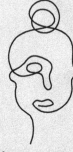

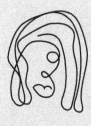

Tim Cunningham
pronouns: He/Him

Tim Cunningham began his professional career as an actor, then a hospital clown. He began doing international humanitarian work with Clowns Without Borders. While a clown, he fell in love with nurses' ability to connect with patients and families, even in times of terrible suffering—so he became an emergency nurse. The rest is history.

Dorrie K. Fontaine
pronouns: She/Her

Dorrie K. Fontaine, a critical care nurse and teacher, has been an academic leader for four decades. While president of the American Association of Critical-Care Nurses, she observed the joys and struggles of bedside nursing. Meditation, yoga, and daily gratitude practice help her overcome the fears and anxieties of our common human existence.

Natalie May
pronouns: She/Her

Natalie May, a writer, researcher, and teacher, collaborates with nurses, physicians, and others to improve patient care and colleague care. An Appreciative Inquiry facilitator, she has focused her research projects on wisdom in medicine and mattering in healthcare. For fun and self-care, she makes quilts.

"I do not trust people who don't love themselves and yet tell me, 'I love you.' There is an African saying which is: Be careful when a naked person offers you a shirt."

–Maya Angelou

When it comes to caring for others, nurses are too often the naked person offering someone else their shirt. We can't—and shouldn't—give something to our patients (and families and friends) that we don't have ourselves. We now know beyond any doubt that stress, and particularly stress in the workplace, has a powerful impact on our mental and physical health. Our goal in this chapter, and this book, is to help you develop an awareness of your in-the-moment risk for the effects of stress and to help you build on the self-care practices that you have most likely begun to develop.

As a nursing student, you already have an intimate knowledge of stress, and you are not alone. Nursing students have "significantly more stress, anxiety, sleep disturbances, and stress-related illnesses than the general student body" (Barlett et al., 2016, p. 87). In addition to the rigors of classwork and exams, you have the added stress of clinicals and, probably for the first time, you are attending to patients and families who are suffering. If you are like most of your nursing school peers, you are also wondering if you will ever be prepared to do the vitally important work of caring for patients. When your non-nursing school friends experience stress, they may have more time to exercise, to go out with friends, and to chill. You, on the other hand, need to get a good night's sleep for tomorrow's 7:00 a.m. clinical.

The good news is that you already have a self-care practice, whether you name it as such or not. You know when you are feeling exhausted. You have probably said to yourself or others, "I just need to take a break and clear my head." Or you know when you need a nap or to go for a run or to call home. And we suspect that you are self-aware enough to feel how the nap, run, or conversation with your family refreshes and restores you.

The goal, however, is to not wait until you're running on empty to take care of your own needs. Don't be the naked person offering someone your shirt. As we wrote in the book's introduction, self-care will involve learning now, while you're a student, which self-care practices work best for you. It will entail *practice* so that self-care behaviors are as hardwired as possible by the time you are a nurse. Most importantly, it will entail a continual monitoring of your mind and body so that you can *choose* in each moment what action will best serve you. It will involve constantly *checking in with yourself*, just as you would check in on a patient.

Personal Perspective

An Inner Energy Gauge

—Anna DeLong, MSW, CEAP (she/her)

A long journey's success will be affected by how well you refuel along the way.

In our culture it is generally accepted mechanical wisdom that if you want to drive across the country in your car, there is no way to do this successfully without pausing to pull over and refuel. Monitoring the gas gauge and refueling accordingly is essential. Neglect refueling, and you end up stuck on the side of the road. While this mechanical wisdom is at times challenged to explore the distance one's vehicle can travel on vapors, it is not questioned. A car requires refueling or recharging in order to sustain progress on the journey.

Can you imagine how your life might be different if you applied this same wisdom to your body? Imagine having an Inner Energy Gauge that monitors not just your physical energy level, but also your emotional energy and your cognitive energy. How might your life be different if you vowed to never go below ¼ tank without refueling? If you were to check your own Inner Energy Gauge right now, what would you discover? Are you running low? Do you know how to refuel? Do you know what nourishes and restores you the most effectively? Do you know your own early warning signs?

Over the past 23 years, I have asked these questions of thousands of dedicated, hard-working healthcare providers. Not only did they indicate they were on empty more often than not, but many also reported they didn't know how to refuel or couldn't remember how they used to do so. I don't believe this is a coincidence. Instead of self-monitoring and honoring one's own needs, it is common in our culture to click into high gear and stay there intending to just "push through" in order to bring a mission to fruition. We often walk around with this unconscious assumption that we will somehow automatically just get what we need for ourselves even as we attend to everyone else. This is a problematic and errant assumption. It is imperative that we intentionally and consciously plan to attend to our own needs along the way.

One of the most debilitating symptoms of depletion is the loss of perspective. Diminished frustration tolerance, lack of empathy, foggy thinking, poor memory, and difficulty problem-solving are also signs of a depleted energy tank. If you find yourself in this brain state, remember this is not an indication of an inadequate person; rather, this is a sign of a person low on energy. An optimal response is one that assesses the inner energy gauge and potential refueling needs with grace and self-compassion.

If the goal is to live and work in a healthy and sustainable way, learning to not only recognize signs you are running low on energy but also to respond in ways that effectively nourish and restore you is essential. Rather than just assume or hope you will get what you need, it is wise to strategize. Looking over your calendar to schedule and protect time for refueling at strategic intervals depending upon the pace and amount of energy you are expending will benefit you as well as those for whom you care.

Check In With Yourself

How do you feel when you are walking to an exam? Are you tense or anxious? Is there any discomfort in your stomach or bowels? A tightness in your neck or shoulders? What are you thinking that makes you feel this way? Could you think differently about the exam, and would that new way of thinking change the way you feel? Can you intentionally release the tension in your shoulders? This begins the process of checking in or noticing; making a choice in the moment about how to proceed; and compassionately caring for yourself by switching to a new thought or behavior.

Much of this book will be about ways to check in with yourself and the myriad responses to what you learn about your physical and mental status when you check in. Try thinking about it this way. If you check in on a patient and she says her legs hurt, you will assess the cause (e.g., DVT, loss of pulse), and then you might try several different things to help her feel better. You may recall something you tried with a patient last month that worked. You might ask a colleague for advice. You might get discouraged, but you'll try again. You may discover there is something she needs, and you'll have to advocate for her to get it. This is a similar process to developing a continual and effective self-care practice. If you check in with yourself and find you're feeling irritated, for example, you might need to try a few things to calm yourself and not let the irritation overtake you.

We suspect you are aware that nurses are likely to face emotional distress while caring for patients who are suffering, injured, or dying. Burnout, professional compassion fatigue, moral distress, posttraumatic stress disorder, and secondary traumatic stress disorder have been studied in the context of nursing for several decades. In writing this book, even we were astonished by the overwhelming research demonstrating the vulnerability of nurses to burnout, anxiety, depression, addiction and substance abuse, and other mental health problems including suicide (American Nurses Association [ANA], 2011; Davidson et al., 2020; Health Policy Institute of Ohio, 2020; Mark & Smith, 2012; Roberts & Grubb, 2014). In fact, nurses have a higher rate of depression than any other profession (Brandford & Reed, 2016; Letvak et al., 2012), and critical care nurses have the highest rates of all (Moss et al., 2016). There is clearly a need for courses, books, and resources to help nursing students prepare to care for their well-being and mental health as they transition to their nursing careers.

In this book, we will also encourage you to check in with and care for your body. Despite the fact that nurses do extraordinary work helping others prevent and mitigate the harm of lifestyle-related disease, nurses are at extremely high risk of developing these diseases themselves, despite having significant knowledge about preventing these diseases (Ross et al., 2017). Nurses have a high prevalence of obesity, poor eating and nutrition, and sedentary lifestyles that result in poor health outcomes such as heart disease and type 2 diabetes (Buss, 2012). They also have high rates of work-related illness, including chronic back pain, headaches, insomnia, tension, fatigue, impaired memory, decreased attention, and injury (Dyrbye et al., 2019; Melnyk, 2020; National Academies of Sciences, Engineering, and Medicine, 2019). Night shifts, evening shifts, and long shifts also have a negative impact on nurses' physical health and even mortality (Books et al., 2017; Melnyk et al., 2018; Stimpfel et al., 2013; Stimpfel et al., 2012). Poor health, in turn, increases nurse absenteeism, job dissatisfaction, and turnover (Dyrbye et al., 2019; Perry et al., 2016; Torquati et al., 2017).

Nurses' poor health also has an impact on patients and their outcomes. Several studies have demonstrated that the physical and mental health of nurses can have a negative impact on the quality of patient care and patient safety (Aiken et al., 2012; Hall et al., 2016; Melnyk et al., 2018). Burnout has demonstrated links to unprofessional clinician behavior and negative patient experiences (Windover et al., 2018). And of great concern, the overall turnover rate in nursing remains high; among early career nurses, one in five new nurses leaves their job within the first year, and one in three nurses leaves within the first two years (Robert Wood Johnson Foundation, 2014).

Your well-being matters. It matters to you in terms of your physical and mental health, and it matters to the patients in your care. In this chapter, we'll discuss why self-care matters and what we know about self-care in nursing, including barriers to self-care that nurses may encounter. We'll begin by exploring stress and the causes of burnout in nursing.

Stress and Burnout in Nursing

We're all up-close-and-personal acquaintances of stress. You couldn't possibly be where you are today without regular encounters with stress, both the good and bad kind, and stressful situations. *Stress* is anything that causes you to have a sudden physical or psychological reaction. It makes sense that some stress and stressors are a good thing. A sports competition, an exam, a first date, and a bear sighting on a hiking trail are all stressful situations, but your body's reaction can heighten your ability to respond effectively, like a jolt of energy and awareness. On the other hand, negative stressors and stress, such as physical danger or a traumatic event, can put your body into overdrive. This "fight or flight" response is a great gift if you are swerving to miss an oncoming car or running from a burning building. But if you are continually bombarded by stressors and you stay in that heightened state, it can cause serious health risks.

If you are not familiar with stress by now, you soon will be. There is no profession that reports a higher level of occupational stress than nursing (ANA, 2011). Hold onto your hat, because the list of factors that cause stress and burnout in nurses is long. Let that sink in while we talk about what we mean by burnout.

A History of Burnout

The term "burnout" was first coined in 1974 by Holocaust survivor and researcher, Herbert J. Freudenberger. While doing volunteer work in a free clinic and substance abuse treatment therapeutic community, Freudenberger began to notice in himself and others a state that he called "burn-out." (The term originated in a 1960 Graham Greene novel, *A Burnt-Out Case*, and had become part of the youth lexicon of the period.) Freudenberger identified the physical and behavioral symptoms of those who had "become exhausted by making excessive demands on energy, strength, and resources" (Freudenberger, 1974, p. 159). The physical symptoms included "a feeling of exhaustion and fatigue, being unable to shake a lingering cold, suffering from frequent headaches and gastrointestinal disturbances, sleeplessness and shortness of breath" (p. 160). Behavioral symptoms included being short-tempered, prone to tears, anger, and emotional outbursts. He argued that the people most susceptible to burn-out were "the dedicated and the committed" (p. 161).

Freudenburger's observations have held up over the years, with many researchers delving deeper into burnout's causes, effects, and remedies. The term has gained traction in multiple fields where employees work closely with other people, such as nursing, social work, ministry, and teaching, to name a few. In 1981, Christina Maslach and Susan Jackson developed a robust and universally used measure of burnout, the Maslach Burnout Inventory (Maslach & Jackson, 1981). The World Health Organization now lists burnout as a work-related syndrome (WHO, 2019). Burnout has become a topic of rigorous and urgent study in healthcare professions as we have recognized the significant role burnout plays in both employee well-being and high-quality patient care (Dyrbye et al., 2019). It is safe to say that burnout in healthcare will remain a priority in the coming decade; its high prevalence has resulted in several high-visibility reports on burnout and clinician well-being in healthcare. As one example, the National Academies of Sciences, Engineering, and Medicine (2019) published an over-300-page report, *Taking Action Against Clinician Burnout,* and the authors point to many signs that momentum is building for us to address the health and safety of healthcare workers and learners. We hope all these efforts will have a significant impact on the epidemic of burnout in healthcare.

What Is Burnout?

Burnout is an employee's response to excessive work-related stress, stress that goes unaddressed for a long period of time. It is not the result of a one-time stressor, such as a difficult shift or an especially challenging patient. Instead, as Maslach describes, burnout stems from one or more "mismatches" between an employee and their work that, if prolonged, result in burnout.

Maslach's (1998) conceptualization of burnout is characterized by three dimensions:

- Emotional exhaustion, or feelings of loss of energy or exhaustion; feeling emotionally drained

- Depersonalization, or feelings of mental distance from one's job, or feelings of negativism or cynicism related to one's job; loss of idealism

- Reduced sense of personal accomplishment, efficacy, or competence

Emotional exhaustion and depersonalization often go hand in hand. If you are feeling emotionally exhausted, you may more readily feel that your patients are less worthy of compassionate treatment. In some cases, depersonalization manifests as the belief that patients are somehow deserving of their bad fortune, or even that they brought it upon themselves (Maslach & Jackson, 1981). Again, it follows that addressing burnout in nursing is critically important in order to ensure high-quality, compassionate care for our patients.

Causes of Burnout

Because unaddressed stressors can lead to burnout, it's important for us to consider the different types of stressors that you will encounter in your future workplace. Let's begin with typical workplace stressors, challenges that anyone can face in any work setting, not just hospitals and healthcare environments. These are the same stressors faced by administrative assistants, piano tuners, librarians, and music producers. Several Stanford researchers conducted a meta-analysis of 228 studies on workplace stressors, and they looked at self-rated physical and mental illness, doctor-reported illness, and mortality rates to determine the significance of workplace stress on health (Goh et al., 2015). The following is a list of workplace stressors they found to have a significantly negative impact on employees' mental health, physical health, and mortality:

- Low job control

- Absence of health insurance

- Work-family conflict

- Lack of perceived fairness in an organization and low organizational justice

- High job demands

- Low social support

- Shift work, long hours, and overtime

- Job insecurity

Stressors That Lead to Burnout in Nursing

While this is a daunting list of factors that increase one's risk of experiencing work-related ill health, they are not the factors unique to nursing. In nursing, whether you are in a small clinic, a large hospital, or anywhere in between, there will be additional workplace stressors resulting from your role in caring for others. In their review of burnout in nursing, Dall'Ora and colleagues (2020) report that:

> Research consistently found that adverse job characteristics—high workload, low staffing levels, long shifts, low control, low schedule flexibility, time pressure, high job and psychological demands, low task variety, role conflict, low autonomy, negative nurse-physician relationship, poor supervisor/leader support, poor leadership, negative team relationship, and job insecurity—were associated with burnout in nursing. (Dall'Ora et al., 2020, p. 13)

There are other stressors in the nursing workplace. In a survey of 14,000 nurses, the ANA (2017) found that:

- "45% of respondents ranked lifting/repositioning of heavy objects as a significant health and safety risk for nurses
- 25% had been physically assaulted at work by a patient or patient's family member
- 9% were concerned for their physical safety at work
- 51% reported experiencing musculoskeletal pain at work
- 56–57% reported often coming in early and staying late and working through breaks to accomplish their work
- About half of the respondents had been bullied in some manner in the workplace
- 59% of respondents reported that they worked 10 hours or longer daily
- 82% said they are at a "'significant level of risk for workplace stress'" (p. 4)

These are just a few of the challenges you will face that can lead to burnout. Many nurses practice in "busy, complex, and demanding work environments" and "are routinely confronted with human suffering, patient morbidity and mortality, complex ethical decision-making, and difficulty conversations with patients and their families" (Cheung et al., 2020, p. 167).

Work-family conflict is also a greater risk among nurses because of the pressures and intensity of our work. Responsibilities of family life often interfere with responsibilities at work, and this was identified among all workers in the Stanford study. In fact, they found that "work-family conflict increases the odds of self-reported poor physical health by about 90%" (Goh et al., 2015, p. 61). However, the nature of our work schedules and the emotionally and physically exhausting nature of nursing exacerbates the workplace-home responsibilities conflict. At least half of nurses report that work chronically interferes with family life, and at least 40% report that family interferes with work (Grzywacz et al., 2006). When there are not enough personal resources—time, energy, and emotions—to go around, this can result in emotional exhaustion, a key component of the burnout triad (Galletta et al., 2019).

Societal Stressors That Affect Nurse Well-Being

There are also larger societal trends that are already having an appreciative impact on the nursing workforce. Buerhaus and colleagues (2017) identified four major trends that will likely affect our ability to thrive in the coming decades. One is the aging of the millions in the baby boom generation that will lead to an increase in the demand, intensity, and complexity of healthcare. The second is the increasing shortage and uneven distribution of physicians. Nurses who practice in rural areas, in particular, will be asked to carry more of the healthcare burden for their populations. Third, just as baby boomer patients are aging, nurses of this generation have begun to retire in extremely high numbers. Since 2012, 60,000 nurses have retired each year, and this number is expected to increase (Auerbach et al., 2015; Staiger et al., 2012). Fourth, the authors identify the persistent uncertainties of healthcare reform as yet another factor that will have an impact on the nursing profession. The increasingly political and unpredictable nature of health policy has implications for patients' health and the care we provide.

Finally, the COVID-19 pandemic is another development likely to have a dramatic effect on the nursing workforce. In one 2020 survey, 61% of nurses responded that they were planning to quit their jobs or leave nursing altogether (Masson, 2020) because they lack personal protective equipment, sufficient safety regulations, and adequate support from administrators. These workforce challenges in the coming decades will have an impact on working nurses, and we will need energy and resilience to address them.

In nursing, given our intimate position beside patients and families, it is our responsibility to *offer compassionate care under all work conditions*. When faced with a bad supervisor or a long shift, nurses cannot dial back the quality of care they provide. Nurses are caught in a particularly stressful circumstance in that workplace stressors are magnified because they impact the quality of care a nurse is able to provide. It's a cruel cycle of stress, and this may be the most important reason why a self-care practice is so important.

Self-Care: Why It Matters

A colleague of ours, Sam, shared the story of her career path. We affectionately call her "the firefighter" because she was a firefighter with her father before she was old enough to drive. She served two military tours as a nurse in Iraq and Afghanistan before returning to the States to work in a busy emergency department. Just like in her firefighter days, she thrived on the pace and the challenge of a war zone and an ED. Reflecting on why she eventually had to leave the ED, she said, "It was so easy to be present [with patients and families] and just be available, but at the same time, that all comes at a price, right? Because every time you're a part of those intense experiences, a little piece of you goes out into the world, your light and your energy. And if you are not working hard to restore that, which I wasn't, it starts to dim."

Sam knew that she was no longer able to provide the kind of care that her patients deserved, and she found a job she loves in interventional cardiology at the same hospital. Her self-awareness allowed her to eventually care for herself, and in her new unit, she provides compassionate care without such a high personal cost. Pamela Ashcraft and Susan Gatto have extensively studied self-care in nursing students, and they express concern that many nursing students may not grasp this "connection between personal self-care and its influence on professional practice" (Ashcraft & Gatto, 2018, p. 140). This harkens back to what we outlined in the introduction of this book, that too often we mistakenly believe that self-care is selfish. The impact of your well-being on your sphere of influence cannot be overstated.

In addition to mental and physical health problems, stress and burnout can have significant consequences to your career, to the patients you care for, and to the organizations you work in. Ashcraft and Gatto have argued that "personal self-care should be an expectation of the professional nursing role," (2018, p. 140) and we cannot agree more. The National Academies of Sciences, Engineering, and Medicine recently published a pivotal document, *Taking Action Against Clinician Burnout: A Systems Approach to Professional Well-Being* (2019), and they summarize the consequences of burnout from personal, patient, and organizational perspectives. We appreciate that this is a lot to take in. We have summarized the consequences of nursing burnout in Table 1.1.

Table 1.1 Impacts of Burnout on Nursing Career, Patient Care, and Healthcare Organizations

Impacts on Nursing Career	Impacts on Patient Care	Impacts on Healthcare Organizations
Job dissatisfaction	Suboptimal quality of patient care	Absenteeism
Intention to leave job	Racial bias toward patients	Lower willingness to lead
Decision to leave job	Increased patient mortality ratios	Lower inpatient satisfaction ratings
Desire to leave profession	Errors and mistakes; patient safety	More healthcare-associated infections

Decline in job performance	Unprofessional behavior by nurses	Increased malpractice claims
Occupational injury	Poor communication between nurses and patients	Presenteeism (working while sick)
Problematic alcohol use	Missed care	High nursing turnover
Suicide risk	Infections	Reduced individual productivity
Career regret	Patient dissatisfaction	
Suboptimal professional development	Patient falls	
Decline in general health	Family complaints	
Decline in mental health		

Vulnerability of New and Early Career Nurses

Health systems have begun to develop transition-to-practice programs to ensure that newly licensed registered nurses (NLRNs) experience a successful transition to their new role. By focusing on maintaining new nurses' physical and mental health, these programs show promise in reducing turnover and slowing job attrition rates (Sampson et al., 2019). While early indications suggest that these programs are beneficial (Edwards et al., 2015), the availability of this support is far from universal. Up to 66% of NLRNs may experience burnout and stress-related ill health in their early years of practice (Laschinger & Fida, 2014). In one study, one in five nurses reported *extremely high levels* of burnout within their first three years after graduation, and the highest risk occurred during the second year of practice (Rudman & Gustavsson, 2011).

In addition to the stressors that nurses at all levels experience, the novice nurse has the added stress of being in a new role, having to master new skills in a high-stakes environment, and becoming socialized into a new profession and workplace. These nurses often face heavy workloads and unsupportive practice environments (Kanai-Pak et al., 2008). They may also find that the daily work of nursing does not match their expectations (Mackintosh, 2006). For these and other reasons, it is critical that novice and early career nurses be equipped to not only care for their patients but also care for themselves.

Defining Self-Care

You have just read an entire chapter about the hazards to your well-being that you will face in the career that you have barely begun. The good news is that you can create, as Dean Cipriano called it in the foreword, your own "personal force field." This force field can be made up of many things, including the qualities that are inherently you, such as your personality, experiences, values, and desires. Your personal force field can also be formed through self-care practices, many of which we will explore in this book. The more we learn about nurses and their self-care practices, the clearer it becomes that these practices are effective. And most importantly, research also demonstrates that the more you *practice* self-care, the more it helps to protect you against the stressors you will face (Frögéli et al., 2020). Self-care will also help you become a more compassionate nurse. There is increasing evidence that "when people increase their own well-being, they usually become more patient, cooperative, and caring in their relationships" (Hanson, 2018, p. 11).

There may be as many definitions of self-care as there are causes of stress and burnout. Researchers Pamela Ashcraft and Susan Gatto (2018) describe self-care as "deliberate decisions made and actions taken by individuals to address their own health and well-being" (p. 140). We underscore that these decisions and actions may be ongoing, or long-term practices (e.g., exercise, healthy nutrition, yoga), as well as in-the-moment awareness and responses to stressors, such as a short-tempered resident or the death of a patient. We have the capacity to decide and to act.

As we wrote in the introduction, self-care is not "one size fits all." It is not selfish. Nurses do not create well-being in themselves simply by caring for others. Self-care is as much about the mind as it is about the body. It is a lifelong practice, something that will take time, patience, self-compassion, and experimentation to develop.

In this book, you will explore a wide variety of self-care practices from many different perspectives. Some will resonate deeply. Others may not be your cup of tea at all. Some might not work for you today, but in a few years, you may revisit them with a different result. We encourage you to try as many as possible, reflect on how effective they were or weren't for you, and begin to build the tool kit that will become your own personal force field.

We invite you to begin with an exploration exercise described in the sidebar, Exploring Self-Care. This activity will give you an opportunity to get a sense of (1) the vastness of the term *self-care* and (2) what practices resonate with you personally.

Exploring Self-Care

Most of our suggested activities will appear in the accompanying workbook. That said, this one is pretty important, and we think spending some time exploring the wide array of self-care practices is the best way to jump into this text or course.

1.   Google the terms "self-care" and "self-care practices." Expand your search if you're feeling especially ambitious or curious.

2.   Grab a pen and paper (or your phone or laptop) and make a list of some of what pops up. You will find memes, posters, infographics, quotes, research articles, and more. Make a list, or a Pinterest board, of things that intrigue you or resonate with your personality and current self-care practices.

Are you an athlete or an artist? Do you recoup your energy by being in nature? Is your highest priority staying connected with family and friends? As you explore, try to imagine yourself engaging in some of these practices.

Which concepts make you think, *"I could get into this?"* Or, *"This makes sense to me?"* What ideas intrigue you or make you want to learn more? These concepts might be your own personal entrées into the study and practice of self-care.

As you are browsing the Internet for self-care practices and ideas, try to categorize each practice into one of the following self-care and wellness categories. Some may fit into more than one category.

• Physical

• Mental

• Emotional

continues

continued

- Spiritual
- Intellectual
- Social
- Financial
- Environmental

What else do you notice about self-care and how it is presented? Do any depictions and practices make you uncomfortale? How do some reinforce or break stereotypes?

Barriers to Self-Care in Nursing

You might be wondering, "If the benefits of self-care are so obvious, why is this such a big deal? Why don't we, as nurses, just take better care of ourselves? We teach our patients how to take care of themselves, so why can't we practice what we preach?" We know from the many studies on nurses' self-care practices that it is not that simple. Alyson Ross and her colleagues conducted a review of barriers to self-care in nursing (2017) as well as a survey of registered nurses (2019) to address those very questions. They wondered why, if nurses possess knowledge regarding health-promoting behaviors, that doesn't translate into their own self-care and well-being. Why is there such a disconnect between what we know to be good for us and what we actually do? Why, for example, are rates of obesity among nurses in the 23%–61.4% range (Buss, 2012), while the prevalence of obesity among adults in the US is 42.4% (Hales et al., 2020).

In Ross and colleagues' examination of current research (2017), they focused on nurses' health-promoting behaviors, such as healthy diet and exercise, stress management, sleep hygiene, and healthy relationship practices. We should note that these behaviors are very synergistic. If you are sleep-deprived, it will be hard to muster the energy to cook a healthy meal or go for a 3-mile run after your shift. If you are constantly stressed, you are more likely to gain weight or be obese. Social support has a strong influence on healthy behaviors, and negative social interactions, such as bullying, increase stress and stress-related illness.

Ross and colleagues (2017) identified barriers to these health-promoting behaviors among nurses. These included intrinsic factors, such as age, sex, past experience, fatigue, anxiety, and depression. Other intrinsic factors included "perceived benefits and barriers" and "self-efficacy." The extrinsic factors that influenced nurses' participation in health-promoting behaviors included "interpersonal influences" such as family, friends, and peers, and "situational influences," which largely fell to the work environment and work schedules, as well as outside demands.

In a later study, Ross and her colleagues (2019) administered a three-item, open-ended survey to over 260 registered nurses in order to identify the influences on their health-promoting behaviors. They identified the following barriers to self-care among nurses:

- **No time/overwork.** "Many participants spoke of commutes in excess of 1 hour that, coupled with shifts of 10+ hours, left precious little time for exercising or preparing healthy meals" (p. 364).

- **Lack of adequate resources/facilities.** This included lack of convenient access to a gym, showers, refrigerators and microwave ovens; reasonably priced healthy snack options; or classes that fit with a nursing schedule.

- **Fatigue/lack of sleep.** Fatigue left nurses "too drained, exhausted, and unmotivated to exercise, to prepare healthy meals/snacks, and/or reduce stress by attending yoga/meditation classes or socializing with family and friends" (p. 364).

- **Outside commitments.** Caring for others doesn't end for nurses when they leave their workplace. Family and community commitments, as well as attending school, left many nurses feeling "overextended."

- **Unhealthy food culture.** Nurses at work face an abundance of junk food, baked goods, and candy as well as frequent occasions (e.g., birthdays, holidays, baby showers, farewells to coworkers) to celebrate with food.

Ross and colleagues (2019) also explored the influence of other individuals in the workplace, mainly coworkers and managers, who had both positive and negative influences on their health-promoting behaviors. Some nurses felt "judged" if they wanted to leave the workplace to take a walk, eat outside, or take a mental-health break. Inflexible scheduling and coverage prohibited many nurses from doing these practices.

On the other hand, coworkers and managers can have a strong positive influence on healthy lifestyles. Positive environment activities included walking with peers, sharing healthy recipes, fitness and weight-loss challenges, and encouragement to eat meals and take breaks. And finally, nurses discussed the power of healthy role models in motivating them to exercise regularly, follow a healthy diet, and craft a healthy work-life balance. Similarly, negative role models can have the reverse effect. Supervisors who did not model healthy behaviors often scheduled regular "working lunch" meetings, encouraged unhealthy food in the workplace, and expected staff to respond to emails on evenings and weekends.

Stressors are everywhere in nursing; they come with the territory. Unfortunately, barriers to self-care are also plentiful, and many of them are found in a nurse's own work environment, the place where we are focused on the health and well-being of others. This is an unsettling conflict and one reason that unhealthy work environments must be called out and addressed.

Healthy Work Environments

Chronic stress and burnout are not necessarily a given. We know that healthy work environments successfully promote well-being among the nurses who work in them (Casalicchio et al., 2017). In a supportive work environment, the average nurse can cope with the necessary stressors of high-acuity patients and adverse events; they are challenging aspects of the job, but a nurse can move through them to the other side and even flourish (Galletta et al., 2019). A supportive work environment also reduces the likelihood that early career nurses will leave their profession (Guerrero et al., 2017). You will read more about healthy work environments in Chapter 18.

If You Only Read One More Thing in This Book...

Self-care for student nurses is a wonderfully broad and exciting topic with the potential to help you flourish and live a life of meaning and compassion. This book is our invitation to you, the student and early career nurse, to build your own tool kit of practices. That said, we believe that the following four practices should be the foundation of whatever tool kit you create for yourself:

1. **Drink water.** In addition to the obvious physiological importance of hydration, water has other restorative properties. What many people don't realize is that when you feel hungry or tired, often a serious drink of water (or sparkling water) will help you regain solid footing. Find a "water transport system" that works best for you. Slap a sticker on it that makes you smile. Keep your bottle full and your water cool. And don't forget to drink.

2. **Unclench.** Right now. Check in with yourself. Are any muscles in your body tightly clenched? Your forehead, jaw, neck, or shoulders? If they are, relax them and notice the difference in how you feel. Pay attention to feelings of tightness as often as you can throughout the day. When you find this physical tension in your body, let it go. Gently. Don't berate yourself for "letting yourself" tighten up again. We get tense. It just happens. But if we notice the tension and release it, we'll feel better. It's a good way to be present with yourself, and that is always a good thing. Neuroscientist Jill Bolte Taylor (2006) recommends that if you're ever having trouble falling asleep, notice if you are clenching your jaw. Release the tension and see what happens.

3. **Take a deep, restorative breath.** Or two or three. A systematic review of interventions using only diaphragmatic breathing for stress reduction supports this self-care practice (Hopper et al., 2019). Restorative breathing is free, can be done anywhere by anyone, involves no pharmaceuticals or calories, has no addictive properties, and works. Deep breaths can effectively lower your respiratory rate and cortisol levels, improve blood pressure, increase concentration and focus, and reduce anxiety and depression. There are many deep breathing practices, including the SKY Breath Meditation

that has shown good results with college students (Seppälä et al., 2020), but one we especially like is the Box Breathing technique, described in the sidebar below.

Box Breathing

Box Breathing is a simple four-part technique that you can do every morning and throughout the day as needed. SEALFIT founder and Navy Seal, Mark Divine, developed the technique, claiming it allowed him to remain calm and focused during the chaos of battle (Divine, 2016). If it can work for a Navy Seal in the middle of combat, we're thinking it can work for a nurse in an ICU. Or anyone who needs a bit of calm.

Begin by expelling all the air from your chest.

Step 1: Keep your lungs empty for four counts.

Step 2: Inhale through your nose for four counts.

Step 3: Hold the air in your lungs for four counts. Don't get tense.

Step 4: Release and exhale smoothly through your nose for four counts.

Divine recommends repeating the cycle five times to get the full effect. This is an excellent technique to share with your patients, too.

4. **Be present.** We will discuss this quite a bit in the next chapter on resilience and throughout the book, but we can tell you now that a "wandering mind is an unhappy mind"(Killingsworth & Gilbert, 2010, p. 932). Killingsworth and Gilbert (2010) conducted a clever study with over 2,000 adult participants and a smartphone app. They contacted participants randomly throughout the day and asked what they were doing at that moment, how they were feeling, and if their minds were wandering. Their study confirmed what philosophical and religious traditions have told us for years, that living in the moment fosters happiness and well-being. They learned that people's minds wander a lot. They also learned that people were less happy when their minds wandered, no

matter what they were doing at the moment. In other words, mind-wandering was the cause, not the consequence, of unhappiness.

Closing Thoughts

This chapter has presented a lot of material, and we admit that it probably hasn't been very uplifting. All jobs have stressors, and people in many lines of work face burnout. You are not alone in this. We believe the good news is that you have chosen a profession that hopefully will provide you with some ballast, that force that gives boats stability and keeps them from tipping over. Your ballast will be many things, including your sense of self, your energy, your sense of humor, and your commitment to your patients and profession. Resilience will be another ballast, and we will explore that in the next three chapters. Our hope is that with your own self-care practices, you will be able to maintain your ballast as well as your balance.

In Real Practice

Yvonne ten Hoeve and her colleagues (2019, 2018) in the Netherlands conducted an interesting study of job turnover, using diary entries of 18 novice nurses. Their research focused on the impact of negative emotions in response to job stressors and whether those resulting negative emotions affected novice nurses' professional commitment. In fact, they found that when lack of support from colleagues, negative experiences with patients, and facing grave illness and death lead to negative emotions, professional commitment decreases. This suggests that it is not the experiences themselves that increase nursing turnover, but the resulting negative emotions. Novice nurses must be supported by supervisors and colleagues and encourage to talk about and process their negative emotions.

Key Points

- Nurses tend to be the "naked person" who tries to give someone else their shirt. Do not be that nurse. Care for yourself so you can better care for others. There is a strong argument to be made that self-care practices should be a professional expectation for all nurses.

- We all face stress, and in general, that isn't a bad thing. The right amount of stress gives us the physiological and psychological boost we need to be at the top of our game. However, too much stress and not having the skills or resources to deal with stress can be a serious threat to well-being.

- Repeated stressors, especially those we have no control over, can lead to burn-out. Burnout in nursing is a significant workforce problem that affects not only the individual nurse, but also patient care, safety, and the organizations where they work.

- There are many causes of burnout in nursing. These include high workload, poor staffing, long shifts, low control, negative relationships with colleagues, and lack of support.

- Nurses face many barriers to self-care practices including lack of time, inadequate resources and facilities, fatigue, outside commitments, and unhealthy food cultures at work.

- Start putting together your tool kit now: drink water, unclench tight muscles, breathe, and be present.

References

Aiken, L. H., Sermeus, W., Van den Heede, K., Sloane, D. M., Busse, R., McKee, M., Bruyneel, L., Rafferty, A. M., Griffiths, P., Moreno-Casbas, M. T., Tishelman, C., Scott, A., Brzostek, T., Kinnunen, J., Schwendimann, R., Heinen, M., Zikos, D., Sjetne, I. S., Smith, H. L., & Kutney-Lee, A. (2012). Patient safety, satisfaction, and quality of hospital care: Cross sectional surveys of nurses and patients in 12 countries in Europe and the United States. *British Medical Journal (Clinical Research Ed.), 344,* e1717.

American Nurses Association. (2011). *2011 health and safety survey.* Author.

American Nurses Association. (2017). Executive Summary: American Nurses Association Health Risk Appraisal. https://www.nursingworld.org/~4aeeeb/globalassets/practiceandpolicy/work-environment/health--safety/ana-healthriskappraisalsummary_2013-2016.pdf

Ashcraft, P. F., & Gatto, S. L. (2018). Curricular interventions to promote self-care in prelicensure nursing students, *Nurse Educator, 43*(3):140–144. doi:10.1097/NNE.0000000000000450

Auerbach, D., Buerhaus, P., & Staiger, D. (2015). Will the RN workforce weather the retirement of the baby boomers? *Medical Care, 53*(10), 850–856. https://doi.org/10.1097/MLR.0000000000000415

Bartlett, M. L., Taylor, H., & Nelson, J. D. (2016). Comparison of mental health characteristics and stress between baccalaureate nursing students and non-nursing students. *Journal of Nursing Education, 55*(2): 87–90. https://doi.org/10.3928/01484834-20160114-05

Books, C., Coody, L. C., Kauffman, R., Abraham, S. (2017). Night shift work and its health effects on nurses. *The Health Care Manager, 36*(4), 347–353. https://doi.org/10.1097/HCM.0000000000000177

Brandford, A., & Reed, D. B. (2016). Depression in registered nurses: A state of the science. *Workplace Health and Safety.* Oct;64(10): 488–511. doi:10.1177/2165079916653415. PMID: 30209987

Buerhaus, P. I., Skinner, L. E., Auerbach, D. I., & Staiger, D. O. (2017). Four challenges facing the nursing workforce in the United States, *Journal of Nursing Regulation, 8*(2), 40–46. https://doi.org/10.1016/S2155-8256(17)30097-2

Buss, J. (2012). Associations between obesity and stress and shift work among nurses. *Workplace Health and Safety, 60*(10), 453–458. https://doi.org/10.1177/216507991206001007

Casalicchio, G., Lesaffre, E., Küchenhoff, H., & Bruyneel, L. (2017). Nonlinear analysis to detect if excellent nursing work environments have highest well-being. *Journal of Nursing Scholarship, 49,* 537–547. https://doi.org/10.1111/jnu.12317

Cheung, E. O., Hernandez, A., Herold, E., & Moskowitz, J. T. (2020). Positive emotion skills intervention to address burnout in critical care nurses. *AACN Advanced Critical Care, 31*(2), 167–178. https://doi.org/10.4037/aacnacc2020287

Dall'Ora, C., Ball, J., Reinius, M., & Griffiths, P. (2020). Burnout in nursing: A theoretical review. *Human Resources for Health, 18,* 41. https://doiorg.proxy01.its.virginia.edu/10.1186/s12960-020-00469-9

Davidson, J. E., Proudfoot, J., Lee, K., Terterian, G., & Zisook, S. (2020). A longitudinal analysis of nurse suicide in the United States (2005–2016) with recommendations for action. *Worldviews on Evidence-Based Nursing, 17*(1), 6–15. https://doi-org.proxy01.its.virginia.edu/10.1111/wvn.12419

Divine, M. (2016, May 4). The breathing technique a Navy SEAL uses to stay calm and focused. *Time.* https://time.com/4316151/breathing-technique-navy-seal-calm-focused/?utm_source=newsletter&utm_medium=email&utm_campaign=time-health&utm_content=20200505

Dyrbye, L. N., Shanafelt, T. D., Johnson, P. O., Johnson, L. A., Satele, D., & West, C. P. (2019). A cross-sectional study exploring the relationship between burnout, absenteeism, and job performance among American nurses. *BMC Nursing, 18*, 57. https://doi.org/10.1186/s12912-019-0382-7

Edwards, D., Hawker, C., Carrier, J., & Rees, C. (2015). A systematic review of the effectiveness of strategies and interventions to improve the transition from student to newly qualified nurse. *International Journal of Nursing Studies, 52*(7), 1254–1268. https://doi.org/10.1016/j.ijnurstu.2015.03.007

Freudenberger, H. J. (1974). Staff burn-out. *Journal of Social Issues, 30,* 159–165. doi:10.1111/j.1540-4560.1974.tb00706.x

Frögéli, E., Rudman, A., Ljótsson, B., & Gustavsson, P. (2020). Preventing stress-related ill health among new registered nurses by supporting engagement in proactive behaviors—A randomized controlled trial. *Worldviews on Evidence-Based Nursing, 17,* 202–212. https://doi.org/10.1111/wvn.12442

Galletta, M., Portoghese, I., Melis, P., Aviles Gonzalez, C. I., Finco, G., D'Aloja, E., Contu, P., & Campagna, M. (2019). The role of collective affective commitment in the relationship between work–family conflict and emotional exhaustion among nurses: A multilevel modeling approach. *BMC Nursing, 18,* 5. https://doi-org/10.1186/s12912-019-0329-z

Goh, J., Pfeffer, J., Zenios, S. A., & Rajpal, S. (2015). Workplace stressors & health outcomes: Health policy for the workplace. *Behavioral Science & Policy 1*(1), 43–52. doi:10.1353/bsp.2015.0001

Greene, G. (1960). *A Burnt-Out Case.* William Heinemann Ltd.

Grzywacz, J. G., Frone, M. R., Brewer, C. S., & Kovner, C. T. (2006). Quantifying work–family conflict among registered nurses. *Research in Nursing Health, 29*(5), 414–426. https://doi.org/10.1002/nur.20133

Guerrero, S., Chênevert, D., & Kilroy, S. (2017). New graduate nurses' professional commitment: Antecedents and outcomes. *Journal of Nursing Scholarship, 49*(5), 572–579. https://doi.org/10.1111/jnu.12323

Hales, C. M., Carroll, M. D., Fryar, C. D., Ogden, C. L. (2020). Prevalence of obesity and severe obesity among adults: United States, 2017–2018. NCHS Data Brief, no 360. Hyattsville, MD: National Center for Health Statistics. https://www.cdc.gov/nchs/products/databriefs/db360.htm

Hall, L. H., Johnson, J., Watt, I., Tsipa, A., & O'Connor, D. B. (2016). Healthcare staff wellbeing, burnout, and patient safety: A systematic review. *PLOS ONE, 11*(7), e0159015. https://doi.org/10.1371/journal.pone.0159015

Hanson, R. (2018). *Resilient: How to grow an unshakable core of calm, strength, and happiness.* Harmony Books.

Health Policy Institute of Ohio. (2020, February 11). A call to action: Improving clinician wellbeing and patient care and safety. www.hpio.net/a-call-to-action/

Hopper, S. I., Murray, S. L., Ferrara, L. R., & Singleton, J. K. (2019). Effectiveness of diaphragmatic breathing for reducing physiological and psychological stress in adults: A quantitative systematic review. *JBI Database of Systematic Reviews and Implementation Reports, 17*(9), 1855–1876. https://doi.org/10.11124/JBISRIR-2017-003848

Kanai-Pak, M., Aiken, L. H., Sloane, D. M., & Poghosyan, L. (2008). Poor work environments and nurse inexperience are associated with burnout, job dissatisfaction and quality deficits in Japanese hospitals. *Journal of Clinical Nursing, 17*(24), 3324–3329. https://doi.org/10.1111/j.1365-2702.2008.02639.x

Killingsworth, M. A., & Gilbert, D. T. (2010, Nov. 12). A wandering mind is an unhappy mind. *Science, 330,* 932. https://wjh-www.harvard.edu/~dtg/KILLINGSWORTH%20&%20GILBERT%20(2010).pdf

Laschinger, H. K. S., & Fida, R. (2014). New nurses burnout and workplace wellbeing: The influence of authentic leadership and psychological capital. *Burnout Research, 1*(1), 19–28. https://doi.org/10.1016/j.burn.2014.03.002

Letvak, S., Ruhm, C., & Gupta, S. (2012). Nurses' presenteeism and its effects on self-reported quality of care and costs. *American Journal of Nursing, 112*(2), 30–38. doi:10.1097/01.NAJ.0000411176.15696.f9

Mackintosh, C. (2006). Caring: The socialisation of pre-registration student nurses: A longitudinal qualitative descriptive study. *International Journal of Nursing Studies, 43*(8), 953–962. https://doi.org/10.1016/j.ijnurstu.2005.11.006

Mark, G., & Smith, A. P. (2012). Occupational stress, job characteristics, coping, and the mental health of nurses. *British Journal of Health Psychology, 17,* 505–521. https://doi.org/10.1111/j.2044-8287.2011.02051.x

Maslach, C. (1998). A multidimensional theory of burnout. In C. L. Cooper (Ed.), *Theories of organizational stress* (pp. 68–85). Oxford University Press Inc.

Maslach, C., & Jackson, S. E. (1981). The measurement of experienced burnout. *Journal of Organizational Behavior, 2,* 99–113. https://doi.org/10.1002/job.4030020205

Masson, G. (May 20, 2020). Nurses say changing guidelines, unsafe conditions are pushing them to quit. *Becker's Hospital Review.* https://www.beckershospitalreview.com/nursing/nurses-say-changing-guidelines-unsafe-conditions-are-pushing-them-to-quit.html

Melnyk, B. M. (2020). Burnout, depression and suicide in nurses/clinicians and learners: An urgent call for action to enhance professional well-being and healthcare safety. *Worldviews on Evidence-Based Nursing, 17,* 2–5. https://doi.org/10.1111/wvn.12416

Melnyk, B. M., Orsolini, L., Tan, A., Arslanian-Engoren, C., Melkus, G. D., Dunbar-Jacob, J., Rice, V. H., Millan, A., Dunbar, S., Braun, L. T., Wilbur, J., Chyun, D. A., Gawlik, K., & Lewis, L. M. (2018). A national study links nurses' physical and mental health to medical errors and perceived worksite wellness. *Journal of Occupational and Environmental Medicine, 60*(2), 126–131. https://doi.org/10.1097/JOM.0000000000001198

Moss, M., Good, V. S., Gozal, D., Kleinpell, R., & Sessler, C. N. (2016). An official Critical Care Societies collaborative statement—burnout syndrome in critical care health-care professionals: A call to action. *Chest, 150*(1), 17–26. https://doi.org/10.1016/j.chest.2016.02.649

National Academies of Sciences, Engineering, and Medicine. (2019). *Taking action against clinician burnout: A systems approach to professional well-being.* The National Academies Press. https://doi.org/10.17226/25521

Perry, L., Gallagher, R., Duffield, C., Sibbritt, D. Bichel-Findlay, J., & Nicholls, R. (2016). Does nurses' health affect their intention to remain in their current position? *Journal of Nursing Management, 24*(8), 1088–1097. https://doi.org/10.1111/jonm.12412

Robert Wood Johnson Foundation. (2014, September 4). *Nearly one in five new nurses leave first job within a year, according to survey of newly-licensed registered nurses.* https://www.rwjf.org/en/library/articles-and-news/2014/09/nearly-one-in-five-new-nurses-leave-first-job-within-a-year--acc.html

Roberts, R. K., & Grubb, P. L. (2014). The consequences of nursing stress and need for integrated solutions. *Rehabilitation Nursing, 39*(2), 62–69. https://doi.org/10.1002/rnj.97

Ross, A., Bevans, M., Brooks, A. T., Gibbons, S., & Wallen, G. R. (2017). Nurses and health-promoting behaviors: Knowledge may not translate into self-care. *AORN Journal, 105*(3), 267–275. https://doi.org/10.1016/j.aorn.2016.12.018

Ross, A., Touchton-Leonard, K., Perez, A., Wehrlen, L., Kazmi, N., & Gibbons, S. (2019). Factors that influence health-promoting self-care in registered nurses: Barriers and facilitators. *Advances in Nursing Science, 42*(4), 358–373. https://doi.org/10.1097/ANS.0000000000000274

Rudman, A., & Gustavsson, J. P. (2011). Early-career burnout among new graduate nurses: A prospective observational study of intra-individual change trajectories, *International Journal of Nursing Studies, 48*(3), 292–306. https://doi.org/10.1016/j.ijnurstu.2010.07.012

Sampson, M., Melnyk, B. M., & Hoying, J. (2019). Intervention effects of the MINDBODYSTRONG cognitive behavioral skills-building program on newly licensed registered nurses' mental health, healthy lifestyle behaviors and job satisfaction. *Journal of Nursing Administration, 49*(10), 487–495. https://doi.org/10.1097/NNA.0000000000000792

Seppälä, E. M., Bradley, C., Moeller, J., Harouni, L., Nandamudi, D., & Brackett, M. A. (2020). Promoting mental health and psychological thriving in university students: A randomized controlled trial of three well-being interventions. *Frontiers in Psychiatry, 11*. https://doi.org/10.3389/fpsyt.2020.00590

Staiger, D., Auerbach, D., & Buerhaus, P. (2012). Registered nurse labor supply and the recession—Are we in a bubble? *The New England Journal of Medicine, 366*(16), 1463–1465. https://doi.org/10.1056.NEJMp1200641

Stimpfel, A. W., Lake, E. T., Barton, S., Gorman, K. C., & Aiken, L. H. (2013). How differing shift lengths relate to quality outcomes in pediatrics. *Journal of Nursing Administration, 43*(2), 95–100. https://doi.org/10.1097/NNA.0b013e31827f2244

Stimpfel, A. W., Sloane, D. M., & Aiken, L. H. (2012). The longer the shifts for hospital nurses, the higher the levels of burnout and patient dissatisfaction. *Health Affairs, 31*(11), 2501–2509. https://doi.org/10.1377/hlthaff.2011.1377

Taylor, J. B. (2006). *My stroke of insight: A brain scientist's personal journey*. Penguin Books.

ten Hoeve, Y., Brouwer, J., & Kunnen, S. (2019). Turnover prevention: The direct and indirect association between organizational job stressors, negative emotions and professional commitment in novice nurses. *Journal of Advanced Nursing, 76*(3): 836–845. doi:10.1111/jan.14281

ten Hoeve, Y., Kunnen, E. S., Brouwer, J., & Roodbol, P. F. (2018). The voice of nurses. Novice nurses' first experiences in a clinical setting. A longitudinal diary study. *Journal of Clinical Nursing, 27*, e1612–e1626. https://doi.org/10.1111/jocn.14307

Torquati, L., Pavey, T., Kolbe-Alexander, T., & Leveritt, M. (2017). Promoting diet and physical activity in nurses: A systematic review. *American Journal of Health Promotion, 31*(1), 19–27. https://doi.org/10.4278/ajhp.141107-LIT-562

Windover, A. K., Martinez, K., Mercer, M. B., Neuendorf, K., Boissy, A., & Rothberg, M. B. (2018). Correlates and outcomes of physician burnout within a large academic medical center. *JAMA Internal Medicine, 178*(6), 856–858. https://doi.org/10.1001/jamainternmed.2018.0019

World Health Organization. (2019). *Burn-out an "occupational phenomenon": International classification of diseases*. https://www.who.int/mental_health/evidence/burn-out/en/

2
The Fundamentals of Resilience, Growth, and Wisdom

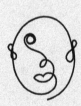

Tim Cunningham
pronouns: He/Him

Tim Cunningham began his professional career as an actor, then a hospital clown. He began doing international humanitarian work with Clowns Without Borders. While a clown, he fell in love with nurses' ability to connect with patients and families, even in times of terrible suffering—so he became an emergency nurse. The rest is history.

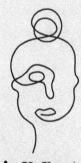

Dorrie K. Fontaine
pronouns: She/Her

Dorrie K. Fontaine, a critical care nurse and teacher, has been an academic leader for four decades. While president of the American Association of Critical-Care Nurses, she observed the joys and struggles of bedside nursing. Meditation, yoga, and daily gratitude practice help her overcome the fears and anxieties of our common human existence.

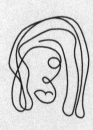

Natalie May
pronouns: She/Her

Natalie May, a writer, researcher, and teacher, collaborates with nurses, physicians, and others to improve patient care and colleague care. An Appreciative Inquiry facilitator, she has focused her research projects on wisdom in medicine and mattering in healthcare. For fun and self-care, she makes quilts.

"So what is it in a human life that creates bravery, kindness, wisdom, and resilience?

What if it's pain? What if it's the struggle?"

—Glennon Doyle

What do you do when things go wrong or even terribly wrong? As you think about your future in nursing, what will you do when you have a string of terrible shifts, when you struggle to work with members of your team, or when you just don't like your patients? How will you respond when one of your patients dies? What will you do if you make a mistake or you lose your job?

Some might take their stress and difficult emotions out on their nursing colleagues, other staff, or even their patients. Others might take their pain home with them and metaphorically kick the dog. Others may self-medicate with shopping, food, alcohol, or drugs. And there are many who decide that the stress and challenges are too difficult to endure, and they leave the nursing profession altogether.

We hope that when you encounter difficulties in your career and life, you will have the capacity to be resilient. There are many definitions of *resilience*, but when we talk about resilience, we are generally referring to one's ability to bounce back from adversity, implying some sort of physical or psychological return to baseline. Resilience is a trait that helps nurses and other clinicians avoid the effects of unmitigated workplace stress, or burnout, as described in the previous chapter. It is not surprising that nursing schools are adding resilience as another skill required of their graduates (Aburn et al., 2016).

Resilience in healthcare has many facets. For example, we talk about our patients' resilience in terms of their recovery from injury or illness. What qualities or factors make some patients more resilient than others? We also talk about a very important aspect of healthcare work: moral resilience. Our colleague, Cynda Rushton, has been committed to studying and nurturing moral resilience in healthcare, and we discuss some of her work in Chapter 11.

In this chapter, we explore the concept of resilience, both as the capacity to recover from adversity or trauma as well as a process of moving beyond resilience to growth and even something that looks like wisdom. More often than we might expect, resilience after trauma results in someone going beyond the traditional idea of returning to baseline, to something more profound. We will also talk about another form of resilience that helps us achieve our long-term goals despite obstacles. That type of resilience is *grit*.

Resilience

Resilience research began with vigor in the 1970s, primarily as a way to better understand and help children who were considered "at risk." Researchers wanted to know why some students overcame adversity and succeeded when others didn't, despite coming from similar circumstances. The hope was that by identifying the magic ingredients that made a child resilient, those ingredients could be nurtured to ensure children's success. In hindsight, and even at the time, the research was problematic (Luthar et al., 2000). Who defines "at risk"? Whose definition of success is appropriate? If resilience is a special characteristic or circumstance, how do we help children who aren't fortunate enough to have those so-called special ingredients?

In 2001, Ann Masten surveyed the three decades of resilience research and proposed that rather than being a rare quality unique to some people, resilience was, in fact, not a magic ingredient or superpower. Instead, resilience was simply the power of the ordinary, a quality that each of us possesses, physically and mentally. Resilience is in everyone; we have the capacity to nurture it and be mindful of its power.

This is a very optimistic place to begin thinking about our own resilience.

There are many definitions of resilience, but they share a common focus on individuals' ability to recover from adversity. Nursing researcher Cynthia Delgado and her colleagues (2017) call resilience "a protective process for the negative effects of emotional labour" (p. 71). There is agreement that resilience is "an innate energy and motivating life force" that is the result of an "accessible inner strength or resource" that can be "enhanced or supported by external resources" (Grafton et al., 2010, p. 700). We have the power of resilience within us, and it can be strengthened or weakened by factors external to us.

Whether it is protecting oneself from the ongoing work of emotional labor or the trauma of a natural disaster or pandemic, resilience is vital to a nurse's well-being. It is clear from current research that nurses with high levels of resilience are less likely to experience burnout, anxiety, depression, and posttraumatic stress disorder (McGarry et al., 2013; Mealer et al., 2012). As we learned in the first chapter, nurses and other healthcare workers face tremendous daily challenges as well as explosive episodes of chaos, such as global pandemics, mass shootings, and natural disasters. In these circumstances, having to bear witness to others' suffering while simultaneously experiencing your own trauma or loss can make for an indescribable burden.

Rewiring Our Brains for Resilience

Much of the self-care advice and information that you encounter will offer great tools and tips to foster your well-being—this book is one of them.

But how does self-care lead to resilience?

It may seem hard to believe that going for a run, getting a massage, or spending time with friends can have much benefit beyond the moment when you are actually doing them. But these self-care activities can benefit your future self in powerful ways.

Many connections between self-care and resilience abide in the science of *neuroplasticity*, your nervous system's ability to change and form new neural pathways. This process is literally the rewiring of your brain, based on your experiences. If you have studied the effects of trauma, you know that traumatic events can change victims' brains in a negative way. Similarly, positive neuroplasticity explains why fostering your own well-being today can have a powerful impact on your well-being months or even years from now when you face adversity. By watching a funny movie or snuggling with your canine or feline companion, you are on your way to building new positive pathways in your brain. Hanson (2018) calls this the ability to "turn passing experiences into lasting inner resources built into your brain" (p. 2).

We appreciate the work of clinical psychologist Rick Hanson because he translates the complex neuroscience of resilience into effective, simple behaviors that anyone can practice. Hanson is the author of *Buddha's Brain* (2009), *Hardwiring Happiness* (2013) and *Resilient: How to Grow an Unshakeable Core of Calm, Strength, and Happiness* (2018), and he describes resilience as follows:

> Mental resources like determination, self-worth, and kindness
> are what make us *resilient*: able to cope with adversity and push

through challenges in pursuit of opportunities. While resilience helps us recover from loss and trauma, it offers much more than that. True resilience fosters well-being, an underlying sense of happiness, love, and peace. Remarkably, as you internalize experiences of well-being, that builds inner strengths which in turn make you more resilient. Well-being and resilience promote each other in an upward spiral. (Hanson, 2018, p. 2)

According to Hanson (2018), the most important method of fostering resilience is to *internalize experiences of well-being*. As we explained in the conclusion of the previous chapter, it is important that we simply be present, paying attention to those experiences that fill us with positive emotions.

Have you ever wondered why walking on the beach, visiting a new city, or hiking a mountain trail makes us feel so good? It makes us feel good in large part because we have to pay attention in these situations. Not paying attention on a mountain trail could mean stumbling over a tree root and tripping into a ravine. We pay attention more when we are in new environments. Our minds are less likely to wander to an upcoming exam or argument with a friend when we're trying not to get lost in the woods. Not only are we focusing our attention on the task at hand (enjoying the scenery, not falling off a cliff or getting lost), we are also enjoying ourselves. We feel better because we're staying in the moment (remember the smartphone experiment at the end of Chapter 1) and because we're having fun.

By savoring these positive moments, you are rewiring your brain, literally changing how you will think and respond to life's highs and lows and everything in between. It's that simple.

Let's explore for a moment why this works. Our brains are designed to be changed based on our experiences, whether they are good experiences or bad ones (Hanson, 2018). This makes sense, especially when you think about children whose brains are especially primed for building neural structures that will form their unique personalities, likes and dislikes, and more. Negative experiences, due to something called the negativity bias, tend to have more power over our brain development.

For example, children must learn not to touch a hot stove for their safety and even survival, so the negative experience of touching the stove is a powerful teachable moment. With intentionality and self-compassion, we can build our own resilience by allowing positive experiences to have the same power as negative ones in terms of our personal neural rewiring.

Two Case Studies in Neuroplasticity: Nevin and Pat

Let's take two nursing students, Nevin and Pat. Both in their early 20s, they each have experienced life's ups and downs.

Nevin's parents announced their divorce when Nevin was 14, after years of fighting and two separations. Pat's mother was diagnosed with cancer 10 years ago and was in and out of hospitals for nearly two years. She recovered and is doing well.

Nevin

Nevin understandably felt anger and sadness over the divorce but never developed the resilience needed to help him flourish as an adult. When something goes wrong—a failed test, a broken friendship, a missed opportunity—Nevin tends to blame others and to dwell for long periods on the disappointment of the moment. Nevin is often the first to point out that something isn't fair or that someone else has made a mistake. Nevin seems to be looking for the world to validate his belief that life is hard, even futile. The result is that Nevin has difficulty dealing with daily annoyances and learning from his mistakes. In truth, he doesn't easily attract others in friendships or even casual relationships. It becomes a self-fulfilling cycle of hardship: Nevin believes the world is harsh, and when he experiences disappointment, that disappointment reinforces his belief that the world is harsh.

Pat

When Pat's mother was ill, Pat remembers that her mom expressed a lot of gratitude for her doctors and nurses and relatives and friends who cared for her and her family. Throughout the experience, Pat noticed the kindness of people who brought the family meals, sent them cards of encouragement, and invited Pat and her siblings on outings so her mom could rest. Several times, Pat went to the clinic to keep her mom company during her chemotherapy treatments. As a young girl, Pat was enthralled by the nurses who efficiently and kindly tended to her mother. They were so expert at the needles and machines, but they seemed approachable, too. They laughed a lot and joked with Pat that someday she might grow up to be a nurse.

Pat's mother never said, "Why me?" at least not in front of her children. In large part because of her mother's attitude, Pat's brain was "wired" to look for silver linings during her family's health crisis. Instead of instilling fear or dread, the clinic inspired awe for the nurses, doctors, and medical technology. Rather than turning her mental eye continually toward her mom's hair loss, hospitalizations, and the disruptions in her own life, Pat learned to see kindness and even delight in some parts of their family's journey. Pat certainly experienced the fear and frustration that any child would in this situation, and some days were terribly hard. But overall, the experience taught her many lessons about resilience, and perhaps most importantly, it led her to a career in nursing.

As a nursing student, Pat has many friends who turn to her for compassion and wisdom. She's fun to be around, in part because she can find the good or goofy in most situations. She attracts like-minded friends, and she has earned the respect of her professors and work colleagues. Nursing school wasn't easy for her. Classes were harder than she expected, and she had a terrible experience with a roommate, just to name two of her struggles. But she came through it all because she had built a network of support, and she had some experience in not letting adversity overwhelm her.

Room for Growth

You may already have an idea of how you will respond to the bad days, or weeks, in nursing. Think about a time in your life when you experienced adversity. Perhaps like Nevin, you went through your parents' divorce, or you have endured the death of a loved one. Hopefully, you have been spared life's worst tragedies, but adversities can be less extreme and still pack a wallop. Have you ever failed an exam? Experienced the end of a romantic relationship? Lost a best friend? Perhaps you didn't get into your first-choice college, or you didn't make a sports team. How you responded in those situations may provide some insight into your default strategies for moving through adversity, whether you are more like Pat or more like Nevin.

The good news is that thanks to the neuroplasticity of our brains, we have the capacity to become more like Pat and build our own reservoir of resilience.

Becoming Resilient

There are several important things to keep in mind about resilience.

First, we must focus on the things that we want more of in our lives. If we want to experience awe, then we focus on awe. If we want to experience compassion, then we look for examples of compassion. In the next chapter, we'll delve into this more deeply, but *our focus is our fate*. If you are like Nevin, it will be easy to find people and experiences around you that reinforce your belief that life is filled with negativity. But it is possible, no matter what your past experiences, to foster a mindset more like Pat's that will ultimately bring you more joy, connection, and satisfaction.

Second, enjoyable experiences reduce stress hormones, strengthen our immune systems, and help you come back to "normal" after you've been angry or upset (Hanson, 2018). As cliché as it sounds, laughter, if not the *best* medicine, is certainly a good one. We're a huge proponent of funny TV shows, movies, and YouTube and TikTok videos because they have a positive psychological and even physical effect on our well-being. There is a considerable body of research supporting this, that positive emotions foster resilience and better mental health (Fredrickson, 2004; Lyubomirsky et al., 2005; Lyubomirsky & Layous, 2013).

Third, it is not enough to simply focus on something; we must truly sit with the experience or feeling long enough (and often enough) to enable that experience to rewire our brains. Remember, our brains are designed to be changed by our experiences, but we need to be intentional about creating positive change. Hanson (2018) argues that this is the weakness in much positive psychology and psychotherapy; they don't place enough emphasis on this essential notion of creating lasting change in our nervous systems, or neuroplasticity. "In order to convert passing experiences into lasting inner strengths, we have to be able to focus attention on an experience long enough for it to start being consolidated into the nervous system." (Hanson, 2018, p. 24)

In other words, for neuroplasticity to take hold, we must *savor* experiences in the moment.

Breathe them in and let them do their work on us. Here's one way to think of it. Do you ever wake up and vaguely remember that you've had a dream? If you race to the coffee pot, the memory of the dream is gone before you've found your mug. But by staying in bed a bit longer and lingering with the dream, it is often possible to make a connection to your waking life that changes you. It is the same with positive neuroplasticity; sitting with and savoring a good feeling has the power to change us.

Imagine going through your day, noticing and savoring the positive moments that you experience but might normally fail to notice.

- Feeling warm and safe in your bed on a cold morning
- The smell of freshly brewed coffee or tea
- The sharp, clean feel of just-brushed teeth
- The smell of your soap or shampoo
- The sound of children laughing at the bus stop
- The rustle of trees on your walk to class or work
- The smile and friendly hello of someone you pass in the hallway

- The smooth feeling of a blank page in your notebook
- Appreciation for a teacher or colleague who worked hard to prepare for this day

This is simply the beginning of an infinite list of moments to savor throughout any given day. Every moment of your day presents an opportunity to create lasting changes in your brain. Do you have a beloved cat or dog? When that fur ball curls up in your lap, don't always be texting or watching Netflix. For just a few moments, notice the cat purring and how happy that makes you feel. Notice how much the dog's snoring makes you smile and feel grateful that you have a pet.

Next time you sit down to a meal, savor the sights, sounds, flavors, and feelings the meal evokes. Is the food delicious? Does it remind you of home? Does it stir gratitude because someone cooked it for you? Are your friends or roommates laughing and making you feel part of a supportive social group?

If you love music, don't simply allow the music to fade into the background. Take time to not only listen intently, but pay attention to how it makes you feel. Does the song make you feel powerful and energized? Does the symphony send you on a whole range of emotions or bring you to tears? Live concerts are the greatest opportunities to truly absorb the sights, sounds, and energy of music.

These experiences and so many others are the fuel for positive neuroplasticity, and this is a key to developing resilience. Your goal is to strengthen the circuits in your brain, specifically the circuits that you *want* to strengthen, such as those that foster positive emotions. Happiness researcher Barbara Fredrickson has identified ten positive emotions to get you started: joy, gratitude, serenity, interest, hope, pride, amusement, inspiration, awe, and love (Cohn et al., 2009). In addition to increasing your resilience, doing simple activities that make you feel good will increase your overall happiness (Lyubomirsky & Layous, 2013) and alleviate depression (Gander et al., 2013).

This takes practice. Your three-pound brain has 1.1 trillion cells, 100 billion neurons, and each neuron fires 5 to 50 times each second (Hanson, 2009). This presents nearly an infinite number of opportunities to strengthen your resilience and fortify your well-being.

Nursing Work Environments That Foster Resilience

The previous chapter laid out all the ways a healthcare work environment can diminish your ability to recover from adversity. The good news is that work environments have the power to support your resilience, too.

Your personal resilience skill development *plus* organizational support are the two primary ingredients that will help determine how you respond to the stressors in your work and life. Both aspects of resilience are mutually important; it's hard to stay resilient if your clinic or hospital does not support individual and organizational well-being. The opposite is also true. You may work in a healthy work environment, but without your own resilience practices, you will be less likely to thrive at work.

Only relatively recently has the healthcare profession acknowledged the importance of workplace factors *in addition to* individual factors in building resilience in nurses (Lowe, 2013; National Academies of Sciences, Engineering, and Medicine, 2019). Lynette Cusack and her colleagues (2016) identified factors that supported nurses' psychological resilience at work, calling it the Health Service Workplace Environmental Resilience Model. The model (see Table 2.1) includes key factors that managers can put in place to support nurses and help them recover from workplace trauma and even flourish. We think this model is an important reminder that you are not alone in your pursuit of well-being. Yes, you have the power of resilience within you, but it can be strengthened or weakened by external factors. This model highlights those supporting factors.

Table 2.1 Health Service Workplace Environmental Resilience Model

Environmental Support	Examples
Policies and structures that enable a nurse to act ethically, respectfully, and benefit patient care	• Explicit lines of communication • Receptive, responsive, understanding, supportive leadership • Timely access to support for ethical guidance • Respectful working relationships
Processes that enable nurses to deliver competent, patient-centered care	• Explicit but flexible role expectations • Appropriate patient allocation • Availability of essential and properly working equipment • Support of interprofessional collaboration
Practices that enable nurses to feel connected, safe, and well	• Culture of kindness and positive staff behaviors • Meetings to address stress and collaboratively create solutions • Workplace violence control • Planned and monitored meal breaks • Scheduling that facilitates rest and time to engage with family and friends • Employee assistance programs • Vacations • Physical space for mindfulness, breathing, and meditation practices
Opportunities for nurses to engage in reflection, career development, and lifelong learning	• Mentoring programs • Review processes that promote staged knowledge and skill development • Opportunities to reflect on practice, feelings, and beliefs and the consequences of these for individuals and groups • Study leave
Opportunities to enhance clinical nursing practice	• Practice development opportunities around clinical knowledge, skills, and problem-solving • Clinical supervision systems that build competence and confidence • Opportunities to debrief and learn from mistakes rather than blaming
Opportunities for nurses to learn resilience skills	• Adaptive coping learning opportunities • Mindfulness and meditation training

Adapted from Cusack et al. (2016)

As teachers and nursing leaders, we feel a responsibility, even an urgency, to foster resilience in our students and new nurses. We have two ways to achieve this; we can:

- Teach you the personal skills you will need, such as those outlined in this book

- Advocate for healthy work environments, workplaces that support the resilience and well-being of everyone who works there

In future chapters we discuss ways that workplaces have the potential to diminish or foster resilience. Throughout the book, we address many of the external forces that can strengthen or weaken your internal resilience resources.

Grit: Another Kind of Resilience

What do you think matters more in life—talent or hard work? If you knew all your classmates' college admissions test scores (such as SAT or ACT), do you think you would be able to predict who would become successful nurses? Conversely, by only observing their behaviors in class (such as focus, passion, work ethic, and effort), would you be able to predict who might leave the nursing profession within two or three years? We can tell you that you will learn more about a person's long-term success in school, work, and even marriage by observing their behaviors rather than knowing their test scores (Eskrels-Winkler et al., 2014).

There is another aspect of resilience that we believe is important to the grueling work of nursing, and that is grit. Not to be confused with talent, grit appears to have more influence on an individual's long-term success than their natural, genetically provided gifts. Over 100 years ago, Galton (1892) studied the biographies of eminent leaders, artists, and athletes and concluded that talent alone did not determine their success. While ability mattered, "zeal" and a capacity for hard work were the factors that outstanding individuals possessed (Duckworth, Peterson, Matthews, & Kelly, 2007).

What Is Grit?

Grit is a relatively recent psychological construct developed by psychology researcher Angela Duckworth. *Grit* is "the tendency to sustain passion and perseverance for long-term goals" (Eskrels-Winkler et al., 2014, p. 1). It may or may not seem intuitive to you, but a person's ability to rise to the occasion, to "never give up," is determined by grit, not talent. We all know individuals who have plenty of natural talent but who get stuck at a certain level, or quit trying when they get bored, tired, or frustrated.

Duckworth began her studies at the United States Military Academy at West Point where students considered the best of the best, both physically and mentally, are admitted and enrolled. Despite an extraordinary admissions process that would put an Ivy League college to shame, 20% of the 1,200 cadets each year drop out, most within their first two months (Duckworth, 2016). Clearly, being physically fit and among the nation's highest academic achievers was not a surefire predictor of success.

West Point, despite its rigorous admissions process, was unable to pin down the "secret sauce" that determined which cadets succeed when others failed. No metrics on file—test scores, fitness measures, recommendations, leadership experience, even something called the Whole Candidate Score—were able to predict a cadet's trajectory.

In 2004, Duckworth developed and administered the Grit Scale to a matriculating class of cadets. When she looked at all the qualities of those who dropped out and those who stayed, *the only predictive measure was grit*. Cadets with more grit were more likely to remain; those with less grit were more likely to drop out.

Duckworth went on to study grit in different populations of individuals who face challenges and setbacks: timeshare salespeople, eleventh graders in Chicago Public Schools, graduate students, Green Berets, and spelling bee contestants. In all populations, grit was a more significant determinant of success than talent, IQ, or measures specific to their subgroup (such as verbal intelligence for spellers) (Duckworth, 2016).

Sharing a conclusion about a study on competitive swimmers, Duckworth writes, "The most dazzling human achievements are, in fact, the aggregate of countless individual elements, each of which is, in a sense, ordinary." (Duckworth, 2016, p. 36).

This to us, is the essence of grit in nursing. Every day, you will perform ordinary acts of duty, caring, and compassion. Many acts will be monotonous. Many will stretch you beyond your limits. Some acts will certainly be extraordinary. One question that will determine your success and career fulfillment will be, "How much grit do you have?" We will revisit grit in Chapter 23, but we'll wrap up our discussion here by listing a few ways that you can grow your grit.

Four Components of Grit

"Mature paragons of grit," according to Duckworth, develop four psychological assets. These assets help them overcome and move past boredom, discouragement, and a willingness to throw in the towel. These gritty paragons embody interest, practice, purpose, and hope.

And the good news is that even if you don't feel like you are an especially "gritty" person today, you can grow your grit by developing these four assets.

Interest

Interest is simply that "I love what I do" feeling that gets us past the tedious chores that are part of our job. It aligns with that advice uttered in every graduation speech we've ever heard: "Follow your passion." It turns out, however, that science backs this up. People are more likely to be successful if they are satisfied with their jobs and engaged with their work. They perform better if their work interests them.

We hope that nursing is your passion, but don't despair if you aren't certain. The nursing profession provides infinite options for those with a broad range of interests or passions. Some students enter nursing school envisioning a career in an emergency department and then fall in love with pediatrics during their clinical rotations. We even know a few who binge-watched *Call the Midwife* and developed an interest in OB-GYN. Others develop a passion for addressing inequality and health disparities and become policy advocates. If you love science, you have the opportunity to flourish in a research or academic position. Don't be afraid to explore whatever aspect of nursing calls you.

Practice

The second asset is practice. *Practice* is our ability to avoid complacency, to build upward from our current skill level. It is our willingness to practice, day after day, until we move from novice to expert. Everything we pursue—from nursing to writing to running to playing the violin—benefits from focused, deliberate practice. Practice is hard. It's uncomfortable and sometimes miserable and frustrating. We bet you can name 20 nursing skills right off the top of your head that were hard and awful the first time you tried them: starting an IV, inserting a Foley catheter, administering an intramuscular injection, suctioning a patient on a ventilator, or getting a frail post-op patient out of bed. You may not be an expert at these skills today, but we suspect that you have progressed. We hope that you can also envision how good it will feel to master those skills with practice, feedback, time, and more practice.

Purpose

As you consider practice and passion, add another "p" to the list—purpose. *Purpose* is the sense that your work matters to others. We'll discuss the importance of mattering in Chapter 20, but for a long career in nursing, we would argue that approaching it as merely a job will not get you through the rough spots. Nurses who bring a sense of purpose to their work and who make an effort to maintain it will have a compelling reason to show up day after day.

Hope

Finally, the fourth asset is hope. Duckworth (2016) claims that hope is not the final stage of grit; it is *all* stages. *Hope* is the belief that you have the power to make things better. It is not the belief that the *universe* will fix things but rather the belief that *you* are the determining factor in making things better. Imagine a violinist who stumbles over the same passage every single time, day after day after day. Without hope, the violinist would simply give up. With hope, the violinist believes that they have it within their power to improve with practice.

You have the power to grow your grit by finding and following your passion, practicing with focus and determination, finding your purpose, and believing in your ability to make things better.

Growth and Wisdom

We all know someone who has faced extreme adversity but who somehow transformed their tragedy or trauma into something meaningful. These may be individuals in our personal lives, or maybe they are people we've read about. The late Congressman John Lewis, Nobel Peace Prize recipient Malala Yousafzai, and the students of Marjorie Stoneman Douglas High School all come to mind. They suffered great violence at the hands of others, but they were able to transform their pain to fight for others and even to change the world.

You have probably heard about, or studied, a condition called *posttraumatic stress disorder*, or PTSD. Posttraumatic stress is essentially the emotional and psychological fallout from traumatic events such as a natural disaster, loss of a loved one, or surviving an act of violence (Davidson & Foa, 1993). PTSD can be caused by a single event or a series of events and exposures to trauma, including systemic racism and discrimination.

In the mid-1990s, Tedeschi and Calhoun developed a different psychological construct for trauma survivors called *posttraumatic growth* (PTG). As you might guess, this refers to a process when individuals experience trauma but change in a positive way. The growth after trauma typically occurs in one or more of five domains: (1) greater appreciation for life and changed sense of priorities; (2) warmer, more intimate relationships with others; (3) recognition of new possibilities or paths for one's life; (4) greater sense of personal strength; and (5) spiritual development (Tedeschi & Calhoun, 1995).

In your career, you will meet patients facing grave health crises who find new meaning and purpose in their lives. You will encounter others who, through illness, are surprised to learn how much inner strength they have. Some reconnect with family, friends, or faith communities as they renew their appreciation for these relationships. It is a privilege to share in these growth experiences with your patients. We will examine posttraumatic growth more closely in Chapter 11, but for now, we offer posttraumatic growth as yet another way to think about resilience.

Many of the survivors of the mass shooting at Marjorie Stoneman Douglas High School in 2018 exemplify posttraumatic growth. Many students, as well as teachers and parents, responded by becoming powerful activists in the gun control movement. Their efforts included confronting lawmakers, leading get-out-the-vote drives, and organizing the March for Our Lives rally in Washington, DC. None of them set out to become the change agents of their generation, but their actions created meaning and growth in the wake of tragedy. In his book *Parkland* (2019) about the events of that day and its aftermath, Dave Cullen shares the community's stories of activism and purpose and how many members found new appreciation for life, more meaningful relationships, and other examples of posttraumatic growth. Many found their life's purpose in some way connected to the event of that terrible day.

Tedeschi and Calhoun gave us a new way to understand adversity and its opportunity to build meaning, connection, and purpose in unlikely circumstances. Just as we seek to understand how we can help individuals build resilience, it is also important for us to know that we can help others and ourselves foster growth in the wake of trauma.

Wisdom in Healthcare

This ability to grow after trauma and transform suffering can be seen in healthcare professionals as well. In an interview study of physicians who had been involved in a serious medical error, we learned that some are too devastated by the experience to remain in medicine (Plews-Ogan et al., 2012). Others self-medicate, become overly cautious in their medical practice, or withdraw emotionally.

There were others, however, who moved through the trauma of making a mistake by eventually becoming better physicians, teachers, and even parents and spouses. As in posttraumatic growth examples, these physicians drew purpose from the trauma of harming a patient. Some became open about sharing their experience of the error so others could learn from their mistake. Others adopted the role of patient safety expert or advocate in order to ensure similar errors would be prevented in the future. And many grew to be more compassionate and less judgmental of others, having themselves experienced shame, the harsh judgment of others, and even legal proceedings (Plews-Ogan et al., 2013).

In this study of physicians and medical error, the authors identified something that looked a lot like wisdom. Although the concept of wisdom is age-old (think Socrates, Job, and Buddha), it has only in the past few decades been studied as a psychological construct. Wisdom researcher Monika Ardelt (2004) has developed a framework that identifies those qualities we typically think of as embodied by "wise" persons. These include (Ardelt, 2004):

- The ability to deal with uncertainty and ambiguity
- Seeing the deeper meaning of things
- An awareness of self and others
- The ability to learn from mistakes
- Compassion and concern for the greater good

Healthcare is beginning to recognize the value of having wise leaders and practitioners and embedding wisdom in our culture as we face today's tremendous challenges (Branch & Mitchell, 2011).

Many believe that wisdom can only be gained through the experience of adversity, that life's challenges force us to find creative coping skills and draw us closer to others who are suffering (Glück et al., 2005). Yet we can hope to attain growth and wisdom in the context of *all* circumstances, as this leaning into wisdom will serve as another form of resilience.

We have observed countless wise nurses throughout the years. Wise nurses are able to navigate the uncertainties and challenges of their jobs with intelligence, reflection, and compassion. They can see situations from multiple perspectives. Wise nurses reflect on their own thoughts and feelings before reacting in the moment. They know how to use their skills in the right way, at the right time, for the right reasons (Schwartz, 2010), and sometimes this may even mean bending the rules a bit.

Finally, a wise nurse is able to demonstrate compassion toward others, to transcend self-centeredness, and make decisions with the greater good in mind. We have seen examples of great wisdom during this time of COVID-19. This compassionate wisdom manifests in the creative ways nurses have found to support their patients who are suffering, in their caring for each other and themselves, and in their willingness to advocate for their patients, health systems, and communities.

> ## In Real Practice
>
> Grit in nursing is a relatively new topic, but there are an increasing number of studies that examine grit in nursing students. In an article that compared grit to the journey of Koi fish, the authors (Terry & Peck, 2020) asked over 2,000 nursing students to complete the short grit scale (Grit-S) to measure their levels of perseverance and passion. Among their findings, grit was lower among students who chose nursing by watching television shows about nursing. (*Call the Midwife* or *Grey's Anatomy*, anyone?) Grit increased significantly with each year of nursing study, and it was higher in students from lower socioeconomic backgrounds and older students.

Closing Thoughts

We encourage you to envision your trajectory through difficulties and adversity now, before you are in the throes of it. We also encourage you to draw on your past encounters with life's challenges and rely on your personal resiliency and grit that you brought to bear on them. Suffering will never be easy, but we each have the capacity to move though suffering and even to transform it into something extraordinary. Cast your eye toward others—patients, colleagues, and friends—to appreciate those who have moved through adversity to growth or even wisdom.

Nurturing your resilience and well-being is critically important. We hope we have presented material here that, rather than feeling burdensome, strikes you as pleasurable, even fun. Finding activities that foster joy and other positive emotions is not the worst assignment you will ever face. Notice what brings you joy and seek it out. Savor the good feelings and let your brain experience the power of positive neuroplasticity.

Key Points

- There are many definitions and forms of resilience, including moral resilience, physical resilience following illness or injury, grit, posttraumatic growth, and wisdom through adversity.

- Resilience is vital to a nurse's well-being. It supports our ability to avoid burnout, maintain our well-being and mental health, and recover from trauma and life's challenges.

- We all have the capacity to be resilient; resilience is not a characteristic unique to a special few. We have the power of resilience within us, and it can be strengthened or weakened by factors external to us.

- You should not be alone in growing your resilience. The Health Service Workplace Environmental Resilience Model identifies key factors that your employer can put in place to support you and help you recover from workplace trauma.

- The key to developing resilience is positive neuroplasticity, our brain's ability to change, or "rewire," from the effects of positive experiences. To encourage positive neuroplasticity, seek out and pay attention to positive experiences; take the time to truly sit with and absorb the positive emotions that these experiences produce.

- Grit, the tendency to sustain passion and perseverance for long-term goals, is a form of resilience that will keep you from quitting when the going gets tough. The four keys to grit are interest, practice, purpose, and hope, and these can all be developed in each of us.

- Posttraumatic growth recognizes that individuals have the capacity to emerge from trauma in a positive way. This growth can include a greater appreciation for life, greater intimacy, discovery of new life possibilities, new personal strength, and spiritual development.

- Wisdom through adversity is another form of resilience. Wise nurses can tolerate uncertainty, put their knowledge and skills to good use, display compassion, and care about the greater good.

References

Aburn, G., Gott, M., & Hoare, K. (2016). What is resilience? An integrative review of the empirical literature. *Journal of Advanced Nursing, 72*(5), 980–1000. https://doi.org/10.1111/jan.12888

Ardelt, M. (2004). Wisdom as expert knowledge system: A critical review of a contemporary operationalization of an ancient concept. *Human Development, 47*, 257–285. https://doi.org/10.1159/000079154

Branch, W. T. Jr., & Mitchell, G. A. (2011). Wisdom in medicine. *Pharos Alpha Omega Alpha Honor 50 Med Society, 74*(3), 12–17. https://pubmed.ncbi.nlm.nih.gov/21877511/

Cohn, M. A., Fredrickson, B. L., Brown, S. L., Mikels, J. A., & Conway, A. M. (2009). Happiness unpacked: Positive emotions increase life satisfaction by building resilience. *Emotion, 9*(3), 361–368. https://doi.org/10.1037/a0015952

Cullen, D. (2019). *Parkland: Birth of a movement*. HarperCollins.

Cusack, L., Smith, M., Hegney, D., Rees, C. S., Breen, L. J., Witt, R. R., Rogers, C., Williams, A., Cross, W., & Cheung, K. (2016). Exploring environmental factors in nursing workplaces that promote psychological resilience: Constructing a unified theoretical model. *Frontiers in Psychology, 7*, 600. https://doi.org/10.3389/fpsyg.2016.00600

Davidson, J. R. T., & Foa, E. B. (Eds.). (1993). *Posttraumatic stress disorder: DSM-IV and Beyond*. American Psychiatric Press, Inc.

Delgado, C., Upton, D., Ranse, K., Furness, T., & Foster, K. (2017). Nurses' resilience and the emotional labour of nursing work: An integrative review of empirical literature. *International Journal of Nursing Studies, 70*, 71–88. https://doi.org/10.1016/j.ijnurstu.2017.02.008

Duckworth, A. (2016). *Grit: The power of passion and perseverance*. Scribner.

Duckworth, A. L., Peterson, C., Matthews, M. D., & Kelly, D. R. (2007). Grit: Perseverance and passion for long-term goals. *Journal of Personality and Social Psychology, 92*(6), 1087–1101. https://doi.org/10.1037/0022-3514.92.6.1087

Eskrels-Winkler, L. Shulman, E. P., Beal, S. A., & Duckworth, A. L. (2014). The grit effect: Predicting retention in the military, the workplace, school, and marriage. *Frontiers in Psychology, 5*(36). https://doi.org/10.3389/fpsyg.2014.00036

Fredrickson, B. L. (2004). The broaden-and-build theory of positive emotions. *Philosophical Transactions of the Royal Society, 359*(1449), 1367–1378. https://doi.org/10.1098/rstb.2004.1512

Galton, F. (1892). *Hereditary genius: An inquiry into its laws and consequences.* Macmillan.

Gander, F., Proyer, R. T., Ruch, W., & Wyss, T. (2013). Strengths-based positive interventions: Further evidence for their potential in enhancing well-being and alleviating depression. *Journal of Happiness Studies, 14*, 1241–1259. https://doi.org/10.1007/s10902-012-9380-0

Glück, J., Buck, S., Baron, J., & McAdams, D. T. (2005). The wisdom of experience: Autobiographical narratives across adulthood. *International Journal of Behavior and Development, 29*(3), 197–208. https://doi.org/10.1080/01650250444000504

Grafton, E., Gillespie, B., & Henderson, S. (2010). Resilience: The power within. *Oncology Nursing Forum, 37*(6), 698–705. https://doi.org/10.1188/10.ONF.698-705

Hanson, R. (2009). *Buddha's brain: The practical neuroscience of happiness, love, and wisdom.* New Harbinger Publications, Inc.

Hanson, R. (2013). *Hardwiring happiness: The new brain science of contentment, calm, and confidence.* Harmony Books.

Hanson, R. (2018). *Resilient: How to grow an unshakable core of calm, strength, and happiness.* Harmony Books.

Lowe, L. D. (2013). Creating a caring work environment and fostering nurse resilience. *International Journal of Human Caring, 17*, 52–59.

Luthar, S. S., Cicchetti, D., & Becker, B. (2000). The construct of resilience: A critical evaluation and guidelines for future work. *Child Development, 71*(3), 543–562.

Lyubomirsky, S., King, L., & Diener, E. (2005). The benefits of frequent positive affect: Does happiness lead to success? *Psychological Bulletin, 131*(6), 803–855. https://doi.org/10.1037/0033-2909.131.6.803

Lyubomirsky, S., & Layous, K. (2013). How do simple positive activities increase well-being? *Current Directions in Psychological Science, 22*(1), 57–62. https://doi.org/10.1177/0963721412469809

Masten, A. S. (2001). Ordinary magic: Resilience processes in development. *American Psychologist, 56*(3), 227–238. https://doi.org/10.1037//0003-066x.56.3.227

McGarry, S., Girdler, S., McDonald, A., Valentine, J., Lee, S.-L., Blair, E., Wood, F., & Elliott, C. (2013). Paediatric health-care professionals: relationships between psychological distress, resilience and coping skills. *Journal of Paediatric Child Health, 49*, 725–732. https://doi.org/10.1111/jpc.12260

Mealer, M., Jones, J., Newman, J., McFann, K. K., Rothbaum, B., & Moss, M. (2012). The presence of resilience is associated with a healthier psychological profile in intensive care unit (ICU) nurses: Results of a national survey. *International Journal of Nursing Studies, 49*(3), 292–299. https://doi.org/10.1016/j.ijnurstu.2011.09.015

National Academies of Sciences, Engineering, and Medicine. (2019). *Taking action against clinician burnout: A systems approach to professional wellbeing.* The National Academies Press. https://doi.org/10.17226/25521

Plews-Ogan, M., Owens, J. E., & May, N. (2012). *Choosing wisdom: Strategies and inspiration for growing through life-changing difficulties.* Templeton Press.

Plews-Ogan, M., Owens, J. E., & May, N. B. (2013). Wisdom through adversity: Learning and growing in the wake of an error. *Patient Education and Counseling, 91*, 236–242. https://doi.org/10.1016/j.pec.2012.12.006

Schwartz, B. (2010). *Practical wisdom: The right way to do the right thing.* Riverhead Books.

Tedeschi, R., & Calhoun, L. (1995). *Trauma and transformation: Growing in the aftermath of suffering.* SAGE Publications.

Terry, D., & Peck, B. (2020). Factors that impact measures of grit among nursing students: A journey emblematic of the Koi fish. *European Journal Investigation in Health, Psychology, and Education, 10*(2), 564–574. https://doi.org/10.3390/ejihpe10020041

The Year of the Nurse/ The Year of COVID-19

—Maggie Beyer, RN, BSN, CCRN

Note to reader:

During the first surge of the COVID-19 pandemic in New York, nurses from around the country volunteered to help on the front lines. Maggie Beyer, a pediatric ICU nurse, and her cousin, Peter Castellano, a nurse in the same unit at Long Island Jewish Hospital, Northwell Health, in Queens, New York, cared for adult ICU patients with COVID-19.

In her own words, Maggie reflects on how the experience strengthened her bond with nursing and with her family.

2020 is the year of the nurse, they said, but who knew what that actually meant.

There was nothing that could prepare you in your career for what we actually witnessed. The heartbreak, the despair, and working tirelessly around the clock. What were we doing? I didn't feel like I was able to take care of my patients like usual. I couldn't get them cleaned and looking nice for family or make sure the room was organized with plenty of supplies. We were always working with limited supplies and machines.

We were the patient's family. No visitors were allowed during this time, but the patients were never alone. We didn't even realize how strong we were, how brave we were, and how resilient we really were as nurses.

I have been a pediatric ICU nurse for six years and have no experience with adult patients. At the time, the virus wasn't affecting kids like it was the adult population. So it wasn't really a question in my mind—I knew I had to help them. That's what nurses do; we help each other. We help each other bathe patients who have just passed; we help each other hang IV bags that are about to run out; and we help each other get through each moment.

A silver lining seemed to be rare in these days of the coronavirus. However, I was able to find one. My cousin is an experienced adult nurse who had recently taken a job in the same pediatric unit as me, working nights. Nurses who had adult experience were asked if they would go over to take assignments with adults. Of course, he accepted right away.

Throughout Long Island Jewish Hospital, there were multiple ICUs filled with COVID-19 patients— multiple units even converted into a makeshift ICU. One night at shift change, I saw my cousin walking into the unit I was on, and sure enough he was taking over my patient assignment for the night.

Growing up we didn't see each other all that much, but working together through this experience brought us closer than ever. I am so grateful for him. He would listen to the hard days I had, and he understood exactly what I was going through. Most times you couldn't even find words to describe the scene you witnessed. But Peter knew. He knew the words I was trying to say but couldn't quite form. I was terrified to work in the new, adult population against this new virus everyone was still learning about. But knowing I had Peter by my side made things seem a little bit easier.

The nursing bond is a strong one, but a family nursing bond is even stronger. Indeed, we will forever remember this time in history as the year of the nurse.

Reprinted with permission from the American Association of Critical-Care Nurses.

Beyer M. (2020). All in the family. American Association of Critical-Care Nurses. Retrieved February 16, 2021. https://www.aacn.org/nursing-excellence/nurse-stories/all-in-the-family

3

Developing a Resilient Mindset Using Appreciative Practices

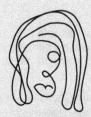

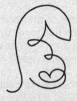

Natalie May
pronouns: She/Her

Natalie May, a writer, researcher, and teacher, collaborates with nurses, physicians, and others to improve patient care and colleague care. An Appreciative Inquiry facilitator, she has focused her research projects on wisdom in medicine and mattering in healthcare. For fun and self-care, she makes quilts.

Julie Haizlip
pronouns: She/Her

Julie Haizlip, a pediatric critical care physician, recognized that she feels most like she matters when she is teaching and personally connected with students. Now teaching at a school of nursing, she is committed to interprofessional education and collaborative practice. She and her family are on a quest to attend a hockey game in all 31 NHL venues.

"What you think, you become. What you feel, you attract. What you imagine, you create."

—Gautama Buddha

In this chapter, we present a set of self-care skills called "appreciative practices." Quite simply, these are tools for well-being that promote a positive and resilient mindset, borne out of the theoretical work of Appreciative Inquiry (May et al., 2020). Appreciative practices are strengths-based. They foster resilience, compassion, and appreciation for others. They are grounded in five core principles that we will explore here. These practices are rooted in the work of positive psychologists, the science of neuroplasticity, and the understanding that we have the power to use our thoughts to shape our feelings and behaviors.

We will invite you to develop your own tool kit of these practices now, while you are a student or new nurse. These practices can be honed anywhere—with your family, your friends, in your dorm, during clinical rotations, or in the Trader Joe's checkout line. Once you become adept at them, they will provide a lift to your work as a nurse on good days and bad, allowing you to provide the high-quality, compassionate care that you strive for without crushing yourself in the process. By practicing them today, they are more likely to be "hardwired" when you need them the most.

The Origins of Appreciative Practices

The term "appreciative practices" grew out of the authors' work with Appreciative Inquiry in healthcare for over a decade. *Appreciative Inquiry* (AI) is a culture change methodology that asks an organization or team, "Who are we when we're at our best, and how do we get more of that?" (Whitney & Trosten-Bloom, 2003) In the AI process, we delve deeply into what is going well in an organization: "What are its strengths? What does it look like when everyone is firing on all cylinders?" Team members dream together about what would be possible if they could maximize these strengths and behaviors. Participants then plot a path forward from where they are today to where they dream they could be. The Appreciative Inquiry process invites all members of a team to become their best selves, together.

What we found in our work with healthcare teams, however, was that the best-laid plans often don't come to fruition. In addition to having a viable plan for change, hospital staff needed to alter the way they interacted with one another. Nurses, physicians, technicians, social workers, chaplains, and others needed to tweak their behaviors to foster an environment conducive to positive change. These behaviors, or appreciative practices, include reframing, assumption of positive intent, constructive communication skills, gratitude practices, and much more (May et al., 2020).

Once the units we worked with began practicing these new behaviors, we found that change happened more readily, and as a bonus, nurses and other staff felt more energized, more eager to come to work, and less burned out (Williams & Haizlip, 2013). It was a win-win, and in the last several years, we have taught workshops and classes on these practices in order to help health system staff and faculty improve their own well-being and to improve the culture of their workplace. These practices have also been integrated into a larger-scale system change at the University of Virginia Health System, a program called "Wisdom and Wellbeing" (May et al., 2020).

A (Very) Brief Introduction to Appreciative Inquiry

Appreciative Inquiry began with a graduate student at the Case Western Reserve School of Business, David Cooperrider. His wife, an artist, asked (so the story goes) her husband why he and his colleagues always focused on what's *wrong* with an organization. She told him that in the art world, there is something known as the "appreciative eye." It means that there is beauty in every piece of art, in *everything*. She wondered why business school students didn't study organizations with an appreciative eye (Wade, 2017).

David Cooperrider's wife posited that there is beauty in everything; it simply depends on how you look at it.

For example, Natalie and her husband have a beloved Christmas-tree topper, a yellow angel made from a plastic party cup, covered in glitter, with pipe cleaner wings, and very crooked eyes and mouth. Their daughter made the angel when she was in preschool, and topping the tree with it each year brings great parental joy. Their daughter, on the other hand, groans and asks why they don't just go to the store and buy a "pretty" tree topper. But her parents think the messy, glittery angel is beautiful. Truth be told, the angel is not at all attractive, but through the eyes of loving parents, it is perfection, and they would never replace it with a store-bought decoration. They are looking at it with eyes of love.

David Cooperrider and his colleagues learned that whatever you look for, you will find, and in their studies, they looked for what they called an organization's "positive core." They flipped organizational study on its head and asked a revolutionary set of new questions. Instead of asking what was wrong or what was broken, they asked what was working well. They began searching for the best in organizations and the people who inhabit them. This new approach unleashed energy, optimism, and creativity that could be harnessed to solve the most challenging organizational problems. Since that time, AI has been used by countless businesses and corporations, nonprofits, cities, health systems, educational institutions, and even the United Nations (Appreciative Inquiry Commons, n.d.).

What Makes Appreciative Inquiry Different?

In the traditional approach to problem-solving, we ask, "What is wrong and how can it be fixed?" It often involves blame and finger-pointing. In contrast, an AI approach asks unconditionally positive questions, such as, "When have I succeeded in the past, and how can I replicate that success now?" It is a strengths-based approach to problem solving, using what is called a "4-D" process. After defining the topic, the process entails Discovery, Dream, Design, and Destiny, or Do (see Figure 3.1).

Let's put Appreciative Inquiry into a real-life context. Imagine that you have failed an exam. Some students might be prone to thinking—

> *I'm a failure.*
>
> *I should never have come to nursing school.*
>
> *It's not my fault.*
>
> *My professor isn't fair.*
>
> *I've never been good at school. I don't belong here.*

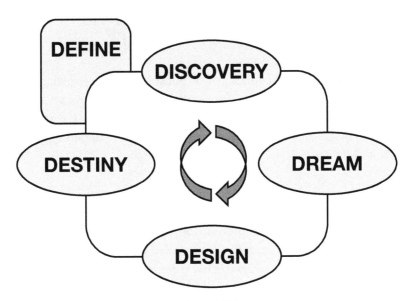

Adapted From: Cooperrider & Whitney,
Appreciative Inquiry: A positive revolution in change, 2005

FIGURE 3.1   The Appreciative Inquiry 4-D cycle.

If you have ever had this experience, you know that this kind of self-talk only takes you further down the road of discouragement, even despair. It's hard to pick yourself up and get back on track. You think that you are somehow broken and need "fixing."

Students using an appreciative mindset would instead begin a process of *discovery* to identify their strengths, abilities, and the circumstances under which they are likely to succeed. The goal is to uncover all the factors that contributed to past success and carry them forward into the present and future. With this approach, a student thinks about a time when they were an academic rock star. What was happening? What were they doing? How did others contribute? These questions would potentially reveal statements such as the following:

> *I get plenty of rest and take care of myself as best I can.*
>
> *I find smart friends to study with. I join a study group.*
>
> *I ask for help.*

I take beautiful, detailed notes. (Or I borrow some.)

I find a way to make the material meaningful to me.

We would argue that this second set of responses is more energizing, even hopeful, and likely to produce more successful results. Also, the statements reveal behaviors that the student already knows how to do. There is no need to learn a new way to study or to care for themselves, just a need to remember these keys to success, dust them off, and use them to face the current challenge.

Appreciative Inquiry also asks participants to build on stories of success by *dreaming* about an ideal future. By asking the question, "What would it look like if we grew the very best of ourselves and our organization?" team members are asked to dream together about the future. In our failed exam example, we suggest that you paint a picture of your success. What is your goal? It could be graduation from nursing school or seeing a passing grade show up on your computer screen. What does it look like when you succeed? How does it feel? In AI, it is very important to visualize this success in as much detail as possible. We'll discuss this more later in the chapter.

The next step is to *design* your strategy for success, to make a plan. If you know that you succeed academically when you can make studies (even pathophysiology) meaningful to you, make a list of how the course material can support your goals of becoming an exemplary nurse. Or, if you succeed academically when you compete with someone a little better than you (in this particular course), identify a classmate to be your friendly competitor. If good self-care helps you shine in the classroom, plan ways to build sleep, exercise, and fun into your daily routine.

The fourth step is to just *do* it. Implement your plan. Ask for help. Get a good night's sleep. Take exquisite notes. Use whatever strategies helped you in the past, see what works, and determine which strategies might need tweaking. And don't forget to keep that detailed dream vision in your head at all times.

Developing an Appreciative Mindset

Our goal in this chapter is to help you develop an appreciative mindset. As humans, and certainly as healthcare professionals, we are prone to a negativity bias (Haizlip et al., 2012). The negativity bias is an evolutionary construct that results in our human tendency to be more strongly influenced by the negative aspects of our environment than the positive (Baumeister et al., 2001). This makes sense from a survival perspective; it's more imperative to notice the hungry predator than the lovely sunset. The negativity bias has remained with us and affected our behaviors in numerous realms, including learning, attention, and how we make sense of the world around us (Baumeister et al., 2001; Vaish et al., 2008). The negativity bias leads us to focus on what is broken or what needs to be fixed.

An appreciative mindset, on the other hand, allows us to focus on more of what we want in ourselves and those around us, while growing the thoughts, feelings, and behaviors that support well-being and happiness. Lyubomirsky & Layous (2013) describe positive activities as "simple, intentional, and regular practices meant to mimic the myriad healthy thoughts and behaviors associated with naturally happy people" (p. 57). The simple, positive activities presented here will also support your overall health, and even success (Lyubomirsky & Layous, 2013). Research in the field of positive psychology has shown benefits to our immune systems (Lyubomirsky, King, & Diener, 2005) and cardiovascular health (Boehm et al., 2020). Numerous studies in positive psychology have shown that positive emotions foster creativity, improve cognition, reduce depression, and increase our ability to cope with stress (Gander et al., 2013; Lyubomirsky & Layous, 2013). By shifting our focus to what we want more of—beauty, joy, kindness, compassion—we most assuredly will create more of it, and creating more will benefit not only ourselves, but those around us, including our patients. Emmons & McCullough (2003) found that participants who wrote about gratitude daily were more likely to offer emotional support to others, and the healthcare field is recognizing the effect of physician emotions on decision-making and patient safety (Croskerry et al., 2010; Estrada et al., 1997).

All the practices that we will describe require some degree of mindfulness practice on your part. By *mindfulness*, we mean a nonjudgmental awareness of the present moment, or the ability to stop yourself in mid-thought or mid-sentence and ask, "Hmmm....I wonder what's up with that? How am I feeling? What other way could I think about this situation?" Be curious. We consider this mindset to be "practical" mindfulness that will foster compassion toward yourself and others.

Personal Perspective

Appreciative Practices and a Breast Cancer Journey
–Natalie May, PhD (she/her)

On the day before my 10th wedding anniversary, I anxiously awaited a call from the hospital with the results of my recent breast biopsy. A week earlier, I had discovered a lump in my left breast; a series of clinic visits ended with the biopsy and several days of worry. When the phone finally rang, I was surprised to hear my primary care doctor's voice, and the words, "Natalie, I am so sorry."

As with most cancer stories, the diagnosis, the confirmation of what you fear, is the beginning of a long journey. Looking back, I am astonished at the confluence of events and circumstances that shaped my cancer experience. Just a few weeks earlier, I had been invited to conduct an Appreciative Inquiry (AI) for our graduate medical education program and was working with a team of thoughtful, humanistic, and brave colleagues who were charged with carrying this important project forward. This team is where I met Julie Haizlip, my friend and co-author. In order to learn more about the AI process, I picked up the book, *Appreciative Living*, by Jackie Kelm and was midway through it when my doctor called.

Kelm's work focuses on the core principles of AI, explaining the science and theory of each and exploring ways the principles can be applied to everyday life. Most of the other AI books on my shelf focused on organizational theory, so this book intrigued me with its personal applications. Kelm writes about how our attention shapes our experience, that our questions are fateful, and ways to harness the power of language and metaphors.

Then I learned I had cancer. Within hours of receiving my diagnosis, I vowed to apply the principles of AI to my cancer experience. Initially, that decision was made as a form of "scholarship," a way to experience firsthand the power of appreciative inquiry so I could better do my job. In the end, the choice to move through cancer intentionally, using the power of appreciative inquiry, was one of the most important decisions of my life. It empowered me to choose my responses in the moment, each day, as my family and I navigated uncertainty, fear, illness, treatments, surgery, and recovery. Looking back, I believe that without an appreciative mindset and the lens it afforded me, I may have missed so many of the lessons, and blessings, that cancer put in my midst.

In this chapter, we use a few aspects of my cancer journey as a way to illustrate appreciative practices and their underlying theories. Navigating illness, or any personal struggle, is something we can all relate to, and we hope that sharing my story will encourage you to think about the potential power of these tools in your own life.

In your years as a nurse, you will encounter many patients experiencing the shock of a cancer diagnosis and the range of emotions and challenges that come with it. You will also walk alongside friends and loved ones as they move through cancer or other grave illnesses. Some patients will say, "Cancer was the best thing that ever happened to me," and others will curse the fact that they were dealt a terrible hand. Holocaust survivor Victor Frankl famously wrote, "Between stimulus and response there is a space. In that space is our power to choose our response. In our response lies our growth and our freedom." We hope that this chapter and others in this book help you to observe how our experiences are shaped and to see that we have choices in how we face life's challenges.

Appreciative Practices—Theory and Practice

Appreciative Inquiry is rooted in five core principles, and these principles are also the underpinning of appreciative practices.

The core principles are:

- Constructionist

- Poetic

- Positive

- Simultaneity

- Anticipatory

Appreciative practices closely mirror the tenets of positive psychology and the exciting research being conducted in that field. If you have studied positive psychology, you will see significant overlap. You will also recognize similarities to other practices described in this book. Others have written extensively about these core principles (Cooperrider & Whitney, 2005; Kelm, 2005), so this is our high-level summary about each principle, followed by the corresponding practices that we think are most effective for fostering well-being and positive interactions in school and work.

The Constructionist Principle

All our work in appreciative practices rests on the foundation of the constructionist principle. Social constructionism suggests that our realities are created by our thoughts, our language, and our interactions with others (Whitney & Trosten-Bloom, 2003). There is no absolute reality. Rather, our conversations, stories, and names for things—the words we use—determine how we perceive and what we believe about the world around us.

If you have not explored social construction in your studies yet, this may seem like a challenging concept. Try for a moment to think about what it means to be a student at your college or university. How much of what it means to be a student there is wrapped up in language: names of buildings and places, nicknames for friends or professors, school traditions, and so on? Think back to your first few days on campus, when you didn't know the names of campus hangouts, buildings, or street names. It was confusing. You didn't know what the words meant. At the University of Virginia (UVA), we have locations that are uniquely ours—the Lawn, the Corner, the Colonnades, the Rotunda, the Beta Bridge. If you were not a UVA student, or if you were brand new to "grounds" (what we call our campus), those names would most likely be meaningless to you. But eventually, after having conversations, hearing stories, reading, and engaging with others, all this new language creates meaning, and the world around you begins to make sense.

The Power of Language

The language of healthcare is often problematic. Imagine, for example, a hospital that does not include signage in languages other than English. What does that omission suggest about the value the hospital places on non-native English speaking patient populations? Doctors, and even nurses, tend to use medicalized language when explaining diagnoses or treatments to their patients, which can result in worsened clinical outcomes (Williams & Ogden, 2004). While talking in medical jargon may just be habit, our failure to speak in an understandable way could convey to our patients that we don't think their understanding of their diagnoses and treatments really matters.

Derogatory language, or language that diminishes patients and their suffering, is another issue in healthcare (Davies, 2007). What about the harried resident who directs a medical student to check on the "frequent flyer in an emergency department"? Or the nurse who tells her replacement on the next shift, "Room 312 is a drug-seeker"?

But just as language can be problematic, it also has the power to transform. We once heard a story of a resident who called a colleague for a consult. Instead of saying, "I have an 86-year-old patient having a heart attack" in his exam room, he told the colleague, "I have a member of the Greatest Generation here who needs your help." Requesting help for a national hero transformed the doctor's perception of the patient in a powerful way that opened him up to compassion and a willingness to help generously.

Language used for the labels or identities that patients choose for themselves or that are used by others also appears to have an impact on their health outcomes. Park et al. (2009) studied different self-identities of cancer survivors—"survivor," "victim," "patient," and "person with cancer." The researchers were interested in how the connotations associated with each identity would "affect personal health behaviors and interactions with one's health care team" (p. S431). They found that identities are complex, overlapping, and fluid over time, but that "identifying as a survivor had a range of apparent advantages in terms of psychological well-being and active involvement" (p. S434).

In the work of making healthcare more patient-centered, we must attend to the language we use. Matson et al. (2019) created a summary of word choices that reflect patient-centeredness, a few of which appear in Table 3.1. The alternative language presented shifts the locus of authority to the patient, places the patient's personhood ahead of the disease, and fosters a therapeutic relationship.

Table 3.1 Conventional Versus Alternative Language

Conventional Language	Alternative Language
Take a history	Elicit/learn the patient's story
Chief complaint	Reason(s) for visit or patient concerns
Diabetic	Person with diabetes
No show	Did not keep appointment
Noncompliant	Nonadherent
Patient refuses	Patient declines

Adapted from Matson et al. (2019)

Appreciative Practice: Choose Language With Care

Given the profound ability of words to shape our reality, we must choose them with great care as we speak to others and ourselves. Our self-talk and the way we talk with others has the tremendous capacity for growth and energy, or for negativity and rumination. This appreciative practice, choosing language with care, requires us to continually pause and reflect upon the power of our words to heal or do harm.

One way to harness the power of language is through the use of metaphor. In Natalie's breast cancer journey, her struggle to navigate the metaphor of illness became a singular experience on its own. It seemed to her that everyone rather unthinkingly used the metaphors "battle with cancer," or "battling the disease." Well-meaning friends sent cards with messages such as, "We're in this battle with you!" or, "We know you'll win this battle!" One day someone delivered a gift basket with a pink book on top, and on the book's cover was a picture of pink boxing gloves. She had a minor meltdown and placed the book, with the entire gift basket, into the trash.

In a discussion with her therapist, she realized that the battle metaphor was simply a poor choice for her. Battles are violent, and Natalie is a strong believer in nonviolence. Battles have winners, but they also have losers; it was unsettling for her to think she might be the loser. The word "battle" connotes masculinity, which was not the source of her power. Eventually, she settled on the metaphor of "cancer as a gift" since her illness was revealing so many remarkable aspects of herself and those around her. For some people, the metaphor of a gift would be inappropriate, but to Natalie, at that time and in those circumstances, the metaphor was transformative. It provided in-the-moment opportunities to seek sources of healing rather than sources of illness.

If language creates our reality, it is important to recognize that the words we choose can become self-fulfilling prophecies (Bushe, 2010; Eden, 1990). "Terrible twos," "an accident waiting to happen," "dumb blonde," and "I'm terrible at math" have a way of setting up expectations, and not necessarily in a good way. If a friend tells you that Professor Smith is boring or unfair, the chances are good that your experience with Professor Smith will confirm those descriptors, simply because your brain is honed to see a dull or unfair teacher rather than one who might, in fact, be interesting and fair. In a clinical setting, if a nurse hands off a patient to you with the warning, "This patient has made my life miserable all day," it is likely that you will approach her as a difficult patient. It becomes a self-fulfilling prophecy. But if the nurse hands the patient off to you with, "This patient is a retired schoolteacher with amazing stories," you are more likely to approach her with curiosity and openness.

We conclude this section with an important caveat: All this discussion about carefully choosing language is *not* the same as the avoidance of naming difficult experiences or emotions when they arise. Naming hard things lets us begin to normalize difficult experiences and facilitate coping. Naming, through writing, speaking, and reflection, is the crucial first step toward learning and growth, or as researcher Brené Brown (2017) calls it, the process of "rumbling," or shaping the stories of our experience.

The Poetic Principle

The poetic principle harkens back to Nancy Cooperrider's "appreciative eye," her statement that there is beauty in everything, depending on how you choose to look. What is most important is that *we have the power to choose*. A rainy day can be depressing, or it can bring life and freshness to the world around us. It can be an opportunity to sleep in or splash in puddles. A long walk to work from your parking spot can be an indicator of your low status in the health system, or it can be an opportunity to get fresh air and exercise or to listen to music or podcasts.

What we choose to focus on becomes our fate (Whitney & Trosten-Bloom, 2003). If we look for problems, we will find problems. If we look for beauty, we will find beauty.

Look for the Orange Backpacks

Have you ever bought something that you thought was unique, say an orange backpack, and suddenly you started seeing orange backpacks everywhere? This is an example of something called the *frequency illusion,* in which you are seeing something more, simply because you are noticing it more. Students aren't suddenly buying more orange backpacks; you are just aware of that specific color backpack because you just got so excited about buying one for yourself.

Often the first thing we hear from people when we teach the poetic principle is that it sounds a lot like we're wearing rose-colored glasses. Does this mean that in looking for the things we want more of we are ignoring the bad and ugly in the world? No, it definitely does not mean that. By learning how to foster an appreciative mindset and an open, curious stance in the world, we are better equipped to encounter life's challenges in creative and meaningful ways.

The fatefulness of our focus can transform a negative circumstance into a positive consequence. An example: A young boy, about age 10, alone in the batter's box of an empty baseball diamond. He enthusiastically shouts, "I'm the greatest batter in the world!" Then he tosses the ball up in the air, swings, and misses. He repeats, "I'm the greatest batter in the world!" tosses up the ball, swings, and misses again.

For a third time, he boasts that he's the greatest batter, tosses the ball, swings, and misses. Three strikes and he's out. But suddenly his face brightens, and the background music blares, and he shouts, "I'm the greatest *pitcher* in the world!" That is the essence of seeking out something positive in a bad situation, or reframing.

Appreciative Practice: Reframing

Reframing is the capacity to intentionally explore new ways of seeing in order to experience the best of what is (Thatchenkery & Metzker, 2006). This practice opens possibilities that may have been hidden to us. Reframing is the "ability to seek out and study a new frame or worldview; to be open to new concepts, ideas, perspectives and possibilities" (A. J. Mann, personal communication, October 22, 2013). In nursing, the technique has been called "positive reappraisal" (Cheung et al., 2020). The Institute for Healthcare Improvement (IHI) has included the practice of reframing in its "Psychological PPE" recommendations for healthcare staff who may be at risk of mental health effects during the COVID-19 pandemic (IHI, 2020). *Reframing* is the ability to view an individual or situation through a new lens. It requires curiosity, creativity, and an openness to new possibilities and ways of understanding the world. As with anything, it requires practice, but the result can be transformative.

We have already given several examples of reframing in our discussion of the poetic and social construction principles. A long walk from a parking spot is an opportunity to listen to podcasts or to exercise. A patient who may be perceived as difficult may also be perceived as in desperate need of compassionate care. Every situation presents an opportunity for reframing, of asking, "What is possible? What do I really want?" (Thatchenkery & Metzker, 2006).

- Being stuck in traffic is an opportunity to practice deep breathing.

- Exercise is a celebration of what your body can do, not a punishment for what you ate.

- We are more likely to succeed if we view stressors and setbacks as challenges, not failures (Achor, 2010).

- It is helpful to think of a chore (e.g., cooking dinner, cleaning house) as an act of caring for yourself or others, rather than a burden.

In 2014, writer Glennon Doyle posted a photo of herself in her kitchen on social media. Almost immediately, followers sent her "helpful" suggestions about how she could tackle some home improvement projects to make her kitchen look better. Glennon says she had always loved her kitchen, but suddenly, through her followers' eyes, it seemed drab. Then she remembered a passage from Thoreau's *Walden*: "I say, beware of all enterprises that require new clothes, and not rather a new wearer of clothes." She looked at her kitchen with "fresh perspecatacles" and saw an appliance that keeps her Diet Coke cold, a faucet that provides clean, running water, and a magical machine that makes coffee. "Every morning. On a timer" (para. 11). And the kitchen floor provides space for her children to dance. In the conclusion, she captures the heart of reframing and appreciative practices, that with a curious and willing mindset, we generate energy that can be turned toward the challenges we face.

> Today I shall keep my perspectacles super-glued to my face and feel insanely GRATEFUL instead of LACKING and I will look at my home and my people and my body and say: THANK YOU. THANK YOU, THANK YOU, THANK YOU. THIS IS ALL MORE THAN GOOD ENOUGH, ALL OF IT. Now. Let us turn our focus *onward and outward*. There is WORK TO BE DONE and JOY TO BE HAD. (Doyle, 2014, para. 19)

The Positive Principle

Appreciative Inquiry practitioners Whitney and Trosten-Bloom (2003) write that "momentum for change requires large amounts of positive affect and social bonding—hope, inspiration, and sheer joy in creating with one another" (p. 67). Think about a class you'll never forget or an extracurricular group that you belonged to; we are willing to bet that you had many positive emotions associated with that experience. Perhaps you looked forward to going to class or you left a group activity feeling better than you did when you arrived. We don't seek positivity simply for the sake of feeling better. Positive psychology and resilience researchers have demonstrated that we are more creative, better able to solve problems, and more open to learning and to new ideas when we are experiencing positive emotions. Positivity begets positive results. Similarly, positivity results in social bonding that feeds our well-being.

As told in the sidebar, when Natalie learned of her breast cancer diagnosis, she was reading Jackie Kelm's book, *Appreciative Living*. She was midway through the "Positive Principle" chapter on the day she received the call from her doctor. Going beyond the "laughter is the best medicine" cliché, the chapter outlined the scientific basis for positivity and positive affect and their relationships to healing, well-being, and resiliency. Positivity, a fundamental element of an appreciative mindset, is a powerful force linked to flexibility, creative problem-solving, recovery from stressful situations, and improved cognitive functioning (Fredrickson, 2009). It is also linked in varying degrees to success in many realms: business and academic success, social relationships, longevity, reducing depression, health behaviors, and overall health (Achor, 2010; Fredrickson, 2004, 2009; Lambert et al., 2012; Van Cappellen et al., 2017). In healthcare practitioners, positive affect and positivity are shown to improve clinical judgment (Estrada et al., 1997), foster resilience (Montero-Marin et al., 2015), and reduce burnout (Cheung et al., 2020).

The research points to the benefit of fostering positive emotions in ourselves and others. Positive psychology researcher Barbara Fredrickson has created a significant body of work on positivity and positive emotions, but we will focus on just a few of them here.

Fredrickson (2004) was the first to establish the "broaden and build" theory of positive emotions. This theory suggests that positive emotions spark, or broaden, our in-the-moment "thought-action repertoire," meaning that when we feel joy, we are more inclined to play. When we feel love, we are more likely to extend kindness to others. Positive emotions expand our menu of responses to daily encounters, unlike negative emotions that tend to shut us down and limit our possible reactions to situations or stressors (Fredrickson, 2004).

Second, Fredrickson determined that not only do positive emotions spark positive thought-action repertoires, they in turn allow us to build and expand our personal physical, intellectual, social, and psychological resources. While a positive emotion may be fleeting, it has power beyond the moment and strengthens our capacity to cope with stress. Remember our discussion of resilience in the previous chapter.

Finally, Fredrickson (2009) has identified and studied what she considers the ten most frequently experienced positive emotions: joy, gratitude, serenity, interest, hope, pride, amusement, inspiration, awe, and love. These positive emotions are correlated with happiness and well-being, and we can foster these emotions in ourselves and others. Again, our goal is to build a reservoir of positive emotions that we can draw upon when faced with daily or intermittent stressors by *savoring* the positive emotion that we are focused on (Hanson, 2018).

For now, let's focus on joy.

Patient safety leader Don Berwick writes in his foreword to an Institute for Healthcare Improvement white paper, *Framework for Improving Joy at Work* (Perlo et al., 2017, p. 4):

> In our work in health care, joy is not just humane; it's instrumental. As my colleague Maureen Bisognano has reminded us, "You cannot give what you do not have." The gifts of hope, confidence, and safety that health care should offer patients and families can only come from a workforce that feels hopeful, confident, and safe. Joy in work is an essential resource for the enterprise of healing.

If, as the white paper claims, "joy is one of healthcare's greatest assets" (Perlo et al., p. 6), how can we get more of it? How can we train our eye to seek out joy so that, like the orange backpacks, we will see more joy simply by looking for it? We have found gratitude journals to be one of the most effective practices, and research has borne this out.

Appreciative Practice: Gratitude

Robert Emmons and Michael McCullough (2003), leading gratitude researchers, write that "an intentional grateful focus is one form of cognitive appraisal of one's life circumstances with the ability to impact long-term levels of well-being" (p. 387). By "cognitive appraisal" they mean that we can judge or determine the value of something, whether it be something done for us by an external source (e.g., another person) or simply an awareness of something such as nature, art, or circumstances. Emmons and McCullough (2003) conducted studies in which participants who wrote daily gratitude lists exhibited higher measures of well-being than study participants who made lists of "hassles" or neutral life events. They also found that the gratitude list makers were more likely to offer emotional support to others.

In numerous studies, gratitude practices are shown to improve happiness, increase well-being, and reduce depression in other populations (Gander et al., 2013; Lambert, Fincham & Stillman, 2012; O'Leary & Dockray, 2015; Seligman et al., 2005; Wood et al., 2010). In a study, 228 healthcare workers who faced high rates of stress were invited to test an intervention to reduce burnout using a well-validated exercise called Three Good Things (Sexton & Adair, 2019). Study participants showed significant improvement in emotional exhaustion, depression symptoms, happiness, and work-life balance for up to 12 months. Three Good Things is a simple exercise that anyone can do, even those with very little time, and the results for nurses, physicians, and others are quite promising.

To practice Three Good Things, commit to taking time at the end of each day to write down three good things that happened to you during the day. These can be exciting events such as acing an exam or receiving a job offer, but most likely, they will be more humble moments. You might appreciate a delicious meal, an unexpected connection with a friend, a nap, or a sunny day. You may choose to write your three good things in a small notebook, or on your phone or laptop. The most important thing is to do it regularly for at least 10 days. You will begin to notice that throughout the day, your attention and thoughts will be drawn toward those good things around you and away from those things that produce negative feelings. If you would like to take this exercise a step further, pick one good thing each day and reflect on the people and events that made that good thing possible. For example, if you are grateful for a hot cup of coffee, think about the barista who made it to work that day and the workers who manufactured the cups; you will increase your sense of connection with the world around you.

Daily Gratitude Practice

—Sarah Franklin, Student Nurse (she/her)

Had taco salad for dinner.

Got 5/5 on quiz.

Walked with friend and her foster dog.

Sometimes the Universe sends you a subtle hint; in Sarah's case, it was a good idea and a blank notebook. When Sarah Franklin began her sophomore year at the University of Virginia School of Nursing, she attended a lecture on appreciative practices as part of the required Foundations of Nursing CARE class. One of the practices she took note of was the Three Good Things, or gratitude, exercise.

A few days later, she joined her class for a day-long mindfulness and meditation retreat. All students were given a new notebook and encouraged to begin their own journaling practice, in any way that was meaningful to them. Sarah decided to use this opportunity to try a gratitude practice. "It seemed like an easy, simple thing to do, to think about the good things that happened during the day."

Just before going to bed each night, she writes down three to six things that she feels thankful for. "I don't write down the big things," she says, meaning the basic needs that she knows she takes for granted, such as food and shelter. Instead, she writes the small things that she notices when she reflects upon her day. "There are definitely themes about eating and relationships, like going for a walk with someone or having a good conversation."

Almost two years later, she continues to make her nightly gratitude list. "It's so easy," she says. "I tried journaling in high school, but it took me so long, it would stress me out. I didn't have time, and I'd get bored with having to write everything down." With a gratitude journal, "it's like a traditional journal, except only the highlights." She adds that it's nice to sometimes flip back through her journal to read some of the things she was grateful for.

Sarah acknowledges that she is a fairly positive person, so this aligns with her values and way of being in the world. But she feels the practice "has kept me a little more accountable, to keep me in this mindset." She says that in addition to supporting her positive outlook, she believes the practice has helped her cope with academics and the rigors of nursing school. "Everyone at some level, on certain days, goes through anxiety and stress, and we can benefit from something like this."

The Simultaneity Principle

The *simultaneity principle* posits that our questions are fateful, that change and our questions are inextricably linked (Whitney & Trosten-Bloom, 2003). Just as David Cooperrider discovered in his studies of organizations, we can harness the power of positive questions in our daily lives. In the earlier blog post by Glennon Doyle, she had a choice of questions to ask herself: "What is wrong with my kitchen and how can I fix it?" or, "What amazing features can be found in my kitchen?" Our questions—in our thinking and in our spoken word—are one of the most powerful tools that we have available to us to shape our lives and experiences. Table 3.2 shows some of our favorite examples.

Table 3.2 Change Your Question, Change Your Mind

Instead of Asking:	Try:
What is wrong?	What is possible?
What are you most worried about?	What are you looking forward to?
Why did this happen?	What can we learn from this?
Why isn't there enough?	What do you want more of?
How will I survive?	How will I find meaning? OR What surprises me about the situation?
Why am I failing?	What can I do to move forward?
What is wrong with this patient?	What are this patient's greatest strengths?
What do I have to do today?	What do I get to do today?

The simultaneity principle provides a path toward curiosity and resilience by pointing us in the direction of creative solutions and new possibilities. The ability to approach situations and others with a stance of curiosity not only expands our options, it also has the power to develop more trusting and collaborative relationships with others (Gino, 2018). Curiosity helps us overcome the trap of *confirmation bias*, or only ingesting evidence that confirms our beliefs rather than exploring information that may contradict them. Studies have shown that curiosity can lessen our defensiveness when we're stressed and can moderate aggressive reactions when we're provoked (Gino, 2018).

Curiosity begins in the form of a question. In writing about design thinking, an exciting, relatively new methodology in healthcare, Professor Liedtka (2018, p. 74) writes, "Defining problems in obvious, conventional ways, not surprisingly, often leads to obvious, conventional solutions. *Asking a more interesting question* can help teams discover more original ideas." We can explore novel ways of moving through the world, simply by asking the right questions. Faced with breast cancer, for example, Natalie asked, "What can I learn from this?" instead of, "Why did this happen to me?"

Curiosity is one of the most valuable tools in your tool kit. Unlocking its power simply takes a moment of awareness to remember that we can choose our questions, and then it requires continued vigilance to keep the guiding question front and center in our mind.

The power of a positive question is available to us beyond our own thoughts. We have seen this play out in patient care settings, in relationships between colleagues, and in our personal lives. The best place to begin is to assume positive intent.

Appreciative Practice: Assumption of Positive Intent

Sociologist Brené Brown, in her book, *Dare to Lead*, shares a client's observation that, "I know my life is better when I work from the assumption that everyone is doing the best they can" (Brown, 2018, p. 215). There is no simpler way, at least in theory, to shift from a stance of judgment to one of curiosity than to assume that others are coming from a place of good intentions. Perhaps the driver who cut you off in traffic is a student driver or a husband trying to rush his pregnant wife to the hospital. Maybe the friend who missed your gym date just learned that a family member was ill and didn't have the bandwidth to reach out to you. Maybe the student who asks "too many" questions in class has learning challenges and is simply anxious about doing well.

For over a decade, we have invited healthcare workers to engage in the practice of assuming positive intent with their patients and colleagues. How might they approach a patient differently if they asked, "I wonder why...?" instead of rushing to judgment? For example, a clinic patient who is always late for appointments or sometimes fails to show up at all can frustrate his entire healthcare team. The natural tendency is to assume that the patient is disorganized or disrespectful of the clinicians' time. But what if clinic staff instead asked, "I wonder why this patient has so much trouble coming to his appointments?" This curious approach might uncover transportation barriers, childcare challenges, or even severe anxiety about a clinic visit. Once discovered, the clinic staff can potentially help the patient address these barriers. Simultaneously, this process of discovery might help staff feel more compassion toward this patient who had previously left them feeling frustrated. This process can also have benefits to a patient who may have felt unseen and judged by his healthcare team.

When faced with any challenge, begin by asking, "I wonder why....?" Notice when you are rushing to make an assumption about something or someone, gently stop that train of thought, and approach the situation with curiosity. As with every activity described in this chapter, it will take awareness on your part and practice, but eventually it will become almost second nature.

The Anticipatory Principle

We move toward the image of the future that we hold in our heads, and the more positive that vision, the more positive our future. This is the essence of the *anticipatory principle*. You may already have some experience with "vision boards." Vision boards are typically collages cut from magazines with images depicting your goals and desires. Many of us use online tools such as Pinterest to collect images to help us plan a future event, such as a vacation, a wardrobe, or a wedding.

There is great power in visualization and our beliefs about the future, and this has been borne out in medical studies. Research on healthy aging reveals that individuals who believe that they will age well are more likely to have lower hospitalization rates, to recover more quickly from a disability, and are less likely to experience cardiovascular events and Alzheimer's disease (Levy et al., 2012; Levy et al., 2009; Sun et al., 2017).

In our work, we encourage individuals and teams to visualize their ideal future, and they must imagine this desired future in great detail. How do things look? How do they feel? What are people doing? Are they smiling, laughing, celebrating? Once we have created this ideal image, our present selves begin to take actions, consciously and unconsciously, to move us toward that ideal future.

Before her cancer diagnosis, Natalie, her husband, and their 10-year old daughter had planned to walk their city's annual 10K race. It was more of an annual party than a race. Rather than give up on their dream of participating in the race, Natalie created a vision of the event that she carried with her through chemotherapy, surgery, and radiation treatments. She imagined how she would feel at the start and finish lines. In her mind, she could see the crowds and the other walkers and runners, some in costumes, some with their children and families. She created a vivid picture of herself, strong and smiling throughout the race. She felt the weight of the finisher's medal around her neck. This vivid mental picture compelled her to walk four miles every single day to and from her radiation treatments. The image of success and completing cancer treatments was her light at the end of the tunnel. After the event, when the race photos were posted online, she was astonished to see a photo of herself, taken at the finish line; the photo looked exactly like she had pictured herself in her imaginings.

Elite golfers Arnold Palmer and Tiger Woods and tennis great Billie Jean King have used visualization techniques for decades. Imagery has been used in nearly every sport, from swimming to ping pong, to help athletes improve their coordination, focus, strength, and flexibility (Schuster et al., 2011). Olympic athletes use imagery to mentally simulate an approaching competition. Team psychologists encourage athletes to create mental images of every aspect of their competitive event, from speaking at news conferences, to riding on the bus, to every twist and turn of the race or event. The imagery must engage all the senses in order to be effective. Emily Cook, an Olympic freestyle aerialist says, "You have to smell it. You have to hear it. You have to feel it, everything" (Clarey, 2014, para. 7). Again, imagery must be positive. Golfers don't visualize their tee shots going into the rough, and tennis players don't imagine their serves landing in the net.

Imagery is a powerful tool for the rest of us as well. Mental imagery mimics the same brain functions as physical actions: motor control, attention, planning, and memory (LeVan, 2009). Positive visualization can enhance confidence, self-efficacy, and motivation (LeVan, 2009). When faced with a public speaking event, many experienced presenters visualize themselves at the venue, giving a flawless and well-received presentation. Visualization has been found effective in reducing public speaking anxiety, even in those with the greatest anxiety (Ayres & Hopf, 1985; Hopf & Ayres, 1992). Various types of motor imagery training have proven effective in music, education, psychology, and medicine (Schuster et al., 2011). Our brains, and our imaginations, are powerful tools that we should harness whenever possible.

A remarkable story about the power of visualization comes from opera singer, Ryan Speedo Green. Green, the subject of the biography, *Sing for Your Life*, was a young man living in the Tidewater region of Virginia. At one time, he was placed in a juvenile correction facility, in solitary confinement. Later, as a student at the Governor's School for the Arts, he went on a class trip to New York's Metropolitan Opera House to see his first opera, and in that one evening, everything changed. In an interview with Terri Gross (Gross & Miller, 2016), he recalled that while in the audience that night, he decided that he, too, was going to sing at the Metropolitan Opera. After the performance, he shared his plan with his teacher, Mr. Brown. Mr. Brown gently explained that Ryan would need to learn to read music, learn to memorize lines, learn a foreign language, go to college, attend a young artist program, and actually get some work singing. If he did all those things, Mr. Brown told him, he might someday be able to audition at the Met. Green concluded the story:

"And then kind of in my mind, I think, I took it all down and made a list. And nine years later, I sang at the Met."

It is certainly astonishing that Green made his way from solitary confinement to the Metropolitan Opera, but we are certain that it would not have happened if he had not held onto a compelling vision of himself performing on that stage. Green's vision had the power to guide his in-the-moment actions, to learn a particular skill, to accept help from a teacher or mentor, and to study with focus and determination.

Appreciative Practice: Visualization

There is a quote often attributed to feminist Gloria Steinem: "Without leaps of imagination, or dreaming, we lose the excitement of possibilities. Dreaming, after all, is a form of planning." We encourage you to harness the power of your imagination as you set goals and plan for your future.

A simple visualization technique can be done before you even get out of bed each morning. Select one or two things that you'd like to accomplish that day and imagine how those activities unfold. Create as much rich detail as you can muster—outline the steps you will take, describe how it looks and feels—and replay these details over and over again in your mind. Some people choose to write down key details or phrases to begin their day, but the most important thing is generating positive, rich details about the activity or end result.

Visualization techniques may be used to achieve larger goals, as in the Ryan Speedo Green example. Focus on a question (What will I do when I graduate?) or a goal (I'd like to find a life partner) and create a block of uninterrupted time (at least an hour) in a quiet, comfortable space. On a piece of paper, or several, make a detailed list. Again, the magic is in the details. If you are thinking about your life after graduation, imagine a day in your post-college life. Write down every single detail, from the moment you wake up until the time you go to bed. Where are you sleeping? What are you wearing? What do you eat for breakfast? How do you get to work? Who do you see when you walk in the door? Are you in the country or the city? Let your mind flow; don't edit your list.

The list of questions (and answers) in this visualization exercise is infinite, but your "map" will come from the seemingly least consequential details. If you are seeking a life partner, for example, make a list of every quality that you seek, the things that you will do together, the place you will live, and more. Engage in all five senses, paying attention to sights, sounds, smells, tastes, and touch. The details generated by this kind of quiet reflection will create a vivid picture of your future that you may begin to move toward in the present moment.

In Real Practice

Let's talk about test anxiety. This is a significant problem affecting an estimated 50%–100% of prelicensure nursing students. Not only may test anxiety diminish learning and test scores, it is also believed to reduce the number of students who go on to graduate nursing programs. Many of the practices outlined in this chapter may be used to help you take texts and exams in a better frame of mind. This 2017 literature review by Brenna Quinn and Anya Peters identified several strategies that can help reduce test anxiety. These strategies include essential lemon oil, listening to classical music, and the presence of a therapy dog. Relaxation techniques, reflective journaling, and a "magic pencil" also reduced test anxiety. In a "Teaching Tip," the review authors also encourage students to write "positive prompts" in the front of their exam books: something you are good at, a personal mantra, or a compliment that made you feel proud (Quinn & Peters, 2019). In another article on NCLEX success, recommendations include visualizing success, maintaining a positive attitude, and diverting yourself with activities that foster positive emotions (Quinn et al., 2018).

Closing Thoughts

We encourage you to adopt one, two, or more appreciative practices. Consider them "self-care superpowers." The most important skill you will need to master appreciative practices is your in-the-moment awareness. Whenever you encounter something potentially stressful or discouraging, in that moment, pause. Notice how you are feeling. Be curious about the situation and your response to it. Why did that happen? Am I missing a piece of the story, perhaps? Why am I responding this way? What is another way I can think about this situation? Am I being influenced by my own thoughts or the language of others? Is there something in this person or situation that I can be thankful for? Once we develop our capacity to notice our reactions to difficult situations, we have taken the first step toward exploring new ways of moving forward. Knowing that we have the capacity to choose our thinking and our response to any given situation is the greatest superpower of all.

Key Points

- Appreciative practices are grounded in the principles of Appreciative Inquiry, an organizational change methodology that uses a strengths-based approach to change.

- A vast amount of research indicates that developing an appreciative mindset can lead to greater happiness, success, resilience, the ability to connect with others, and creative means to solve problems.

- There are five core principles that support the behaviors prescribed in appreciative practices: constructionist, poetic, positive, simultaneity, and anticipatory.

- There are many appreciative practices to foster resilience and well-being. In this chapter we focused on intentional use of language, reframing, gratitude, assumption of positive intent, and visualization.

- Appreciative practices can be done by anyone with no special training or materials. Like muscle strength, an appreciative mindset can be developed with regular daily practice.

References

Achor, S. (2010). *The happiness advantage*. Crown Business.

Appreciative Inquiry Commons. (n.d.). *Applications of AI*. https://appreciativeinquiry.champlain.edu/learn/appreciative-inquiry-introduction/applications-of-ai/

Ayres, J., & Hopf, T. S. (1985). Visualization: A means of reducing speech anxiety. *Communication Education, 34*(4), 318–323. https://doi.org/10.1080/03634528509378623

Baumeister, R. F., Bratslavsky, E., Finkenauer, C., & Vohs, K. D. (2001). Bad is stronger than good. *Review of General Psychology, 5*, 323–370. https://doi.org/10.1037/1089-2680.5.4.323

Boehm, J. K., Chen, Y., Qureshi, F., Soo, J., Umukoro, P., Hernandez, R., Lloyd-Jones, D., & Kubzansky L. D. (2020). Positive emotions and favorable cardiovascular health: A 20-year longitudinal study. *Preventive Medicine, 136*, 106103. https://doi.org/10.1016/j.ypmed.2020.106103

Brown, B. (2017). *Rising strong: How the ability to reset transforms the way we live, love, parent, and lead*. Random House.

Brown, B. (2018). *Dare to lead: Brave work, tough conversations, whole hearts*. Random House.

Bushe, G. R. (2010). *Clear leadership: Sustaining real collaboration and partnership at work*. Davies-Black.

Cheung, E. O., Hernandez, A., Herold, E., & Moskowitz, J. T. (2020). Positive emotion skills intervention to address burnout in critical care nurses. *AACN Advanced Critical Care, 31*(2), 167–178. https://doi.org/10.4037/aacnacc2020287

Clarey, C. (2014, February 22). Olympians use imagery as mental training. *The New York Times*. https://www.nytimes.com/2014/02/23/sports/olympics/olympians-use-imagery-as-mental-training.html

Cooperrider, D. L., & Whitney, D. (2005). *Appreciative inquiry: A positive revolution in change*. Berrett-Koehler Publishers.

Croskerry, P., Abbass, A., & Wu, A.W. (2010). Emotional influences in patient safety. *Journal of Patient Safety, 6*(4), 199–205. https://doi.org/10.1097/pts.0b013e3181f6c01a

Davies, P. (2007). The language of health care: The alienating language of health care. *Journal of the Royal Society of Medicine, 100*, 6–9. https://doi.org/10.1177/014107680710000104

Doyle, G. M. (2014, August 11). Give me gratitude or give me debt. *Momastery*. https://momastery.com/blog/2014/08/11/give-liberty-give-debt/

Eden, D. (1990). *Issues in organizational management series. Pygmalion in management: Productivity as a self-fulfilling prophecy*. Lexington Books/D. C. Heath and Com.

Emmons, R. A., & McCullough, M. E. (2003). Counting blessings versus burdens: An experimental investigation of gratitude and subjective well-being in daily life. *Journal of Personality and Social Psychology, 84*(2), 377–389. https://doi.org/10.1037//0022-3514.84.2.377

Estrada, C. A., Isen, A. M., & Young, M. J. (1997). Positive affect facilitates integration of information and decreases anchoring in reasoning among physicians. *Organizational Behavior and Human Decision Processes, 72*, 117–135. https://doi.org/10.1006/obhd.1997.2734

Fredrickson, B. L. (2004). The broaden-and-build theory of positive emotions. *Philosophical Transactions of the Royal Society B, 359*, 1367–1377. https://doi.org/10.1098/rstb.2004.1512

Fredrickson, B. L. (2009). *Positivity*. Crown Publishing.

Gander, F., Proyer, R. T., Ruch, W., & Wyss, T. (2013). Strengths-based positive interventions: Further evidence for their potential in enhancing well-being and alleviating depression. *Journal of Happiness Studies, 14*, 1241–1259. https://doi.org/10.1007/s10902-012-9380-0

Gino, F. (2018, Sept/Oct). The business case for curiosity. *Harvard Business Review*, 48–57.

Gross, T., & Miller, D. (Producers). (2016, September 20). Opera singer Ryan Speedo Green. *Fresh Air* [Audio podcast]. NPR. https://www.npr.org/2016/09/20/494770846/opera-singer-ryan-speedo-green

Haizlip, J., May, N., Schorling, J., Williams, A., & Plews-Ogan, M. (2012). The negativity bias, medical education, and the culture of academic medicine: Why culture change is hard. *Academic Medicine, 87*(9), 1205–1209. https://doi.org/10.1097/ACM.0b013e3182628f03

Hanson, R. (2018). *Resilient: How to grow an unshakable core of calm, strength, and happiness*. Harmony Books.

Hopf, T., & Ayres, J. (1992). Coping with public speaking anxiety: An examination of various combinations of systematic desensitization, skills training, and visualization. *Journal of Applied Communication Research, 20*(2), 183–198. https://doi.org/10.1080/00909889209365328

Institute for Healthcare Improvement. (2020). *"Psychological PPE": Promote health care workforce mental health and well-being.* IHI. http://www.ihi.org/resources/Pages/Tools/psychological-PPE-promote-health-care-workforce-mental-health-and-well-being.aspx

Kelm, J. B. (2005). *Appreciative living: The principles of appreciative inquiry in personal life.* Venet Publishers.

Lambert, N. M., Fincham, F. D., & Stillman, T. F. (2012). Gratitude and depressive symptoms: The role of positive reframing and positive emotion. *Cognition and Emotion, 26*(4), 615–633. https://doi.org/10.1080/02699931.2011.595393

LeVan, A. (2009, December 3). Seeing is believing: The power of visualization. *Psychology Today.* https://www.psychologytoday.com/us/blog/flourish/200912/seeing-is-believing-the-power-visualization

Levy, B. R., Slade, M. D., Murphy, T. E., & Gill, T. M. (2012). Association between positive age stereotypes and recovery from disability in older persons. *JAMA, 308*(9), 1972–1973. https://doi.org/10.1001/jama.2012.14541

Levy, B. R., Zonderman, A. B., Slade, M. D., & Ferrucci, L. (2009). Age stereotypes held earlier in life predict cardiovascular events in later life. *Psychological Science, 20*(3), 296–298. https://doi.org/10.1111/j.1467-9280.2009.02298.x

Liedtka, J. (2018, September/October). Why design thinking works. *Harvard Business Review,* 72–79.

Lyubomirsky, S., King, L., & Diener, E. (2005). The benefits of frequent positive affect: Does happiness lead to success? *Psychological Bulletin, 131*(6), 803–855. https://doi.org/10.1037/0033-2909.131.6.803

Lyubomirsky, S., & Layous, K. (2013). How do simple positive activities increase well-being? *Current Directions in Psychological Science, 22*(1), 57–62. https://doi.org/10.1177/0963721412469809

Matson, C. C., Beck, L. A., & Rajasekaran, S. K. (2019). Using language that reflects who is the center of our care. *Academic Medicine, 94*(9), 1400. https://doi.org/10.1097/ACM.0000000000002799

May, N. B., Haizlip, J., & Plews-Ogan, M. (2020). Changing the conversation: Appreciative inquiry and appreciative practices in healthcare. In S. McNamee, M. M. Gergen, C. Camargo-Borges, & E. F. Rasera (Eds.), *The SAGE handbook of social construction practice* (pp. 464–475). SAGE Reference.

Montero-Marin, J., Tops, M., Manzanera, R., Piva Demarzo, M. M., de Mon Melchor, A., & García-Campayo, J. (2015, December 17). Mindfulness, resilience, and burnout subtypes in primary care physicians: The possible mediating role of positive and negative affect. *Frontiers in Psychology.* https://doi.org/10.3389/fpsyg.2015.01895

O'Leary, K., & Dockray, S. (2015). The effects of two novel gratitude and mindfulness interventions on well-being. *Journal of Alternative and Complementary Medicine, 21*(4), 243–245. https://doi.org/10.1089/acm.2014.0119

Park, C. L., Zlateva, T., & Blank, T. O. (2009). Self-identity after cancer: "Survivor", "victim", "patient", and "person with cancer." *Journal of General Internal Medicine, 24,* S430–S435. https://doi.org/10.1007/s11606-009-0993-x

Perlo, J., Balik, B., Swensen, S., Labcenell, A., Landsman, J., & Feeley, D. (2017). *IHI Framework for Improving Joy in Work.* [White paper]. Institute for Healthcare Improvement. http://www.ihi.org/resources/Pages/IHIWhitePapers/Framework-Improving-Joy-in-Work.aspx

Quinn, B. L., & Peters, A. (2017). Strategies to reduce nursing student test anxiety: A literature review. *Journal of Nursing Education, 56*(3), 145–151. https://doi.org/10.3928/01484834-20170222-05

Quinn, B. L., & Peters, A. A. (2019). Positive prompts: A quick exercise to reduce test anxiety. *Nurse Educator, 44* (5), 249. doi:10.1097/NNE.0000000000000641

Quinn, B. L., Smolinski, M., & Peters, A. B. (2018). Strategies to improve NCLEX-RN success: A review. *Teaching and Learning in Nursing, 13*(1), 18–26. https://doi.org/10.1016/j.teln.2017.09.002

Schuster, C., Hilfiker, R., Amft, O., Scheidhauer, A., Andrews, B., Butler, J., Kischka, U., & Ettlin, T. (2011). Best practice for motor imagery: A systematic literature review on motor imagery training elements in five different disciplines. *BMC Medicine, 9*, 75. https://doi.org/10.1186/1741-7015-9-75

Seligman, M. E., Steen, T. A., Park, N., & Peterson, C. (2005). Positive psychology progress: Empirical validation of interventions. *The American Psychologist, 60(5)*, 410–421. https://doi.org/10.1037/0003-066X.60.5.410

Sexton, J. B., & Adair, K. C. (2019). Forty-five good things: A prospective pilot study of the Three Good Things well-being intervention in the USA for healthcare worker emotional exhaustion, depression, work-life balance and happiness. *BMJ Open, 9*(3), e022695. https://doi.org/10.1136/bmjopen-2018-022695

Sun, J. K., Kim, E. S., & Smith, J. (2017). Positive self-perceptions of aging and lower rate of overnight hospitalization in the US population over age 50. *Psychosomatic Medicine, 79*(1), 81–90. https://doi.org/10.1097/PSY.0000000000000364

Thatchenkery, T., & Metzker, C. (2006). *Appreciative intelligence: Seeing the mighty oak in the acorn.* Berrett-Koehler.

Vaish, A., Grossmann, T., & Woodward, A. (2008). Not all emotions are created equal: The negativity bias in social-emotional development. *Psychological Bulletin, 134*, 383–403. https://doi.org/10.1037/0033-2909.134.3.383

Van Cappellen, P., Rice, E. L., Catalino, L. I., & Fredrickson, B. L. (2017). Positive affective processes underlie positive health behaviour change. *Psychology & Health, 33*(1), 1–21. https://doi.org/10.1080/08870446.2017.1320798

Wade, H. (2017). *Time to appreciate appreciative inquiry.* https://innovativethoughts.net/2017/08/25/time-to-appreciate-appreciative-inquiry/

Whitney, D., & Trosten-Bloom, A. (2003). *The power of appreciative inquiry: A practical guide to positive change.* Berrett-Koehler Publishers, Inc.

Williams, A., & Haizlip, J. (2013). Ten keys to the successful use of appreciative inquiry in academic healthcare. *OD Practitioner, 45*(2), 20–25.

Williams, N., & Ogden, J. (2004). The impact of matching the patient's vocabulary: A randomized control trial. *Family Practice, 21*, 630–635. https://doi.org/10.1093/fampra/cmh610

Wood, A. M., Froh, J. J., & Geraghty, A. W. A. (2010). Gratitude and well-being: A review and theoretical integration. *Clinical Psychology Review, 30*(7), 890–905. https://doi.org/10.1016/j.cpr.2010.03.005

4

The Community Resiliency Model (CRM)® Approach to Mental Wellness for Nursing Students and New Graduate Nurses

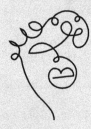 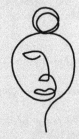

Linda Grabbe
pronouns: She/Her

Linda Grabbe has been a nurse in Honolulu, Kazakhstan, and Cote d'Ivoire. Her original passion was teaching resiliency skills to women with addictions and homeless youth in her Atlanta patient population, but she recognized the profound need of nurses and other frontline workers—as well as her own need—to learn these skills. She has been an indefatigable teacher of the Community Resiliency Model (CRM)® ever since.

Kate M. Pfeiffer
pronouns: She/Her

Kate M. Pfeiffer, an advanced practice nurse in mental health and a nursing instructor, is a passionate advocate for optimal mental health and agency for students and new nurses alike. In addition to CRM skills for fun self-care, she runs, hikes, and knits.

"When we bring awareness to the inner wisdom of our bodies, well-being can grow, even in times of great suffering. Moments of gratitude can be seen and sensed."

—Elaine Miller-Karas

Note to reader:

The authors would like to acknowledge Drs. Sandra Dunbar and Laura Kimble, Elaine Miller-Karas, and Connie Buchanan for their valuable insights and support.

The Community Resiliency Model (CRM)® is an innovative self-care model that entails simple sensory awareness practices to improve functioning in personal, family, professional, and community life (Miller-Karas, 2015). CRM skills can be used in day-to-day minor challenges, or in difficult circumstances—even in acute clinical situations. CRM presents a novel framework to help you understand your varying mental states through its resilient zone concept (Miller-Karas, 2015). We can train ourselves to notice when we are in a functioning resilient state, or, in reaction to stress and trauma, leaving that state, either in a hyper- or hypo-aroused state. As you understand this new perspective, you are more likely to view yourself compassionately, and this very awareness will interrupt some of the default negative circuitry that comes naturally to the brain. You can create powerful and resilient neurocircuitry instead.

Why is "community" in the title of this practice? CRM naturally lends itself to community settings and group teaching. CRM supports communities experiencing stress and trauma by increasing the resiliency of its members (Miller-Karas, 2015). As individuals create meaning from their struggles, the life of a community can also be transformed. Resiliency-informed individuals create resiliency-informed communities. While individual nurses can practice CRM for their own well-being and create a ripple effect by sharing the skills with friends, family, coworkers, and patients one-on-one, some nurses will want to share the model with their communities or patient populations. The Community Resiliency Model is culturally sensitive and adaptable to any ethnicity and developmental age, and it may be taught in an accessible peer-to-peer group format. CRM is "not only an innovative intervention that can be used for large numbers of people to build a prevention infrastructure for mental health challenges, but to create capacity" (Miller-Karas, 2015, p. 148). Any practitioner who wishes to formally teach a CRM class is required to become a Certified CRM Teacher with the Trauma Resource Institute (https://www. traumaresourceinstitute.com).

By practicing CRM's body-awareness skills, you will become sensitive to body sensations and be able to distinguish between internal sensations of distress and those of well-being (Miller-Karas, 2015). This awareness will give you a sense of control, and it will help you maintain emotional self-regulation during stressful clinical experiences, traumatic events, and day-to-day challenges. By learning and practicing these skills, you can develop an integrated mind-body balance that will promote attunement and resilience. For example, when interactions with your patients are tense or stressful, these skills will be helpful for your own emotional balance. This balanced state will affect your interactions with others as they sense your calm and attune to you. Additionally, CRM can be used directly with distressed patients, which will further enhance the therapeutic relationship and the patient's healing experience. We co-author this chapter as both researchers (Grabbe et al., 2020) and practitioners of CRM.

The Community Resiliency Model

The wellness skills of CRM focus on simple sensory awareness practice; using these skills will enhance your resiliency. We define *resiliency* as "an individual's and community's ability to identify and use individual and collective strengths in living fully in the present moment, and to thrive while managing the activities of daily living" (Miller-Karas, 2015, p. 6). Resiliency is the ability to withstand or cope with stress, trauma, and adversity, while maintaining mental well-being (Haglund et al., 2007). When we are resilient, we can manage significant sources of stress or trauma by accessing assets and resources within ourselves, our lives, and our environment in order to adapt and bounce back from adversity; this capacity will vary across the life course (Windle, 2011).

There are many mindfulness or meditation approaches to self-care, and these can be enormously beneficial. CRM is unique as a simple and purely body-based approach to well-being. In this chapter, we will use awareness of normal, everyday sensations already occurring in the body to develop a language of sensations and to understand their link to our body's autonomic nervous system responses to stress, perceived threats, or trauma. These responses emanate from the autonomic nervous system's sympathetic ("fight or flight") and parasympathetic (restoration of energy and balance) responses (Miller-Karas, 2015). Figure 4.1 shows the body's responses to the autonomic nervous system.

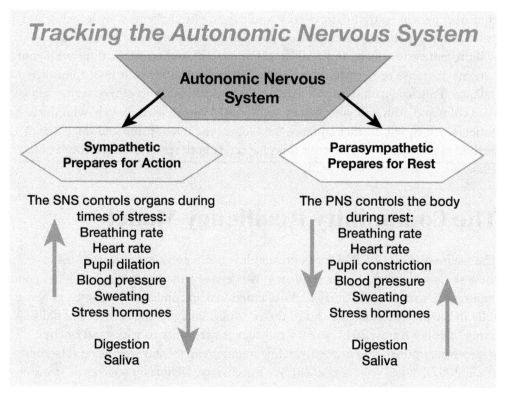

FIGURE 4.1   Tracking the autonomic nervous system.

Our bodies are naturally attuned to internal physical sensations such as thirst, hunger, and fatigue. This is known as *interoception*, or "felt-sense." Our bodies send messages about pleasant, unpleasant, or neutral sensations all the time, and this nervous system messaging system protects us and promotes homeostasis. In chaotic clinical situations, it can be easy to tune out interoceptive signals, like needing to use the restroom or taking a lunch break. But we can use this same felt-sense to "sync" our mind-body connection and regulate our emotional state (Miller-Karas, 2015).

Secondary Stress and Trauma

It is clear that nurses need to practice self-care in order to reduce their vulnerability to secondary or vicarious stress due to work. *Vicarious stress* (or trauma) is a type of cumulative trauma that comes from caring for and witnessing the stress and trauma of patients and families as they navigate illness and loss (Beck, 2011). Trauma, stress, and adversity can lead to emotional dysregulation and feelings of burnout, overwhelm, or general difficulties in work, school, and social relationships.

It is perfectly normal that our nervous system becomes highly activated as a normal response to trauma and stress. This is our body's way of protecting us and keeping us safe, but this can sometimes feel distressing or uncomfortable. We may feel edgy, irritable, or have difficulty concentrating, or we may feel isolated, sad, numb, or tired. As nurses, working with injured or ill patients can bring about these stress-related responses in our own bodies and take a toll on our overall well-being and the quality of our professional and personal lives. Using our interoceptive capacity will help us tune into body clues that we are experiencing in reaction to stress.

The Community Resiliency Model takes advantage of our tremendous capacity to pay attention to our body's internal state. But instead of focusing only on sensations such as fatigue, cold, pain, hunger, or a full bladder, CRM heightens our awareness of a full range of sensations and teaches us to identify them as pleasant, unpleasant, or neutral. The act of naming these physical sensations in our own body strengthens our capacity to self-regulate (Miller-Karas, 2015).

CRM Origins in Trauma Survivor Support

The Community Resiliency Model was initially developed by Elaine Miller-Karas with her colleagues Genie Everett and Laurie Leitch as a means of helping survivors of natural disasters reset their emotional state under devastating circumstances (Miller-Karas, 2015). It is based on widely accepted sensory-motor, or somatic, psychotherapy principles (Heller & LaPierre, 2012; Levine, 2010; Ogden, 2015). While CRM draws on these psychotherapeutic techniques, it is not psychotherapy. Put very simply, it is a form of self-care. CRM's self-regulation skills are used by psychotherapists to help clients self-regulate to process trauma, but CRM may also be learned and practiced as a stand-alone model. As a disaster relief tool, these easily and quickly taught, body-based self-regulation strategies demonstrated a reduced incidence of posttraumatic stress disorder in survivors (Leitch, 2007; Leitch, Vanslyke, & Allen, 2009; Parker et al., 2008).

Practitioners recognized that these mental well-being strategies were an effective self-regulation tool for persons suffering from the residual effect of acute trauma, those with chronic or cumulative trauma (Citron & Miller-Karas, 2013), and for care providers working with disaster victims (Leitch & Miller-Karas, 2009). The model's value was also recognized among people who routinely deal with traumatic or highly stressful circumstances in their professional roles, such as nurses, physicians, paramedics, social workers, therapists, and police (Miller-Karas, 2015; Grabbe et al., 2020).

The Resilient Zone

The cornerstone concept of CRM is the resilient zone (RZ). The *resilient zone* (RZ) is an internal state of well-being where individuals can function to their fullest capacity. It is where we are best equipped to think clearly, manage daily challenges, make decisions, engage fully in relationships, and be our most productive (Miller-Karas, 2015). It is where we feel most fully alive. It is possible to be in the resilient zone and feel sad or irritable, but we are still able to cope and function. Figure 4.2 illustrates the resilient zone.

The bandwidth of the zone varies among individuals. People who chronically experience emotion dysregulation may have a narrower zone than people who typically tolerate stress well. Everyone, however, has times when they experience a narrowed resilient zone and increased vulnerability to stress. This narrowing can occur due to many reasons including hunger, fatigue, boredom, pain, loneliness, or internalization of external stressors (Miller-Karas, 2015).

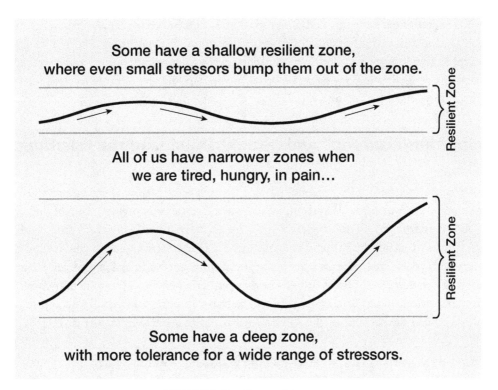

FIGURE 4.2 The resilient zone.

Let's Practice! Awareness of Our Resilient Zone

Take a few moments to think about your personal resilient zone. What does it feel like? Perhaps you are in the resilient zone now. If you've experienced some bumps in your day, are you still managing? Are you still in the zone? Maybe something wonderful happened today, or maybe you got a great night's sleep, or you went for a run this morning. Maybe these accomplishments make you feel like your best self. Now that you are aware of your resilient zone, check in periodically throughout the day to see where you are.

The wavy line within the resilient zone in Figure 4.2 corresponds to the rise and fall of energy in the body, which is also the normal alternation between sympathetic and parasympathetic dominance in the nervous system (Haglund et al.,

2007). Much like a car's gas pedal (sympathetic) and brake (parasympathetic), these are the balancing forces in our nervous system. The mere awareness of these normal body changes and the learned ability, with intention, to bring awareness to sensations of well-being are potent factors in rebalancing the nervous system and in withstanding the stress of nursing.

Being "Bounced Out" and "Stuck" Outside of the Resilient Zone

A traumatic or stressful experience may lead to over-activation of the gas or the brake pedals in our nervous system. When the accelerator is pressed, our bodies rev up our *sympathetic nervous system* with a rise in heart rate, respiratory rate, and muscle tension. The sympathetic nervous system is the component of the autonomic nervous system that prepares the body for action; you've heard it referred to as our *"fight or flight"* response. When the sympathetic nervous system is activated, you may notice anxiety, anger, irritability, or hyperactivity, and you'll know that you have been pushed out of the top of your resilient zone (Miller-Karas, 2015).

The *parasympathetic nervous system* is the brake, the autonomic nervous system's complement to the fight or flight response. Parasympathetic nervous system activation is restorative and calming, slowing breathing and heart rates, reducing blood pressure, and increasing digestion and muscle relaxation. This brake pedal, however, gets stuck sometimes, and we experience fatigue, depression, heavy limbs, and feeling disconnected or numb (Miller-Karas, 2015).

Figure 4.3 illustrates how stress, trauma, and negative events can disrupt the natural rebalancing of the nervous system.

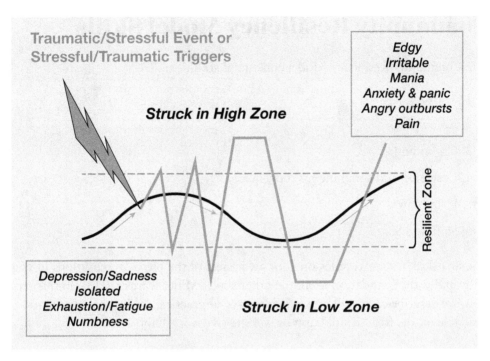

FIGURE 4.3 Outside the resilient zone.
Note: Graphic adapted from an original graphic of Peter Levin/Heller, original slide design by Genie Everst.

When our nervous system's gas or brake pedals are stuck, and we are out of our resilient zone, this imbalance makes it difficult to think clearly and make good decisions. In this state, we may feel uncomfortable, unsettled, or just yucky. It is important to clarify that there is nothing *wrong* with this; it is simply our body's signaling system notifying us to bring our awareness back to a state of well-being. It is human nature to desire this state of well-being, and we naturally engage in behaviors that return us there, such as exercise, rest, journaling, eating comfort foods, and other adaptive coping strategies. Alternatively, we may engage in unhealthy or maladaptive behaviors such as lashing out, overeating, or using substances. Understanding the connection between stressors and our *natural* physical and emotional responses to them goes a long way toward self-compassion and resilience (Miller-Karas, 2015).

Community Resiliency Model Skills

The Community Resiliency Model consists of six skills:

1. Tracking

2. Resourcing

3. Grounding

4. Gesturing and spontaneous movement

5. Help Now!

6. Shift and Stay

The first skill, tracking, relies on your awareness of the physical sensations in your body and is the foundation of all the other skills (Miller-Karas, 2015). In this section, we describe each skill and provide ways to practice. Additional information is available on the free "iChill" app or website (www.ichillapp.com).

Skill 1: Tracking

The first and foundational skill of CRM is tracking, and we will use tracking as we practice all the CRM skills. Because our bodies naturally relay messages of discomfort, such as pain, hot or cold temperatures, and hunger to keep us safe and out of danger, we tend to listen very closely to these signals. But tracking in CRM directs our conscious awareness toward *positive or neutral sensations* in our body (Miller-Karas, 2015). We can practice by simply shifting our awareness and paying attention to our five senses: sight, sound, smell, taste, and touch. Identifying and sensing these pleasant or neutral sensations helps to decrease the body's tendency to focus so closely on the discomfort messages.

Let's Practice! Tracking Using the Five Senses

To hone your tracking skills, try to practice each of the following:

1. Notice a few things you can *see.* Pay special attention to something you do not normally notice in the space you are in right now.

2. Notice a few things that you can *hear.* Listen for and notice sounds in the background, steady or sudden sounds, and loud or quiet sounds.

3. Notice *smells.* Perhaps there are smells associated with the room you are in, food or drink nearby, or your skin and clothing.

4. Notice *taste.* Take a sip of a drink or a bite of food and notice the taste in your mouth. Perhaps you can even sense taste without ingesting anything.

5. Notice a few things you can *feel.* Bring your attention to the texture of this book, the feel of your clothing against your skin, or your toes inside your socks or shoes.

Continue tracking by noticing stimuli coming from *inside* your body. This could be tension, muscle aches, thirst, or tingling. Use words to describe these sensations—tight, loose, twitching, trembling, throbbing, mild, intense, jittery, calm—as many labels and descriptors as you can. Finally, determine if each of the sensations is pleasant, unpleasant, or neutral.

We should note that sometimes people cannot sense well inside their bodies, and for others, noticing internal sensations might cause distress (Miller-Karas, 2015). That's perfectly fine and doesn't mean there is anything wrong with you. If you feel any distress or if you cannot feel anything, as sometimes happens, see if you can sense your heartbeat or your breathing. Are they slow or fast? Deep or shallow?

We can also become aware of our own body's sensations that are associated with stress, resilience, and release. A fascinating signal called *release sensations* occurs when the body re-equilibrates after a significant stressor and we reenter the resilient zone (Miller-Karas, 2015). These release sensations are automatic processes that can include shaking or trembling, even burping or yawning. Figure 4.4 shows the flow of sensations during and following a traumatic or stressful experience.

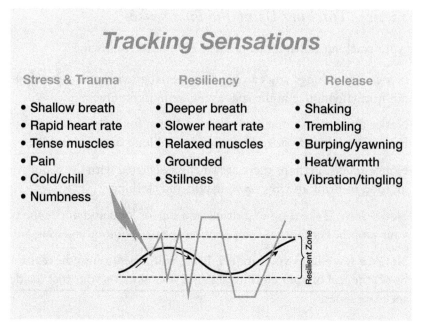

FIGURE 4.4 Tracking sensations following stress and trauma.

Skill 2: Resourcing

Resourcing uses the first skill, tracking, to help you build a sense of internal strength. A powerful tool, resourcing is like a strong muscle that helps you reinforce your own sense of capability and purpose. Your *internal resources* can be many things: your values or beliefs; a wonderful quality, talent, or ability; or a significant experience or moment in your life. Your *external resources* may include happy memories, people, places, or things that bring you support, calm, or peace (Miller-Karas, 2015). They could be hobbies, social groups, and animals. *Imagined resources* are those that are brought to mind from experiences yet to be, like a daydream or a wished-for image or thought.

Resourcing is akin to establishing a new pathway in the limbic system or etching a positive template in the mind. We are essentially using our own nervous system to calm our nervous system. A resource is like a template you can access anytime, and like a muscle, its strength grows with repeated use. You can draw on your resource any time, and under times of stress, you can use your resource to counter any existing negative templates that are the natural stress default in our brain (Vaish et al., 2008). When you experience future stress, you can purposefully access your resource and return to the RZ as your central nervous system begins to reset and release tension.

Let's Practice! Identify a Resource

Take a moment to identify a resource that you'd like to try out. It could be a memory, idea, place, or person associated with calm, comfort, and safety. Maybe it is walking along a beach or jogging through a park. If you're a musician, maybe your resource is mentally rehearsing a song or remembering a time you played music with friends. For artists, a resource might be visualizing the next painting or sculpture you will create, or walking through a museum. Everyone's resource is different, but it should evoke calm and pleasant feelings.

Now that you have decided on a resource to try, take a moment to describe three or four aspects of the resource in your mind. Write down what comes to mind. As with the visualization exercise in the previous chapter, it is important to be as descriptive and detailed as possible. Your goal is to paint a rich picture that touches all your senses. This elaboration is called *resource intensification*, a way to deepen the resource with sensory details that help the resource become more potent. As you think about your resource, what do you notice happening on the inside of your body (*heart rate, breathing, changes in muscles, fullness, warmth, lightness*)? Do you notice any movement on the outside of your body (*smiles, gestures, posture changes*)? Notice if the sensations are pleasant, unpleasant, or neutral.

Once you have found these pleasant or neutral sensations, stay with them for about 12–20 seconds. There is no rush to get back to daily life. Rather, take your time to firmly establish this resource. Staying with it for a period will strengthen your newfound resilience pathway. Revisit your resource periodically to get used to relying on it. Resourcing is a muscle you can stretch and strengthen anytime you want to stay in your RZ or get back inside your best self.

Even when someone is experiencing crisis, stress, or grief, resourcing is possible. For example, you can ask, "What is it about you that helps when you are going through such a hard time?" A painful experience should be briefly acknowledged, but CRM's *focus is on resources and strengths*. Helpful CRM questions might be: "What was the moment you knew you would survive?" or, "Tell me about who (or what) helped you get through it?" This simple, positive approach may allow for a shift from a negative state to a state of resilience, with the accompanying ability to withstand stress and adapt to change.

Another consideration we should note is that sometimes a resource has both a pleasant and an unpleasant component, perhaps tinged with loss. An example is a loving memory of a grandmother that can simultaneously evoke feelings of sadness or grief if the grandmother is deceased. Here we encourage you to acknowledge the sadness but focus on the pleasant and calming aspect of that resource. For example, "If your grandmother were here now, what might she say to you?" Or "What did you love best about her?" Or "Do you remember a moment with her that was special for you?" Any of these questions will result in resource intensification. Be sure to notice what happens in your body when you think or talk about this kind of dual-sided resource.

Skill 3: Grounding

Grounding is a CRM skill that "settles" the nervous system through somatic awareness of the sensations of support, security, and safety—gravitational and environmental security. Again, it uses tracking to generate sensory awareness, in this case, a conscious focus on the body in contact with itself or something in the environment (Miller-Karas, 2015). Grounding brings our attention away from worries about the past or future, and into the present moment. Bringing our present moment awareness to our body in contact with a surface is a shortcut to a sense of safety.

When we are grounded, we have a sense of self in relation to the present, the earth, to time and space. We do not worry about past or future. By bringing attention to our body's relationship to the present moment, we communicate a greater sense of safety to our nervous system.

You can practice grounding through your hands, feet, or any other area of your body that feels safe. Grounding can be done quickly and without drawing any attention to yourself. And grounding can take place anywhere or anytime: during physical movement, while sitting or lying down, or engaging in daily activities like driving a car, walking, or even swimming. While grounding, track sensations that are pleasant or safe in the present moment.

Skill 4: Gesturing and Spontaneous Movement

Gesturing and spontaneous movements are natural, involuntary actions of the body that occur as expressions of internal sensations of distress or well-being (Miller-Karas, 2015). We do them all the time, often without noticing. Gestures are universally recognized nonverbal expressions that indeed have a powerful purpose. Examples of natural positive gestures and spontaneous movements include open, relaxed postures, smiling, taking a deep breath, and hand movements such as restful folding or opening of the hands. Most people use calming gestures or postures that help bring them back to their RZ, often unknowingly.

It is important to be aware of your own involuntary positive gestures and movements when you are in your resilient zone, and to intentionally use one or more of these gestures as a resource when needed in times of stress or reduced resiliency. When you are at your best, how do you breathe? Is your breath steady and calm? How about your shoulders? Are they relaxed? Are your fingers clenched or loose? By noticing and absorbing the sensations of your calming gestures, postures, or movements, you can be intentional about replicating them when you experience stress. You already know how to do these things, so you won't have to learn anything new. These gestures or postures may serve as hefty "resiliency collateral" (backup) in times of distress.

Let's Practice! Identify a Gesture or Movement

Take a moment to find a gesture that engenders a sense of calm. It could be a posture or a hand movement that, for you, brings about a peacefulness—maybe crossed or open hands or a relaxed body posture. Become aware of your internal sensations as you make the gesture. Sometimes making a gesture slowly and repeating it can be quite soothing. You may enjoy observing not only your own gestures throughout the day, but also the calming gestures made by others.

Skill 5: Help Now!

Help Now! (also called Reset Now!) skills are quick strategies for those distressing moments when you bounce out of your resilient zone. Help Now! techniques include a quick, focused activation of the senses by tuning in to environmental stimuli through grounding or via the five senses (Miller-Karas, 2015). The Help Now! skills take advantage of the anchoring effect of *sensory awareness*, or attention to visual, auditory, tactile, and other details experienced via external senses. These quick skills can help you shift back into the RZ by drawing attention away from unpleasant sensations and emotions and shifting your focus to positive and neutral body sensations or stimuli in the room or environment (Miller-Karas, 2015). They can also help you remain present in the moment through grounding, movement, or physical release.

The menu of Help Now! strategies includes:

- Noticing the temperature, texture, color, or shape of objects in the room

- Noticing sounds in the environment

- Drinking a glass of water

- Counting steps while walking

- Opening your eyes wide

- Counting backward from 20 (to yourself or aloud)

- Slowly pushing the arms against a hard, flat surface such as a wall or a door, in a plank-like fashion, noticing the sensation of engaging the large muscles in the arms and legs

These strategies may be accompanied by noticing what is happening in the body as we perform them and the resulting change in mood or internal state of distress. When we pay attention to sensation, in that moment, we are less likely to be angry, ashamed, or anxious.

Let's Practice! Try a Help Now! Skill

Choose one or two of the Help Now! tools or make up your own. If you are upset or sad, activities that engage the large muscles in the arms and legs may be quite beneficial, such as pushing up against the wall. As you engage in the Help Now! skill, notice how you feel. How long do you need to practice the skill before the change occurs? As with all the CRM skills, practice them throughout the day to see what works for you.

These simple skills may be used as an immediate self-help intervention, but you can also use them to help others when they appear stuck in the high zone or low zone. These strategies are always offered in an invitational manner, to help the anxious, hyper-aroused individual to calm down, or help the depressed, exhausted, hypo-aroused individual to gain more energy.

Skill 6: Shift and Stay

Shift and stay is the technique of selecting from the menu of grounding, tracking, resourcing, gesturing, or Help Now! skills depending on the needs of the situation and your preference. When you use a skill and experience a resultant shift, you may notice greater comfort and well-being. It is important that you linger with those new, more pleasant sensations. The selection of a CRM technique may be made anytime you are experiencing unpleasant emotions and sensations, such as feeling distressed, emotionally unstable, overwhelmed, or disconnected. Using a CRM skill at that moment will allow for a purposeful shift to a more pleasant or neutral state. We encourage you to notice as the unpleasant sensation and emotion abate. Once the shift occurs, intentionally linger and absorb the more neutral or pleasant state. Shift and stay is a purposeful action that can become an automatic response when practiced over time. It is essential to stay with the pleasant or neutral sensations for approximately 12 seconds to experience the shift successfully and to transfer the experience into long-term memory (Hanson, 2016). The continued practice of intentional shift and stay may widen your resilient zone over time.

Considerations When Using CRM

We recognize that, as with other self-care approaches, CRM may not be effective for everyone. Tracking internal sensations may be unpleasant, or even triggering for some people. It may be uncomfortable to sense-in to your body's "internal climate" for many reasons (Miller-Karas, 2015, p. 37). It is possible that you may associate some "felt" sensations with a past traumatic or stressful event. If this is something you struggle with, we suggest tracking neutral (or less unpleasant or painful) internal sensations, or noting muscle tension, heartbeat, or breathing, if those are acceptable to you. A shift to a more neutral sensation or even to an area of the body where there is less pain may be helpful. If you are triggered by sensing neutral or even pleasant sensations, the Help Now! skills can be useful. If at any time discomfort with skill use occurs, CRM should be stopped.

CRM in Clinical Settings

It is critical that nurses engage in protective, preventive practices for their own resiliency, but a resilient workforce will have a multiplicative effect on patient care. A nurse who practices CRM may make a habit of "CRMing" patients, and these patients will have the empowering experience of finding within themselves their own "best medicine." CRM is never meant to take the place of therapy or medication, but as a self-care modality, CRM can have a powerful effect on one's sense of well-being.

You may find it tempting to practice "conversational CRMing," when a simple question such as, "Tell me about your favorite vacation," can evoke a treasured experience and bring a sense of pleasure or hope to the person you are speaking with. Healthcare institutions are responsible for creating healthy, supportive work environments where nurses and other providers can thrive. Nurses can share CRM's resiliency skills with patients and other care providers and help organizations learn how best to create settings where systemic empathy is the norm.

CRM is a psychosocial intervention that has a developing evidence base and shows promise for the enhancement of mental wellness. Nurses, because of their numbers and the public's confidence in the profession, are in a unique position to consider innovations that can potentially influence public good and mental well-being. Nurses who are trained in CRM may be able to use CRM to anchor themselves as they navigate through their important, but stressful, work. If nurses who practice CRM skills can integrate the CRM principles in their clinical interactions with coworkers, patients, and families, there may be a corresponding increase in professional fulfillment and quality of patient care.

In Real Practice

One of the articles cited in this chapter caught our attention. Linda Grabbe and her colleagues (2020) conducted a study with hospital-based nurses, randomly placing 40 volunteers in a CRM intervention and 37 in a nutrition group. Both workshops were 3 hours in duration, and the study looked at the nurses' well-being over a 1-year period. The CRM group showed improved well-being, resiliency, secondary traumatic stress, and physical symptoms over time. Nurses said they used the techniques for self-stabilization during stressful times at work, and they shared the techniques with patients, friends, coworkers, and family.

Closing Thoughts

The Community Resiliency Model is an innovative, elegantly simple self-care practice that you can draw on anytime, anywhere. It complements and can even deepen other self-care modalities, such as appreciative practices (Chapter 3), exercise, meditation, mindfulness, and yoga. You may practice as little or as much as you like. CRM takes advantage of mechanisms that are already within our bodies to interrupt the hijacking of the brain by strong emotions or stress reactions. It enables us to maintain or return to a resilient state via a momentary, brief, and unnoticeable CRM self-care skill. For this reason, you may choose to add CRM to your toolbox of skills to enhance your ability to be your best-nurse self.

Key Points

- The Community Resiliency Model is a set of skills and concepts that support emotion self-regulation by accessing the autonomic nervous system.

- The cornerstone concept of CRM is the resilient zone; we can notice if we or others are outside of this bandwidth of stress tolerance and use CRM skills to reduce the impact of stress and trauma.

- Each of the CRM skills is based on *tracking*, the intentional awareness of external and internal body sensations.

- Additional CRM skills include *resourcing, grounding, gesturing, shift and stay*, and *Help Now!*

- CRM complements other self-care modalities and can enrich patient care experiences.

References

Beck, C. T. (2011). Secondary Traumatic Stress in Nurses: A Systematic Review. *Archives of Psychiatric Nursing, 25*(1), 1–10. https://doi.org/10.1016/j.apnu.2010.05.00

Citron, S., & Miller-Karas, E. (2013). *Community resiliency training innovation project: Final CRM innovation evaluation report*. Department of Behavioral Health, San Bernardino County, CA.

Grabbe, L., Higgins, M. K., Baird, M., Craven, P. A., & San Fratello, S. (2020). The Community Resiliency Model to promote nurse well-being. *Nursing Outlook, 68*(3), 324–336. https://doi.org/10.1016/j.outlook.2019.11.002

Haglund, M. E. M., Nestadt, P. S., Cooper, N. S., Southwick, S. M., & Charney, D. S. (2007). Psychobiological mechanisms of resilience: Relevance to prevention and treatment of stress-related psychopathology. *Development and Psychopathology, 19*(3), 889–920. https://doi.org/10.1017/S0954579407000430

Hanson, R. (2016). *When good is stronger than bad*. http://www.rickhanson.net/teaching/tgc-public-summary/

Heller, L., & LaPierre, A. (2012). *Healing developmental trauma: How early trauma affects self-regulation, self-image, and the capacity for relationship*. North Atlantic Books.

Leitch, L., & Miller-Karas, E. (2009). A case for using biologically-based mental health intervention in post-earthquake China: Evaluation of training in the trauma resiliency model. *International Journal of Emergency Mental Health, 11*(4), 221–233. https://www.ncbi.nlm.nih.gov/pubmed/20524507

Leitch, M. L. (2007). Somatic Experiencing treatment with tsunami survivors in Thailand: Broadening the scope of early intervention. *Traumatology, 13*(3), 11–20. https://doi.org/10.1177/1534765607305439

Leitch, M. L., Vanslyke, J., & Allen, M. (2009). Somatic experiencing treatment with social service workers following Hurricanes Katrina and Rita. *Social Work, 54*(1), 9–18. https://somaticexperiencing.dk/wp-content/uploads/2017/02/Social_Work_Journal_Article.pdf

Levine, P. A. (2010). *In an unspoken voice: How the body releases trauma and restores goodness.* North Atlantic Books.

Miller-Karas, E. (2015). *Building resilience to trauma: The trauma and community resiliency models.* Routledge.

Ogden, P. (2015). *Sensorimotor psychotherapy: Interventions for trauma and attachment.* https://www.overdrive.com/search?q=38DE9EBE-52F5-485F-821C-CC33BABDAA80

Parker, C., Doctor, R. M., & Selvam, R. (2008). Somatic therapy treatment effects with tsunami survivors. *Traumatology, 14*(3), 103–109. https://doi.org/10.1177/1534765608319080

Vaish, A., Grossmann, T., & Woodward, A. (2008). Not all emotions are created equal: The negativity bias in social-emotional development. *Psychological Bulletin, 134*(3), 383–403. https://doi.org/10.1037/0033-2909.134.3.383

Windle, G. (2011). What is resilience? A review and concept analysis. *Reviews in Clinical Gerontology, 21*(2), 152–169. https://doi.org/10.1017/S0959259810000420

section II
The Mind of a Nurse

5

Self-Care, Communal Care, and Resilience Among Underrepresented Minority Nursing Professionals and Students

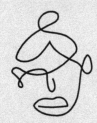

Ebru Çayır
pronouns: She/Her

While a young clinician at a preventive care clinic in Istanbul, Ebru Çayır became interested in how the organization of society shapes individual well-being and the use of social justice-based and intersectional public health approaches to reduce suffering in vulnerable communities. More recently, she explored contemplative practices in improving clinician well-being. She is a nature lover, tree and people hugger, art maker, and choir singer.

"My mission in life is not merely to survive, but to thrive; and to do so with some passion, some compassion, some humor, and some style."

–Maya Angelou

Note to reader:

The term *underrepresented minority* (URM) used in this chapter is based on the National Institutes of Health definition that includes racial and ethnic categories of Black or African American, Asian, Latinx, American Indian or Alaska Native, Native Hawaiian or Other Pacific Islander (National Institutes of Health, 2020). Although I acknowledge that other nursing professionals and students such as LGBTQ+ individuals or those living with a disability are among the minorities within the nursing profession, and these identities intersect with race/ethnicity to shape their experiences in unique ways, experiences of these groups are beyond the scope of this chapter. You will see that we dedicate the following chapter to LGBTQ+ individuals.

Underrepresented minority (URM) nursing professionals and students have historically served important roles within the United States healthcare workforce. However, the unique workplace stressors they face due to longstanding social and structural inequities—such as institutional and interpersonal racism, discrimination, and stereotyping—often remain invisible and unaddressed. This chapter focuses on URM nursing professionals' and students' training and workplace experiences and discusses the role of self-care and communal care in offsetting the negative health and well-being impact of work-related stressors; promoting resilience; and developing a sustainable, fulfilling professional identity.

Stressful Workplace Experiences

We begin with three examples of stressful workplace experiences faced by underrepresented minority nurses and nursing students.

Example 1

> So I knew somebody was coming, so I was trying to get her [the patient] done, and the lady came in, and, since the way she walked into the room, my back was to her, she couldn't see my badge the

way I [was] standing because I was facing the patient. And she said, "Oh, what is she here to do? Give you your bath or something?" And, no, she said, "Who is this? What, is she here to do your bath?" And the patient said, "No, she's the one in charge of everybody else!" (Tamara [pseudonym], a Black nurse; Cottingham et al., 2018. p. 151)

Example 2

I don't think people always understand, you know. I've seen [nursing] students come from the reservations to State University or one of the big universities. It's a culture shock to put it mildly. But it's also, um, they expect the students to be independent. You know, come down there, get themselves enrolled and all of this. Native culture doesn't value independence. They value interdependence. So you help each other. It's a group, um, they think in groups, not individualistic and developing independence. So when students come down from the reservation and the faculty were like, "Well, you know, you have to take care of yourself." But you can't do that or you're going to lose the students. They're just going to go back home. (Faculty of color employed at predominantly White school of nursing; Hassouneh & Lutz, 2013, p. 160)

Example 3

One classmate, when I first met her, she kept putting on accents purposely when she spoke, of different races and minorities. To her, I guess it's a joke, but to me it wasn't. I don't think that she understands that when you are a minority, when you make simple little things like that, or a little joke, it actually does affect the people around you. (Chan, a Chinese nursing student; Gardner, 2005a, p. 158)

These three experiences reflect the daily exposure to racism and microaggressions in the educational and work lives of many URMs in the healthcare workforce. The 2003 report by the Institute of Medicine, "Unequal Treatment: Confronting Racial and Ethnic Disparities in Health Care," called for "increasing the proportion of underrepresented minorities in the healthcare workforce, integrating cross-cultural education into the training of all health care professionals" as an integral part of eliminating healthcare disparities (Smedley et al., pp. 21 & 186). In the aftermath of this report, the US has witnessed significant efforts by healthcare organizations, as well as medical and nursing schools, to increase the recruitment of URM populations and improve their training and work experiences.

Racial Disparities in the Healthcare Workforce

Racial disparities in the US healthcare workforce continue to be a critical public health problem. Figure 5.1 summarizes race/ethnicity distribution of all active physicians in the US in 2018 (Association of American Medical Colleges, 2019).

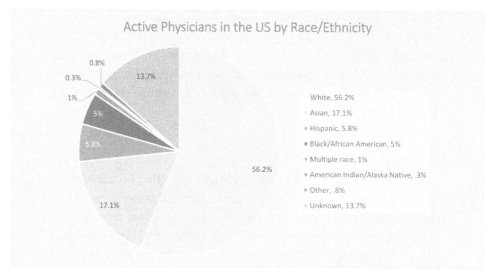

FIGURE 5.1 Active physicians in the US by race/ethnicity (Association of American Medical Colleges, 2019).

The disparities were even larger among registered nurses: Race/ethnicity of registered nurses in the US as documented by the National Nursing Workforce Study in 2017 is depicted in Figure 5.2 (Smiley et al., 2018).

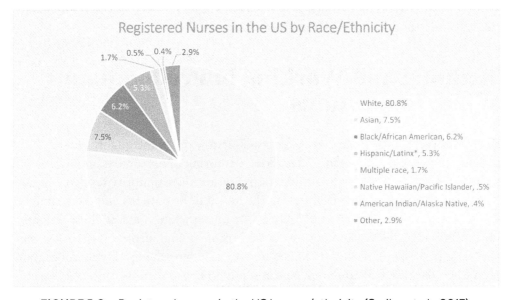

FIGURE 5.2 Registered nurses in the US by race/ethnicity (Smiley et al., 2017).
Hispanic or Latinx origin was asked in a separate question, thus potentially including some respondents in the multiple race or other race category.

While racial and ethnic minorities consisted of 38.7% of the US population in 2017 according to the US Census Bureau, they represented only 19% of the registered nurse workforce (Smiley et al., 2018).

Accompanying the efforts to close the gap in numbers across different racial and ethnic groups, there has been more research within the past few decades that examines experiences of URM healthcare students, trainees, educators, and professionals. Understanding the factors that shape URM nurses' job engagement and fulfillment is essential to develop institutional climates that support inclusion, equity, and diversity, and, in turn, improve retention (Diefenbeck et al., 2016; Xue, 2015). These studies show that increasing the proportion of the minority workforce in healthcare alone is not sufficient to transform work experiences of URM providers and to improve retention rates among them. Despite the increase in the recruitment of URM students and professionals in healthcare, URMs continue to report institutional discrimination, interpersonal racism, and microaggressions. Thus, it is not surprising that attrition rates remain higher among URM nursing students (Diefenbeck et al., 2016; Gipson-Jones, 2017).

Training and Working in Predominantly White Institutions

Significant racial and ethnic disparities continue to exist in the quality and experience of medical and nursing education, mentoring opportunities, as well as professional quality of life after graduation. For instance, minority residents report "being mistaken for nonmedical staff in the hospital, by patients and their families, and sometimes ancillary staff" despite "wearing white coats, stethoscopes and identification badges" as an indicator of their professional identity (Osseo-Asare et al., 2018, p. 4). Their names are mixed up and used interchangeably by colleagues, even when they are from different cultures and do not look alike (Osseo-Asare et al., 2018).

Black nursing students who receive education in predominantly White institutions (PWIs) report feeling isolated, struggling to belong and fit in (White & Fulton, 2015). They feel invisible and voiceless in the multirace study groups and in their classrooms (Coleman, 2008). They often experience an alienating divide between how they express their authentic selves within their family and community versus how they have to present within the PWIs to confront the stereotypes of being not as hard-working or smart as their White peers (Durkee & Williams, 2015).

Code-Switching

To navigate this stressful identity separation in their private and professional lives, Black nursing students may be forced to go in and out of their authentic selves and adjust their language in an effort to "act White" and fit in with the White students, and then "talk Black" when they are with family and friends (Durkee & Williams, 2015; Horvat & Lewis, 2003). Labeled as *code-switching*, this practice refers to the use of more than one language, or different subsystems of a language with different speech styles, during one conversation, or multiple conversations that take place in different sociocultural contexts (Nilep, 2006).

Code-switching can have complex implications: it may help URMs be more resilient and advance in their careers more easily because they often work for PWIs. But it may also take an emotional toll by requiring a constant awareness and monitoring of how they present in professional contexts and among White colleagues (Durkee & Williams, 2015; Horvat & Lewis, 2003). Perceived as "other," URM healthcare students and professionals constantly negotiate their professional identity and belonging to the organizations they work for, while trying to remain authentic to themselves (Osseo-Asare et al., 2018).

Social Exclusion

Experiences of minority nursing students reveal that race-driven subgroups and cliques in the academic and clinical environment pose a barrier to social cohesion, interpersonal trust, and intercultural exchange. Latinx, Asian, Native American, and Eastern Indian nursing students report feeling excluded in group lab projects, experiencing isolation and loneliness during educational activities within and outside of their classrooms (Evans, 2008; Gardner, 2005b; Hassouneh & Lutz, 2013; Weaver, 2001; Xu et al., 2005). Due to a lack of understanding of cultural differences among White peers and educators, URM students and residents can involuntarily find themselves in situations where they have to correct misunderstandings, confront prejudice, and educate others about their culture, while carrying the burden of having to represent their whole community and taking on the role of "race/ethnicity ambassador" (Osseo-Asare et al., 2018, p. 3). Even when they take on this role willingly and serve in diversity initiatives within their institutions, it can be a struggle to obtain the adequate resources for the tasks they are being given, such as developing curricula to promote diversity and inclusion, or specific programs that address the needs of URM students (Osseo-Asare et al., 2018).

Equity, Diversity, and Inclusion in Educational Settings

The unique challenges that URM nursing students face during their education require a different approach to mentoring. In addition to providing diversity and inclusion trainings for faculty and receiving student feedback on whether these trainings are having the expected impact on mentor-student relationships and classroom environment, nursing schools are employing strategies to recruit and retain more faculty of color (Hamilton & Haozous, 2017). Seeing URM individuals among faculty and having the opportunity to be mentored by them sends a message to URM students that they are valued members of the nursing community and they too can excel in clinical practice or nursing research as these faculty members have (Hassouneh & Lutz, 2013). When the schools lack faculty diversity and genuine efforts to promote diversity, inclusion, and equity, it is challenging for URM students to imagine a fulfilling professional experience for themselves in the future and develop a feeling of professional belonging (Diefenbeck et al., 2016).

It is important to ensure that the responsibility of developing a more diverse and inclusive educational space and workplace to retain URMs does not fall disproportionately on URM individuals. White faculty and students also need to be involved in these efforts. URM faculty and students may already feel more vulnerable in terms of the time and energy these efforts require and the consequences of engaging in this work on their educational advancement, employment, or tenure achievement. URM faculty and students, particularly those who are in earlier stages of their training or academic positions, may need additional support and mentoring to protect their time and energy so they do not have to sacrifice academic and professional development while investing heavily in transforming the racial climate of their institutions (Beech et al., 2018; Campbell & Rodríguez, 2018; Phillips et al., 2016).

Compassionate Care and Gender

Healthcare systems have been going through a rapid transformation to achieve greater financial profit while using fewer resources (Waitzkin, 2018). Prioritizing "customer satisfaction," this change has shaped patient-provider interactions to be more transactional. The transactional approach treats patient-provider interactions the same way other service industries prioritize profits, overlooking the human aspects of providing care to people who are vulnerable and suffering. Transactional interactions concern the exchange of health services for the "customer's" money (or insurance compensation) and satisfaction (Waitzkin, 2018).

Not surprisingly, the patient expectation of being cared for by not only competent but also compassionate healthcare providers has not diminished. As Erickson and Grove highlighted: "Ironically, the economic rationalization of health care and the increasing use of advanced technology have occurred at the same time that social and medical scientists have expressed a growing interest in the more human(e) facets of provider–patient interaction" (2008, p. 705). Within the prevalent social structures of the US healthcare system, which are male-dominated, paternalistic, and hierarchical, emotional labor and provision of compassionate care mostly fall on the shoulders of female healthcare providers, particularly nurses (Bell et al., 2014; Erickson & Grove, 2008). The traditional image of a nurse is a woman who is capable of and enjoys providing tender care.

Compassionate Care and Race

Nurses' experiences of emotional labor are not only gendered but also racialized. Another challenge URM nurses may face is having to engage in a disproportionate amount of emotional labor when they care for patients (Cottingham et al., 2018). Systems of power and domination, including but not limited to racism, sexism, and class inequalities, mutually interact with one another to shape the ways in which practices of emotional labor are distributed disproportionately among nurses of different social locations. Race-related emotional experiences (e.g., facing microaggressions, stereotype threat), on top of daily work stressors, exhaust URM nurses' emotional capital, and in turn, negatively affect their ability to engage in self-care and care for their patients (Cottingham et al., 2018).

Analyzing data from audio-recorded diaries completed by 48 nurses practicing in two US Midwestern cities, Cottingham, Johnson and Erickson (2018) explored how gender and race interacts to shape daily emotion practices of nurses, as well as nurse well-being and patient care. The authors argued that nurses of color engage in "emotional double shift" (Evans, 2013, p. 12) due to navigating everyday racial microaggressions and facing negative stereotype threat. One of the participants in their study, a Black nurse in her 50s who cared for psychiatric patients, shared:

> This man has a diagnosis of schizophrenia and he was a very diffi-
> cult patient in that he was racially and sexually inappropriate with
> staff...he called me a "nigger," a "humpbacked monkey" several
> times. He called one of the other nurses a "White nigger" (...) all
> we could do to not retaliate and even if you—it started like my re-
> sponse was to start to sing a hymn under my—in an undertone and
> of course he caught on to that and said "you a Christian nigger?"
> ...and it was just awful, awful things and when you have a patient
> like who's having a crisis, it is very difficult on the staff emotionally
> (Cottingham et al., 2018, p. 150).

Engaging in race-related emotional labor leaves nurses of color with diminished resources for self-care and reduces their ability to provide compassionate care to patients. In PWIs, nurses of color feel that they have to keep up with the emotional labor required from them to avoid stereotypes such as "angry Black woman" from their colleagues and administrators (Dickens & Chavez, 2018, p. 768). In addition, clinical experiences of URM nursing students and registered nurses can be affected negatively by patients' racism when patients request a White nurse to care for them (Paul-Emile et al., 2016). Paul-Emile et al. argued that "For many minority health care workers, expressions of patients' racial preferences are painful and degrading indignities, which cumulatively contribute to moral distress and burnout" (2016, p. 710).

Similarly, non-White immigrant nurses experience systemic and sociocultural barriers to their integration into the workplace and job satisfaction (Xiao et al., 2014).

Since its founding, the US has been shaped and defined by immigrants and thus, its healthcare workforce has long consisted of immigrant nurses from non-Western countries such as the Philippines, South Korea, China, and India (Ghazal et al., 2020). Internationally educated nurses (IENs) migrate to the US to benefit from more educational and career opportunities, lower workloads, and greater workplace resources. However, they also face institutional discrimination, inadequate acknowledgement and underuse of their expertise and previous work experience, lack of understanding and ignorance about their sociocultural background, and communication difficulties with their colleagues and patients (Ghazal et al., 2020; Xiao et al., 2014). For instance, IENs who migrate to the US are less likely to serve in management positions, less likely to receive promotions, and more likely to be paid less than nurses trained in the US (Moyce et al., 2016). They can be employed for lower-level positions compared to their level of education due to the stigma and distrust about the educational preparation they received in their home countries (Ghazal et al., 2020; Rosenkoetter et al., 2017).

Encouraging the contributions of racial and ethnic minority and immigrant nurses to the US health system while simultaneously promoting their well-being and resilience is more important than ever. This is true, in part, given the US census population projections indicating that racial and ethnic minorities will form the majority of American citizens by the mid-21st century (Frey, 2018). In the following sections, we define and discuss the role of self-care and communal care in allowing URM nursing professionals and students to fulfill their potential and maintain a healthy professional identity.

Self-Care and Communal Care

Self-care can be defined as the "proactive strategies, or routines" adopted by caregiving professionals such as nurses to reduce the negative physical, mental, and spiritual health effects of working with human beings who suffer, and to promote well-being (Wasco & Campbell, 2002, p. 734). When you serve as a provider in a healthcare institution in any capacity—as a nurse, physician, social worker, a chaplain—the practice of self-care is essential to your ability of sustaining a fulfilled, engaged, and resilient professional identity (Cunningham et al., 2017).

Healthcare providers face stressors such as high workload, time pressure, lack of control over work schedule, diminished work-life balance, changing payment and service delivery approaches, and exposure to patients' physical and psychological trauma (Shanafelt & Noseworthy, 2017). Even when they work for organizations that prioritize creating a healthy work environment, engaging in professional care-giving work often includes treating human beings who suffer and takes a toll on the caregivers' own psychosocial health and well-being in the long term. For this reason, self-care skills are now considered crucial for nursing students and professionals.

There are multiple perspectives on the overall notion of self-care and what self-care practices involve. In her article "The Politics of Self Care and Feminism," Sharanya Sekaram discusses how in today's context caring for ourselves is often treated as a performance materialized by individual consumption: "A $10 billion-dollar [*sic*] industry has led us to believe that in order to be practicing self-care we need to take a spa trip, go on a vacation, or purchase a box of indulgence items" (Sekaram, 2018, para. 4). This industry has grown exponentially since Sekaram reflected on the issue in 2018.

Self-Care Can't Be Accomplished Alone

On the other hand, self-care recommendations that appear in healthcare literature as well as blog posts and social media essays can reduce the source of overall wellness to individual health behaviors such as having a regular sleep schedule, eating nutritious meals, meditating, and spending time in nature (Spicer, 2019). Indeed, these behaviors need to be promoted among nursing professionals and students since they contribute to health and wellness. However, conceptualizing self-care as a solely individual responsibility to protect and improve one's health and well-being overlooks the social determinants of health, such as the risks to health and well-being that are posed by educational or workplace structures, practices, and cultures (Pappas & Rushton, 2020).

When we think about self-care, structural and sociocultural factors that shape nurses' workplace experiences also come into play, particularly for URMs. As we discussed earlier, URM nursing students and professionals may experience significant stressors other than those related to the medical tasks they perform, such as institutional discrimination, racism, and microaggressions perpetrated by teachers, coworkers, or patients, which cause exclusion from the social fabric of the organization and lack of access to power (Griffith et al., 2007). URM nurses are often underrepresented in management positions, thus lacking the resources and social networks that are necessary to influence organizational structures and practices (Griffith et al., 2007).

For all these reasons, engaging in self-care may have a far-reaching meaning and purpose in the lives of URM nursing students and professionals.

In "A Burst of Light," Audre Lorde tells us: "Caring for myself is not self-indulgence, it is self-preservation, and that is an act of political warfare" (Lorde, 1988, p. 205). Reflecting on Audre Lorde's work, Sara Ahmed discusses why those who do not have the social privileges that act as a natural support system—such as being White, heterosexual, and able bodied—need to engage in this important act of political warfare. Even though "privilege does not mean we are invulnerable," it can, however, "reduce the costs of vulnerability, so if things break down, if you break down, you are more likely to be looked after" (Ahmed, 2014, para. 12). Therefore, for URM nursing students and professionals, engaging in self-care serves a purpose beyond the prevention of burnout; it is necessary for their survival in majority PWIs, which are often not designed to meet their needs.

Communal Care

Here, I would like to offer another term: "communal care." Informed by the work of scholars such as Billings (2018), and Wever and Zell (2017), who called for a shift in our understanding of how to better support psychosocial well-being in caregiving professionals, I use this term to contextualize individual wellness within our communities. For the nursing community, *communal care* is a collective practice through which nurses can develop a multitude of strategies to care for each community member's well-being by mobilizing not only the individual, but also interpersonal, organizational, and systems-level resources in reciprocal ways. This approach to cultivating health and wellness engages all constituents of a community, highlighting the interdependence between them and holding them responsible for each other's well-being. Communal care also acknowledges the diversity of health and wellness needs among nurses, aiming to create space for diverse, equitable, and inclusive approaches to addressing the problems of the most vulnerable members in the nursing community.

Wever and Zell (2017) argued that when individual self-care is proposed as "an antidote" for the negative impacts of the work within human service organizations, it "places the responsibility of managing the effects of social, cultural and organizational injustices squarely on the individual worker" (p. 210). Without ignoring the necessity for each advocate (*or nurse, in our case*) to be cognizant of their own well-being needs and to be proactive, they called for "a movement of caring for and acknowledging each other in human service organizations" (Wever & Zell, 2017, p. 211).

Nurses who identify with more collectivistic cultures (e.g., most communities from Asia, Central America, South America, and Africa) may be more familiar with this notion, and their well-being needs may be better served by taking a communal approach (Hassouneh & Lutz, 2013). For instance, Latinx writer and activist Angie Jamie highlights how individual wellness in communities of color is inextricable from the social relationships, interdependent with others' wellness (2019, para. 4):

> I was raised by a clan of Mexican women, mothers, sisters, and cousins who assured me I was capable of anything, as well as a neighborhood of working-class immigrants whose watch maintained our mutual safety. Caring for myself was built on caring for others, for all living things, in an interdependent relationship that our communities had maintained for generations.

As a woman of color who grew up in a communal culture, Jamie experiences her "self" as more fluid, constantly in relationship with the world around her, and her vision of self-care is interwoven into the well-being of her community.

For caregiving professionals, having strong interpersonal relationships with colleagues is one of the most important protective factors in sustaining an engaged, fulfilled professional life (Çayir et al., 2020). This applies to not only addressing the common factors that lead to high burnout and turnover rates among nursing professionals regardless of their social location, but also addressing the mental, physical, and spiritual effects of feeling as "the other" due to multiple mechanisms of structural inequality such as racism, nationalism, and sexism (Osseo-Asare et al., 2018; Cottingham et al., 2018).

Engaging in communal care means to "cultivate a culture of care" (King, 2018, p. 131) to tend to "collective, social forms of suffering" (Walsh, 2017, p. 2). Taking a collectivistic approach that emphasizes the interconnectedness of the individual and the community is even more important when we are confronting racism within the communities of healthcare provision.

Along with reflecting on the historical roots and contemporary social structures perpetuating racism in our society, Ruth King, a meditation teacher and author, ponders the inner world experience of racism and describes racism as a disease of our hearts (King, 2018). To heal our communities from the long-lasting impacts of racism, whether these communities are within our neighborhoods, classrooms, or inside the hospitals as our workplaces, we need to remember the responsibility we have to each other. Fulfilling the responsibility of recognizing each other's suffering, identifying its sources, reflecting on our own potential contribution to ongoing oppressive practices, and intentionally acting to transform the sources of this suffering is the true act of caring for each other.

Transforming our communities to create equitable, diverse, multicultural workplaces requires that we transform ourselves, too. The notion of communal care does not have to be in contradiction with self-care; rather, the two can co-exist and complement each other. As we strive to deliver quality and compassionate healthcare in a world where institutional racism and discrimination affect our workplaces, we need to remember our common humanity and interconnectedness.

Contemplative Practices as Self-Care for URMs

Contemplative practices are practical and transformative experiences that help cultivate a state of calm centeredness, which promotes meaning and purpose in life (The Center for Contemplative Mind in Society, 2020). They can take different forms and have a long history in many different cultures around the world. These practices include a wide range of traditions that are based in movement, stillness, creativity, activism, and relational engagement, among others. They are shown to improve physical and mental health by a growing number of research studies, and they are wonderful self-care tools for nursing students and professionals (Lomas et al., 2018; van der Riet et al., 2018).

Offering a multitude of nurturing experiences, contemplative practices can address a variety of self-care needs among nurses. It is important to highlight the diversity and flexibility of contemplative practices because within the last decade, some of these practices, such as yoga and mindfulness, have been highly commercialized and promoted as the new solution to all ailments. For some people, these practices are indeed very helpful in restoring balance, bringing flexibility of body and mind, coping with physical pain, and shifting perspective on life and work challenges; they may be less effective for others. I encourage you to try what works best for you.

I would like to emphasize that when it comes to self-care for nurses and nursing students, one size *does not* fit all. Yes, there is a common wisdom to eating nutritious and balanced meals, exercising regularly, and trying to get enough sleep. But self-care practices that work for you will not come from a generic formula that could be applied to everyone. What helps you relax and replenish while bringing your work life more meaning is very much embedded in your social background, cultural traditions, and lifestyle. If you enjoy taking time to prepare a beloved dish for family gatherings, forgetting about anything else as you add the spices, there is your meditation! When you are able to engage in and fully focus on an activity that allows you to experience a calm, nonjudgmental awareness while nourishing you, that serves as a meditation. If this is an activity that you particularly find meaningful and enjoy, even better!

Self-care is not about forcing yourself to engage in what others are doing to remain healthy and replenished. You may not like exercising in a gym, for instance, but enjoy taking walks in the woods by your house. That is your way of moving your body mindfully. You may be volunteering at your church, mosque, or temple because it brings you a sense of connection, wholeness, and joy.

A survey of nurses from a rural, level-one trauma center showed that nurses engaged in a broad range of self-care practices: prayer, music, breathing exercises, yoga, meditation, writing, visual arts, reading, gardening, sewing crafts, travelling, dancing, horseback riding, and knitting (Cunningham et al., 2017). Results of this study provided two important insights. First, these nurses were very intentional about incorporating activities into their lives to replenish and recharge from work, even though they did not necessarily perceive it as engaging in self-care. Second, these activities were more diverse than the conventional conceptualizations of self-care in the clinician well-being literature. It is important to learn about, acknowledge, and support the multi-tude of self-care practices nurses adopt to cultivate well-being and resilience.

Self-care and communal care practices are often interwoven, rather than being mu-tually exclusive. An example would be creating dedicated spaces for URM nurses to get together and share their workplace experiences and seek solutions from within their community. Also, creating organizational initiatives led by URM nurses and nursing students serves as an act of communal care necessary for transforming the social fab-ric of healthcare institutions to be more inclusive and equitable. At my institution, the nurses in rehabilitative medicine organized monthly potlucks, and each nurse brought a favorite dish from their country of origin. It became a fun way to share backgrounds and celebrate the diversity of the nursing team.

Diversity, Inclusion, and Equity in Contemplative Spaces

It is important to consider issues of diversity, inclusion, and equity when designing and delivering mindfulness-based, contemplative practices as self-care techniques for nurses. Within the mindfulness community in the US, scholars and practitioners such as Rhonda Magee, Ruth King, Zenju Earthlyn Manuel, and Lisa M. Campbell have long been scrutinizing these issues, because people of color have not always felt welcome or fully included in the movement.

Magee discussed the tendency within mindfulness communities to see themselves as immune to social identity–based biases, and the desire to create "colorblind" spaces: "We are comfortable with the belief that bias isn't much of a problem, and that the demographics of our teaching settings, even if worthy of some note, are not really relevant to our experience of them" (Magee, 2016, p. 226).

Yet, her own embodied experiences within the mindfulness community, as well as the experiences of other people of color, tell a different story. Instead of ignoring the issues of race and ethnicity within mindfulness communities in the US, Magee suggests that we first turn to this side of ourselves with compassion, the side that struggles with openly facing how social identity–based bias operates even within the communities that highlight teachings of Buddhism, so that we can understand it better (Magee, 2016). Then we can use mindfulness "as a means of understanding racial- and social identity-based suffering more effectively" (Magee, 2016, p. 226) and, in turn, transform ourselves and our communities to eliminate this suffering.

In addition, the ways in which mindfulness programs are often conceptualized and marketed can lead to the exclusion of lower-income, URM communities. In a study conducted with majority low-income, single Black women, researchers documented that barriers to practicing yoga and mindfulness in this sample included the high cost of yoga classes, the perceived pressure to dress in a certain way, such as wearing expensive yoga pants, shirts, and accessories, and the common representation of thin bodies in yoga classes (Tenfelde et al., 2018).

Researchers also observed that older Black women described their relationship with faith as a way of engaging in self-care through praying, which was experienced in similar ways to meditating. Black women in this study suggested that the mindfulness practitioners need to "acknowledge deep faith traditions in the community," while "demystifying the mind/body/spirit connection" (Tenfelde et al., 2018, p. 233) to focus on the health benefits of yoga and mindfulness. They also suggested the provision of free programs in community spaces to make these practices more accessible (Tenfelde et al., 2018). These suggestions are crucial to developing and implementing mindfulness programs that address health and well-being needs of Black communities. If these practices are to address social and health inequities, they need to be promoted in a way that recognizes the institutional and environmental causes of suffering (Walsh, 2017).

Mindfulness, Religion, and Culture

Sometimes mindfulness can be perceived as an alternative to religion and religious practices, or in conflict with religion, which may alienate Black communities from exploring what mindfulness has to offer as a self-care practice (Woods-Giscombé & Gaylord, 2014). This could be addressed by raising awareness that these practices are not tied to any certain religious belief and meant to be adopted by people from diverse religious and spiritual backgrounds (Woods-Giscombé & Gaylord, 2014).

In addition, many cultures have traditionally adopted practices that function in similar ways with mainstream mindfulness, such as the collective experience of "meditative drumming and other forms of music" and dancing within African cultures (Woods-Giscombé & Gaylord, 2014, p. 151). Prayers and stories in different Native American cultures that illustrate values such as interconnectedness of all beings and nature, humility, kindness, nonstriving, and nonjudgmental awareness are another example of how contemplative practices are integral to different cultures. There is a need to acknowledge and promote these practices among URM nurses (Harrell, 2018).

Contemplative practices may support the acknowledgment and acceptance of the present moment, including the situations posed by an unjust social environment. Exploring the role of contemplative practices in reducing health disparities, Bruce et al. stated: "Contemplative practices can also empower people who are disadvantaged, marginalized, or under-resourced to respond to the stresses that surround them (e.g., racism, poverty) in ways that serve their spiritual, emotional, mental, and physical health needs" (Bruce et al., 2018, p. 2).

This may also apply to URM nursing students and professionals since they may be receiving education or working in institutions that still have a long way to go toward establishing inclusive and equitable organizational practices. This does not mean that URMs need to accept their educational and professional social environments as they are; however, contemplative practices can provide culturally meaningful tools that help cope with "the dissonance between one's actual condition vs. one's desired condition" (Bruce et al., 2018, p. 1).

Why do we need to develop healthy behavioral responses to such a dissonance? Experiencing a dissonance between the actual world we live in and what we think of as a moral and just world triggers stress response and can lead to negative health outcomes in the long term (Geronimus et al., 2006). Contemplative self-care practices are important tools for URM nursing professionals and students because the social change required to make their training and working conditions inclusive and equitable takes a long time and occurs simultaneously with the daily experiences of racism and discrimination. Contemplative practices might also promote tolerance, compassion, and active listening skills among nursing professionals and students of different social backgrounds, resulting in more authentic interpersonal relationships and deeper understanding of each other's cultural background and workplace experiences (Bruce et al., 2018; King, 2018).

Closing Thoughts

Similar to other institutions in the United States, healthcare organizations are not immune to the historical legacies and contemporary practices of racism and discrimination. How these dynamics take place in an organization, and how they are addressed by the leaders, shapes the overall organizational culture, in turn determining the interactions between healthcare providers of different social locations, as well as patient-provider relationships.

URM nursing students and professionals experience unique workplace stressors that are based in social identity–based bias and discrimination. These sources of workplace stress need to be considered by leaders of healthcare organizations when developing and offering self-care and communal care practices to prevent burnout and promote retention among URMs.

In Real Practice

When we consider diversity, the nursing profession will ideally reflect the population that it serves. It follows that nursing schools should also reflect the population of the community where the nursing school sits. In the U.S., this is rarely the case despite the fact that we live in an incredibly diverse country. Jessica Alicea-Planas (2017) addresses this concern in her qualitative study examining, phenomenologically, factors that may influence minority students' decisions to remain in nursing programs or leave them. She focuses her study on Hispanic nursing students at Jesuit University. The following themes, all centered on an idea of connectedness, emerged: journey into the unknown, creating a culture of acceptance, and keeping on course in uncharted territory (Alicea-Planas, 2017, abstract).

Key Points

- The field of nursing in the US has been working toward more diverse, inclusive, and equitable workplaces and educational spaces. However, URM nursing professionals and students continue to face differential treatment (from their leaders, educators, colleagues, and patients) on the basis of their racial/ethnic identity.

- Experiences of institutional discrimination, interpersonal racism, and stereotype threat contribute to high rates of isolation in the workplace, moral distress, burnout, and attrition among URM nurses.

- Self-care and communal care practices that are informed by the unique needs of URM nursing professionals and students can support them in navigating workplace stressors and cultivating a sustainable professional identity.

- Healthcare organizations have a responsibility to create opportunities and allocate resources for diversity and inclusion initiatives that focus on transforming discriminative structures and policies that compromise URM nurses' well-being, resilience, and professional fulfillment. These initiatives need to be led or coled by URM nursing professionals and students to truly address the needs of this community.

References

Ahmed, S. (2014, August 25). Selfcare as warfare. *Feminist Killjoys.* https://feministkilljoys.com/2014/08/25/selfcare-as-warfare/

Alicea-Planas, J. (2017). Shifting our focus to support the educational journey of underrepresented students. *Journal of Nursing Education, 56*(3), 159-163. https://doi.org/10.3928/01484834-20170222-07

Association of American Medical Colleges. (2019). *Diversity in medicine: Facts and figures 2019.* https://www.aamc.org/data-reports/workforce/interactive-data/figure-18-percentage-all-active-physicians-race/ethnicity-2018

Beech, B. M., Bruce, M. A., Thorpe, Jr, R. J., Heitman, E., Griffith, D. M., & Norris, K. C. (2018). Theory-informed research training and mentoring of underrepresented early-career faculty at teaching-intensive institutions: The obesity health disparities PRIDE program. *Ethnicity & Disease, 28*(2), 115–122. https://doi.org/10.18865/ed.28.2.115

Bell, A. V., Michalec, B., & Arenson, C. (2014). The (stalled) progress of interprofessional collaboration: The role of gender. *Journal of Interprofessional Care, 28*(2), 98–102. https://doi.org/10.3109/13561820.2013.851073

Billings, D. L. (2018). *Manual de habilidades y herramientas para la vida de mujeres sobrevivientes de violencia intrafamiliar* [Manual of skills and tools for the lives of women survivors of intrafamilial violence].

Bruce, M. A., Skrine Jeffers, K., King Robinson, J., & Norris, K. (2018). Contemplative practices: A strategy to improve health and reduce disparities. *International Journal of Environmental Research and Public Health, 15*(10), 2253. https://doi.org/10.3390/ijerph15102253

Campbell, K. M., & Rodríguez, J. E. (2018). Mentoring underrepresented minority in medicine (URMM) students across racial, ethnic and institutional differences. *Journal of the National Medical Association, 110*(5), 421–423. https://doi.org/10.1016/j.jnma.2017.09.004

Çayir, E., Spencer, M., Billings, D., Hilfinger Messias, D. K., Robillard, A., & Cunningham, T. (2020). "The only way we'll be successful": Organizational factors that influence psychosocial well-being and self-care among advocates working to address gender-based violence. *Journal of Interpersonal Violence.* https://doi.org/10.1177/0886260519897340

The Center for Contemplative Mind in Society. (2020). *What are contemplative practices?* https://www.contemplativemind.org/practices

Coleman, L. D. (2008). Experiences of African American students in a predominantly White, two-year nursing program. *ABNF Journal, 19*(1), 8–13. http://www.tuckerpub.com/ABNF2008Index.pdf

Cottingham, M. D., Johnson, A. H., & Erickson, R. J. (2018). "I can never be too comfortable": Race, gender, and emotion at the hospital bedside. *Qualitative Health Research, 28*(1), 145–158. https://doi.org/10.1177/1049732317737980

Cunningham, T., Inkelas, K. K., Trail., J. (2017). *Pilot data addressing the use and impacts of self-care, resilience and compassion at a level-one trauma center and school of nursing* [Conference presentation abstract]. CENTILE Conference, Washington, DC, United States.

Dickens, D. D., & Chavez, E. L. (2018). Navigating the workplace: The costs and benefits of shifting identities at work among early career U.S. Black women. *Sex Roles, 78*(11–12), 760–774. https://doi.org/10.1007/s11199-017-0844-x

Diefenbeck, C., Michalec, B., & Alexander, R. (2016). Lived experiences of racially and ethnically underrepresented minority BSN students: A case study specifically exploring issues related to recruitment and retention. *Nursing Education Perspectives, 37*(1), 41–44. https://pubmed.ncbi.nlm.nih.gov/27164777/

Durkee, M. I., & Williams, J. L. (2015). Accusations of acting White: Links to Black students' racial identity and mental health. *Journal of Black Psychology, 41*(1), 26–48. https://doi.org/10.1177/0095798413505323

Erickson, R. J., & Grove, W. J. C. (2008). Emotional labor and health care. *Sociology Compass, 2*(2), 704–733. https://doi.org/10.1111/j.1751-9020.2007.00084.x

Evans, B. C. (2008). "Attached at the umbilicus": Barriers to educational success for Hispanic/Latino and American Indian nursing students. *Journal of Professional Nursing, 24*(4), 205–217. https://doi.org/10.1016/j.profnurs.2007.06.026

Evans, L. (2013). *Cabin pressure: African American pilots, flight attendants, and emotional labor.* Lanham, Maryland: Rowman & Littlefield.

Frey, W. H. (2018). The US will become "minority White" in 2045, census projects: Youthful minorities are the engine of future growth. *Brookings.* https://www.brookings.edu/blog/the-avenue/2018/03/14/the-us-will-become-minority-white-in-2045-census-projects/

Gardner, J. (2005a). Barriers influencing the success of racial and ethnic minority students in nursing programs. *Journal of Transcultural Nursing*, *16*(2), 155–162. https://doi.org/10.1177/1043659604273546

Gardner, J. (2005b). Understanding factors influencing foreign-born students' success in nursing school: A case study of East Indian nursing students and recommendations. *Journal of Cultural Diversity*, *12*(1), 12–17. Retrieved from http://www.ncbi.nlm.nih.gov/pubmed/15918248

Geronimus, A. T., Hicken, M., Keene, D., & Bound, J. (2006). "Weathering" and age patterns of allostatic load scores among Blacks and Whites in the United States. *American Journal of Public Health*, *96*(5), 826–833. https://doi.org/10.2105/AJPH.2004.060749

Ghazal, L. V., Ma, C., Djukic, M., & Squires, A. (2020). Transition-to-U.S. practice experiences of internationally educated nurses: An integrative review. *Western Journal of Nursing Research*, *42*(5), 373–392. https://doi.org/10.1177/0193945919860855

Gipson-Jones, T. L. (2017). Preventing program attrition for underrepresented nursing students. *Journal of Cultural Diversity*, *24*(4), 111.

Griffith, D. M., Childs, E. L., Eng, E., & Jeffries, V. (2007). Racism in organizations: The case of a county public health department. *Journal of Community Psychology*, *35*(3), 287–302. https://doi.org/10.1002/jcop.20149

Hamilton, N., & Haozous, E. A. (2017). Retention of faculty of color in academic nursing. *Nursing Outlook*, *65*(2), 212–221. https://doi.org/10.1016/j.outlook.2016.11.003

Harrell, S. P. (2018). Soulfulness as an orientation to contemplative practice: Culture, liberation, and mindful awareness. *Journal of Contemplative Inquiry*, *5*(1).

Hassouneh, D., & Lutz, K. F. (2013). Having influence: Faculty of color having influence in schools of nursing. *Nursing Outlook*, *61*(3), 153–163. https://doi.org/10.1016/j.outlook.2012.10.002

Horvat, E. M. N., & Lewis, K. S. (2003). Reassessing the "burden of 'acting White'": The importance of peer groups in managing academic success. *Sociology of Education*, *76*(4), 265–280. https://doi.org/10.2307/1519866

Institute of Medicine. (2003). Unequal treatment: Confronting racial and ethnic disparities in health care. The National Academies Press. https://doi.org/10.17226/12875

Jamie, A. (2019, August 8). True self-care is not about you. *Vice*. https://www.vice.com/en_us/article/ywazwb/true-self-care-is-not-about-you

King, R. (2018). *Mindful of race: Transforming racism from the inside out*. Sounds True.

Lomas, T., Medina, J. C., Ivtzan, I., Rupprecht, S., & Eiroa-Orosa, F. J. (2018). A systematic review of the impact of mindfulness on the well-being of healthcare professionals. *Journal of Clinical Psychology*, *74*(3), 319–355. https://doi.org/10.1002/jclp.22515

Lorde, A. (1988). *A burst of light: Essays*. Firebrand Books.

Magee, R. V. (2016). Teaching mindfulness with mindfulness of race and other forms of diversity. In D. McCown, D. K., Reibel, & M. S. Micozzi (Eds.), *Resources for teaching mindfulness* (pp. 225–246). Cham: Springer International Publishing. https://doi.org/10.1007/978-3-319-30100-6_12

Moyce, S., Lash, R., & de Leon Siantz, M. L. (2016). Migration experiences of foreign educated nurses: A systematic review of the literature. *Journal of Transcultural Nursing*, *27*(2), 181–188. https://doi.org/10.1177/1043659615569538

National Institutes of Health. (2020). Diversity Matters—Underrepresented Racial and Ethnic Groups. Retrieved November 25, 2020, from https://extramural-diversity.nih.gov/diversity-matters/underrepresented-groups

Nilep, C. (2006). "Code switching" in sociocultural linguistics. *Colorado Research in Linguistics*, *19*(June), 1–22. https://www.researchgate.net/publication/239461967_Code_Switching_in_ Sociocultural_Linguistics

Osseo-Asare, A., Balasuriya, L., Huot, S. J., Keene, D., Berg, D., Nunez-Smith, M., Genao, I., Latimore, D., & Boatright, D. (2018). Minority resident physicians' views on the role of race/ethnicity in their training experiences in the workplace. *JAMA Network Open*, *1*(5), e182723. https://doi. org/10.1001/jamanetworkopen.2018.2723

Pappas, S., & Rushton, C. (2020, February 8). Leading the way to professional well-being. *American Nurse Journal*, *15*(2), 28–31. https://www.myamericannurse.com/leading-the-way-to-professional-well-being/

Paul-Emile, K., Smith, A. K., Lo, B., & Fernández, A. (2016). Dealing with racist patients. *New England Journal of Medicine*, *374*(8), 706–708. https://doi.org/10.1056/NEJMp1514939

Phillips, S. L., Dennison, S. T., & Davenport, M. A. (2016). High retention of minority and international faculty through a formal mentoring program. *To Improve the Academy*, *35*(1), 153–179. https://doi.org/10.1002/tia2.20034

Rosenkoetter, M. M., Nardi, D., & Bowcutt, M. (2017). Internationally educated nurses in transition in the United States: Challenges and mediators. *Journal of Continuing Education in Nursing*, *48*(3), 139–144. https://doi.org/10.3928/00220124-20170220-10

Sekaram, S. (2018, October 18). *The politics of self care and feminism*. Genderit.org. https://www. genderit.org/feminist-talk/politics-self-care-and-feminism

Shanafelt, T. D., & Noseworthy, J. H. (2017, January). Executive leadership and physician well-being: nine organizational strategies to promote engagement and reduce burnout. In *Mayo Clinic Proceedings* (Vol. 92, No. 1, pp. 129-146). Elsevier.

Smedley, B. D., Stith, A. Y., & Nelson, A. R. (2003). *Unequal treatment: Confronting racial and ethnic disparities in health care*. The National Academies Press.

Smiley, R. A., Lauer, P., Bienemy, C., Berg, J. G., Shireman, E., Reneau, K. A., & Alexander, M. (2018). The 2017 National Nursing Workforce Survey. *Journal of Nursing Regulation*, *9*(3), S1–S88. https://doi.org/10.1016/S2155-8256(18)30131-5

Spicer, A. (2019, August 21). 'Self-care': how a radical feminist idea was stripped of politics for the mass market. *The Guardian*. https://www.theguardian.com/commentisfree/2019/aug/21/self-care-radical-feminist-idea-mass-market

Statistic Stats. (2019, August 8). *Male nursing statistics*. https://www.statisticstats.com/health/male-nursing-statistics/

Tenfelde, S. M., Hatchett, L., & Saban, K. L. (2018). "Maybe Black girls do yoga": A focus group study with predominantly low-income African-American women. *Complementary Therapies in Medicine*, *40*, 230–235. https://doi.org/10.1016/j.ctim.2017.11.017

van der Riet, P., Levett-Jones, T., & Aquino-Russell, C. (2018). The effectiveness of mindfulness meditation for nurses and nursing students: An integrated literature review. *Nurse Education Today*, *65*, 201–211. https://doi.org/10.1016/j.nedt.2018.03.018

Waitzkin, H. (2018). *Health care under the knife: Moving beyond capitalism for our health*. NYU Press.

Walsh, Z. (2017). Contemplative praxis for social-ecological transformation. *The Arrow*, *4*. https:// doi.org/10.1029/2002GL014657

Wasco, S. M., & Campbell, R. (2002). A multiple case study of rape victim advocates' self-care routines: The influence of organizational context. *American Journal of Community Psychology, 30*(5), 731–760. https://doi.org/10.1023/A:1016377416597

Weaver, H. N. (2001). Indigenous nurses and professional education: Friends or foes? *Journal of Nursing Education, 40*(6), 252–258. https://doi.org/10.3928/0148-4834-20010901-05

Wever, C., & Zell, S. (2017). Re-working self-care: From individual to collective responsibility through a critical ethics of care. In B. Pease, A. Vreugdenhil, & S. Stanford (Eds.), *Critical ethics of care in social work: Transforming the politics and practices of caring* (pp. 207). Routledge.

White, B. J., & Fulton, J. S. (2015). Common experiences of African American nursing students: An integrative review. *Nursing Education Perspectives, 36*(3), 167–175. https://doi.org/10.5480/14-1456

Woods-Giscombé, C. L., & Gaylord, S. A. (2014). The cultural relevance of mindfulness meditation as a health intervention for African Americans: Implications for reducing stress-related health disparities. *Journal of Holistic Nursing, 32*(3), 147–160. https://doi.org/10.1177/0898010113519010

Xiao, L. D., Willis, E., & Jeffers, L. (2014). Factors affecting the integration of immigrant nurses into the nursing workforce: A double hermeneutic study. *International Journal of Nursing Studies, 51*(4), 640–653. https://doi.org/10.1016/j.ijnurstu.2013.08.005

Xu, Y., Davidhizar, R., & Joyce, N. G. (2005). What if your nursing student is from an Asian culture? *Journal of Cultural Diversity, 12*(1), 5–11.

Xue, Y. (2015). Racial and ethnic minority nurses' job satisfaction in the U.S. *International Journal of Nursing Studies, 52*(1), 280–287. https://doi.org/10.1016/j.ijnurstu.2014.10.007

Younas, A., Sundus, A., Zeb, H., & Sommer, J. (2019). A mixed methods review of male nursing students' challenges during nursing education and strategies to tackle these challenges, *Journal of Professional Nursing, 35*(4), 260–276. https://doi.org/10.1016/j.profnurs.2019.01.008

Men in Nursing School: A Conversation With Ryan Thomas, University of Virginia

Fourth-year nursing student, Ryan Thomas, always felt pulled to be a "helper." Whether that meant doing community service in his hometown of Lovettsville, Virginia, or taking on leadership roles in high school student government, he knew that helping others was the path he would follow. He just wasn't certain what specific path he would take.

In his junior year of high school, he tagged along with a classmate who volunteered for a nearby rescue squad. After completing his requisite physicals and trainings, he remembers his very first day as a rescue squad volunteer. In a six-hour shift, "We ran two calls. It was the coolest experience of my life. Everyone was so nice. These were the kind of people I wanted to be with. People who were down-to-earth, who just wanted to help people."

In a later EMT class, he had the flash of insight he had been looking for. Students were required to do clinicals, to see what happened to patients after the ambulance pulled away. Ryan had the opportunity to shadow a nurse who also happened to volunteer with the same rescue squad. "By the end of the night, it was like, 'You're a guy in healthcare, making a difference for a lot of people. Your job is very cool.' It's like everything I've wanted to be, and finally there's a word for it—being a nurse."

Fast-forward four years, and Ryan is months away from completing his nursing degree at the University of Virginia (UVA). He calls his years there "a phenomenal experience," but he has been in the gender minority at the nursing school. Only 11.4% of all BSN candidates in the United States are men, and in the 2019 nursing workforce, only 12% are men (Statistic Stats, 2019). This gender imbalance is an international phenomenon; the highest percentage of male nurses is found in Saudi Arabia (32%) and Italy (21%) (Younas et al., 2019).

Ryan acknowledges that being a man in nursing brings unique challenges. First, there are the assumptions that a man in nursing isn't "smart enough" to get into medical school. When he began sharing his decision to go into nursing, countless times he heard, "But why don't you go to medical school?" or, "You can go to medical school when you finish nursing school, right?"

Ryan also observes that there is an assumption that all men in nursing are gay, and this prompts a discussion about pervasive masculine stereotypes. This assumption, he says, "points to the masculine stereotype that heterosexual men are incapable of selfless compassion, kindness, and caring. In a larger sense, it speaks to toxic masculinity, all the different gender norms that make masculinity so toxic. I'm still combatting it and learning. As a heterosexual male, you're not the person you go to for emotional support because that's not what masculinity is all about. My masculinity has changed here. I define a lot of my masculinity as being kind, caring, and compassionate."

He also found that his predominantly female clinical instructors never talked about how male nurses should interact with patients. "As a man, you can't just put your hand on someone's shoulder without making sure they're okay with it. It could be triggering." Ryan says there are a lot of little tips and tricks that he was grateful to learn from a male clinical instructor. For example, "You don't roll the patients toward you because you don't want your genitalia in their facial region. It's not something a woman would think about. For them, it's not a sign of disrespect. As a man, you either roll the patient from their feet or on the other side."

As a way to help himself and other male nursing students, Ryan took over the leadership of the Men and Nursing (MAN) club at UVA. The club has two goals—to provide a community for men in nursing and to put themselves out there, to "remind people that guys can be nurses." They learn from each other in addition to doing community service, such as handwashing seminars in elementary schools. "If you're confused about something, a way to act, an experience you've had, the club is a way to help you process through it." He emphasizes that the club is also not about "men being better than women in nursing. It's about diversity."

Ryan made the fateful decision to become a "guy in healthcare" where he could make a difference and live his passion for helping others, while also having time to pursue his other interests. His advice to others following in his footsteps: Don't play into others' notions of masculinity and be sure to seek out male nursing mentors and a community of peers.

It Takes a Village to Raise a Nurse

—Ren Capucao (he/him)

My mother was born as "Julie" in the Philippines in 1954. Yet the midwife misinterpreted the name my grandmother had said and officiated my mother's legal name as "Jolly." While she went by the former in the Philippines, she used the latter upon immigrating to the US in 1986. Throughout her nursing career, and in life, she has lived up to her name of "Jolly" in the midst of adversity.

One challenge Filipina/o nurses, like my mother, faced was the taking of the Nursing Certification Licensure Examination (NCLEX). Limited English proficiency and multiple-choice test-taking experience left these potential nurses faced with questions that were hard to interpret. Many of these nurses were more familiar with open-response questions alongside oral and practical examinations. Imagine taking a test when your past experience with all tests had been short-answer and now, all of a sudden, you are faced with a multitude of multiple-choice questions. That was the experience of my mother and her nursing friends. Regardless of the number of years they spent working as nurses in the Philippines, the NCLEX determined their fate of working as nurses in the US.

Born in a provincial town as one of nine siblings, my mother dreamed of becoming a nurse at a young age. During the mid-century, while typhoid vaccines were prevalent in the US, the geography and healthcare infrastructure in the Philippines prevented equitable access to healthcare. My maternal grandmother contracted typhoid fever, developed a stage-four pressure ulcer followed by sepsis, and died shortly thereafter. The death of my grandmother made my mother even more determined to become a nurse. At the age of fourteen, my mother became the maternal figure of the family. Despite this obstacle, she received help from the community in not only caring for her siblings but also funding her nursing education.

When she arrived in the United States, my mother worked as a nurse's aide alongside other Filipina/os, biding time while they studied for the NCLEX. Through shared goals and cultural values, they formed long-lasting friendships. Together, they drove four hours to a testing site in Baltimore, Maryland. There, they failed the exam together, over and over again.

Yet in the face of defeat, my mother knew that she was not a failure, as she had practiced nursing almost her entire life, from caring for her siblings to practicing as a trained nurse. In addition, her devout faith in Catholicism steeled her for hard times. After traveling thousands of miles across the sea, she would not let any circumstance diminish her dream of becoming a nurse. In 1990, after taking the test a fourth time, she passed. My mother's Filipina/o support system played a vital role in her and her friends' eventual success in receiving their nursing licenses.

6
Self-Care for LGBTQ+ Nursing Students

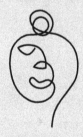

Kimberly D. Acquaviva
pronouns: She/Her

Kimberly Acquaviva is a social worker committed to making healthcare—and nursing education—more LGBTQ+ inclusive. As a lesbian, she believes it's important for nursing students to be taught by a diverse group of faculty—including "out" LGBTQ+ faculty members. When she isn't teaching or writing, she enjoys hiking, playing with her dogs, and making letterpress stationery using her 1894 Chandler and Price 8 × 12 Old Style printing press.

"Caring for myself is not self-indulgence, it is self-preservation, and that is an act of political warfare."

–Audre Lorde

This chapter focuses on the additional stressors that lesbian, gay, bisexual, transgender, gender nonconforming, queer, or questioning (LGBTQ+) nursing students may experience and offers suggestions for self-care strategies to address them.

To Begin, A Note About Language

In the other chapters of this book, you've learned about common stressors for nursing students as well as about self-care strategies that can be helpful regardless of the identities you hold. This chapter focuses on the additional stressors that lesbian, gay, bisexual, transgender, gender nonconforming, queer, or questioning (LGBTQ+) nursing students may experience and offers suggestions for self-care strategies to address them. As an LGBTQ+ person myself, I remember going through my undergraduate and graduate programs without ever coming across a chapter in a textbook that was written for me. There was no shortage of textbook chapters *about* me, though—chapters that talked about LGBTQ+ people under that ubiquitous catch-all heading, "Special Populations." For this reason, I've written this chapter specifically for LGBTQ+ people. When I use the word "you," I'm talking to LGBTQ+ readers. If you don't identify as LGBTQ+ but you're reading this chapter, this is an opportunity to experience what it might feel like to navigate a world in which the default assumptions about your identities are wrong.

Acknowledging How Far You've Come

Your journey to get to nursing school wasn't easy. Whether you came out to your family a long time ago, came out to them recently, haven't come out to them yet, or have decided you're never going to come out to them, you've gone through life carrying something that most of your nursing school classmates haven't had to: the knowledge that your sexual orientation or gender identity are "different" than most of the people around you. Even if your family has been loving and accepting of who you are, you may have struggled to love and accept yourself. The fact that you're here today pursing a degree in nursing, or you're a new nurse just beginning this professional trajectory, is something you should feel incredibly proud of. So, before we jump into talking about self-care in nursing school, take a minute to appreciate how well you've taken care of yourself on your journey to get here.

"Straight Talk" About Stressors

As an LGBTQ+ nursing student, you're going to be exposed to many of the same stressors as your peers: piles of reading, assignment deadlines, tests, and clinical skills to master. In addition to the usual stressors, however, you're likely to encounter a few that your non-LGBTQ+ classmates will not. The following are some of the stressors you may encounter in nursing school and beyond.

Family Expectations

There's probably a disconnect between who your family thought you'd grow up to be and who you actually are. At first glance this may not seem like a nursing school–related stressor, but it is: Your relationship with your family can be a source of support or a source of stress as you progress through nursing school. When you were born or adopted into your family, they probably didn't think you would grow up to be LGBTQ+. Some families navigate this disconnect with ease, lovingly accepting their LGBTQ+ child unconditionally, and other families struggle to reconcile their expectations with their new reality. Some families are unaware there even is a disconnect because their LGBTQ+ child has not "come out" to them. If your family is aware of your LGBTQ+ identity/ies, they may express concern about your safety and about whether you should be "out" at school. Regardless of what you've told your family about your identity/ies and how accepting they've been, managing your relationships with your family can be challenging at times.

Social Norms and Assumptions

Odds are that most of your classmates in nursing school are heterosexual and cisgender. The social norms in nursing school are similar to those found in other groups of mostly heterosexual and cisgender young adults. For undergraduate nursing students at residential colleges or universities, social life may seem to revolve around parties, hanging out with friends, and "hooking up" with romantic partners. (For undergraduate nursing students at community colleges or graduate nursing students in any educational setting, a school-centered social life may feel nonexistent.) Regardless of the setting or educational level, nursing students will generally assume everyone they meet is cisgender and heterosexual unless they're told otherwise. This is because nursing students have been raised and educated in an environment that is heteronormative, meaning an environment in which heterosexuality and the gender binary are considered to be the norm and, as such, are the default assumption. For LGBTQ+ nursing students, the heteronormativity of nursing school can translate into some uncomfortable situations; your fellow nursing students might:

- Ask you on a date while making an incorrect assumption about your sexual orientation

- Ask questions about your weekend that clearly convey an incorrect assumption about the gender identity of the people you date

- Refer to you using the wrong pronouns because they made an incorrect assumption about your pronouns based on their visual assessment of you

Invisibility

Where there's heteronormativity, there's invisibility. Unless you tell the people you interact with in nursing school that you're LGBTQ+, they're probably going to assume that you aren't. In my 20s I remember feeling like no one could see me—my long hair and makeup were interpreted by others to mean "straight." Being invisible can seem like a good thing: If no one knows you're LGBTQ+, you may feel somewhat shielded from homophobia (or transphobia). After all, if people don't know you're LGBTQ+, how can they treat you badly because of it? Over the long haul, though, the feeling of being invisible may weigh you down, and you may begin to feel as though that invisibility isn't a superpower, it's a prison.

Legally Sanctioned Discrimination, Hate, and Violence

With "outness" comes the risk of discrimination, hate, and violence. As an LGBTQ+ nursing student, you face a very real risk of legalized discrimination in half of the states in the United States (Movement Advancement Project, 2020). When you graduate and pass the NCLEX, your gender identity or sexual orientation can be used against you when you try to rent an apartment, attempt to buy a house, or try to enter a public business. In fact, until June 2020, it was completely legal to fire someone for being LGBTQ+ in 25 states and three territories in the United States because there were "no explicit prohibitions for discrimination based on sexual orientation or gender identity in state law" (Movement Advancement Project, 2020). On June 15, 2020, the US Supreme Court issued a ruling that the 1964 Civil Rights Act protects employees from being fired because of their sexual orientation or gender identity. While this landmark ruling protects LGBTQ+ people from employment discrimination, LGBTQ+ people are still vulnerable to discrimination in other aspects of their lives (Movement Advancement Project, 2020):

- In 25 states and five territories, it's completely legal to evict someone or refuse to rent or sell housing to someone solely because they are LGBTQ+.

- In 26 states and five territories, it's completely legal to deny entry or refuse to serve someone in a restaurant, hotel, doctor's office, bank, or park because they are LGBTQ+.

- In 17 states and three territories, assaulting or killing an LGBTQ+ person because of their sexual orientation or gender identity would not be considered a hate crime even if the person who committed the assault or murder explicitly said—in front of hundreds of witnesses—that they were beating you up because you were LGBTQ+.

Self-Care Strategies for LGBTQ+ Nursing Students

Given the plethora of stressors that LGBTQ+ nursing students face, practicing self-care is vitally important. The following self-care strategies are designed to complement the strategies provided elsewhere in this book.

Explore "Outness" in Your Own Time and Your Own Way

There is no "right" way to be an LGBTQ+ person in nursing school. You can choose to share your LGBTQ+ identity/ies with some, all, or none of your classmates, instructors, and preceptors. Give yourself permission to share your LGBTQ+ identity/ies only when and where you feel safe doing so. If coming out to your parents/family of origin may put your physical safety, mental health, or source of financial support at risk, allow yourself the time and space to come out to them only if and when you feel safe doing so.

Find a Mentor Who Shares Your Identity/ies

A good mentor can help you navigate nursing school as well as your career in the coming years. Mentors don't have to be LGBTQ+ in order to be effective, but you may find it helpful to work with someone who shares your identity/ies. LGBTQ+ mentors have likely experienced some of the challenges you're going to encounter—as such, they're uniquely qualified to give you helpful guidance. If you also identify as Black, Latinx, Indigenous/Native, or a member of another under-represented group, you may find it helpful to also have a mentor who shares that identity. You can never have too many mentors!

Seek Out Healthy Ways of Being in Community With Other LGBTQ+ People

As an LGBTQ+ nursing student, you may be unsure of how to meet other LGBTQ+ people. If you're an undergraduate student, this may be the first time in your life that you've had the freedom to construct a social life for yourself without your parents/guardians watching your every move. This can be both exciting and terrifying, especially if you don't know where to find other LGBTQ+ people in your college/university community. It can be tempting to think that dating apps like Tinder, Grindr, and Bumble are the answer to this dilemma, but "finding community" is more complicated than finding someone to hook up with. As a starting point, make a list of the activities in your life that bring you joy. Do you enjoy hiking? Dancing? Photography? Basketball? Attending religious services? Cooking? Once you've put together your list, look for LGBTQ+ clubs for these activities.

For example, if you're LGBTQ+ and you love playing basketball, do a Google search for the name of your town and the words "basketball" and "LGBT." (Not everyone uses the term LGBTQ+, so the term LGBT when used as a search term may give you more "hits.") Pick one activity and make a commitment to yourself that you'll set aside time for it each week. Spending time with other LGBTQ+ people in settings other than bars will help you envision what your life as an LGBTQ+ adult can be like.

Focus on What Your Body Can Do, Not on Who Your Body Can Attract

The LGBTQ+ community isn't immune to the pressures experienced by cisgender, heterosexual people regarding physical appearance and weight. Rather than see your body as something that needs to be shaped or constricted or shrunk to make you attractive to other people, try to see your body as a vehicle that's going to get you from Point A to Point B in life. What does your body need from you in terms of food, sleep, and exercise in order to function at its very best? If you focus on treating your body like a racecar that needs premium gas instead of like a fixer-upper that's never good enough, you'll feel a lot more joy in life. If you're interested in dating during nursing school, you can find someone who appreciates your body just as it is. You don't need to make yourself smaller or prettier or stronger—you are perfect exactly as you are.

> ### In Real Practice
>
> You've heard of professional organizations like Sigma Theta Tau International (STTI) and the American Nurses Association (ANA), but did you know there's an organization for LGBTQ+ nurses? Founded in 2013, GLMA Nursing: Nursing Advancing LGBTQ Health Equity was established to serve as a "home" for LGBTQ+ nurses and allies who are actively engaged in improving LGBTQ+ health and LGBTQ+ issues in nursing. Now or when you graduate, join professional organizations like STTI and ANA and get involved as a member. If you're LGBTQ+ or an ally committed to advancing LGBTQ+ health, consider also joining GLMA Nursing and getting involved as a member. Participation in events like GLMA Nursing's annual summit can be incredibly energizing and affirming for LGBTQ+ nurses. Many national nursing organizations have taken steps in advocating for LGBTQ+ health. For a complete list of supportive statements and actions from national nursing organizations, check out Table 26.2 in Zollweg et al. (2020).

Queering Self-Care: The Daily Becoming the Sacred

–Dallas Ducar, MSN, RN, PMHNP-BC, CNL, NREMT-B, NP (she/her)

I felt an incredible sense of loneliness as a nursing student, especially when being perceived as male. After graduating, and becoming a nurse, I embarked on a new journey; I allowed myself to be authentic and the world to see me as I truly was, female. No self-care book could have prepared me for this.

Transitioning gender is an unfolding process, an intentional act of noticing the self and how people react to the changing self. When I started to transition, patients no longer assumed I was the doctor; they assumed I was the nurse. When a patient was agitated, I was no longer on the frontline; I stood in the back. (It seems to frequently be the case that cis men—and many cis women—generally operate from the mental schema that men should be in the front when confronting an agitated patient, as that is what is traditionally expected of them as men.)

To be sure, I was White in the southern United States. I was not the subject of the same discrimination that the QTBIPOC (Queer, Trans, Black, Indigenous People of Color) community bore. Still, this was an act of losing privilege. My muscles waned, my physical strength disappeared, my frame slightened, and my voice softened. With this, I also gained a supreme sense of self-confidence. My transition was an existential quest—to proclaim myself and know myself.

Traditional, Western self-care involves sitting on the meditation cushion, in silence, alone. Emerson and Thoreau both retreated in solace to discover their own self. Self-care for the queer community, like many marginalized communities, is relational, to learn you are not alone, or the only one. Queering self-care involves connecting with others and knowing those compartmentalized and closeted spaces of your self do not need to stay hidden. It involves deep listening, storytelling, sacred spaces, bearing witness, and organizing together. These rituals open space for voices that have not been heard, to welcome stillness, generativity, and activism.

I was supported by strong allies in my workplace. This was crucial. However, self-care had to be communal.

Self-care would not have been possible without other queer folks. I had to know queer people who were not suicidal. Being together was a chance to escape "flight or fight mode," even when it served someone to survive. It was an opportunity to no longer need to fight to survive and be seen. It was a chance to be vulnerable enough to allow others to see me. Once I could truly experience others seeing me, I could then see myself, and care for my self.

I continue to queer self-care by organizing collectively against systems of oppression today, the social, cultural, economic, and political forces that are dedicated to suppressing queer voices and identities. My very expression of being is a radical act of self-care. Painting my nails, braiding my hair, buying a dress, dancing to pop music. It is through loving traditional forms of gender expression and femininity that I am able to live authentically and queer self-care. Living into my identity becomes a radical act to turn oppression into liberation. In this way, the daily becomes the sacred, and self-care becomes a radical act of social justice. Most importantly, that loneliness is gone, and the community has taken its place.

Key Points

- LGBTQ+ students have gone through life carrying something that most of their nursing school classmates haven't had to: the knowledge that their sexual orientation or gender identity are "different" from most of the people around them.

- LGBTQ+ nursing students are exposed to many of the same stressors as their heterosexual, cisgender peers: piles of reading, assignment deadlines, tests, and clinical skills to master. In addition to the usual stressors, however, they're likely to encounter stressors related to family expectations, social norms and assumptions, invisibility, and legally sanctioned discrimination, hate, and violence.

- Given the plethora of stressors that LGBTQ+ nursing students face, practicing self-care is vitally important. Four self-care strategies are presented here to complement the strategies provided elsewhere in this book.

References

Movement Advancement Project. (2020). *Nondiscrimination laws.* https://www.lgbtmap.org/equality-maps/non_discrimination_laws

Zollweg, S. S. F., Tobin, V., Goldstein, Z. G., Keepnews, D. M., & Chinn, P. L. (2020). Improving LGBTQ+ health: Nursing policy can make a difference. *Policy & Politics in Nursing and Health Care-E-Book,* 211.

7

Nursing Our Identities: Self-Compassion and Intersectionality

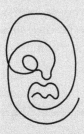

Reynaldo (Ren) Capucao, Jr.
pronouns: He/Him

Ren Capucao is a nurse historian on a never-ending quest of self-discovery and battling the effects of historical traumas on well-being. He views every experience with childlike curiosity and welcomes learning from those of different walks of life. While his mind tends to be in the past, his mantra is to use his gained insight and knowledge to keep moving forward and help others along their own journeys.

"I think you travel to search and you come back home to find yourself there."

—Chimamanda Ngozi Adichie

Cultural diversity within the nursing profession greatly pales in comparison to the US population. By 2045, the US census projects the non-Hispanic White population to fall below 50% of the total population (Frey, 2018). So, what is the forecast for the nursing profession? Historically, the American nursing profession developed under social values that centered nursing education around White middle-class women. This legacy remains prominently visible as over three-fourths of the nursing workforce racially identifies as "White" (see Figure 7.1).

Because nursing schools serve as the direct pipeline of nurses into the workforce, low enrollment of prospective nurses of color (NOCs), particularly those from non-Western backgrounds, directly affects the cultural diversity of the nursing workforce (Graham et al., 2016). Recruitment depicts one-half of the issue, while retention represents the other. The latter involves an intricate relationship between nursing students inside the structures of nursing schools and hospitals (Loftin et al., 2012). Taking a closer look at the personal level, race and ethnicity represent just one dimension to understand the unique experiences felt by NOCs navigating historically White spaces.

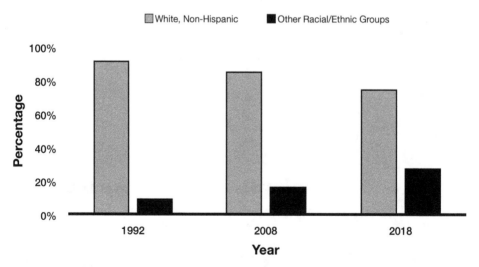

FIGURE 7.1   Racial and ethnic composition of the US nursing workforce through the decades.

(U.S. Department of Health and Human Services, Health Resources and Services Administration 1992, 2010, and 2020)

Intersectionality explains how cultural, historical, and social inequalities and their associated structural differences among identities affect NOCs' access to power and resources (Crenshaw, 1989). *Identities* are social constructions of ourselves and can be viewed temporally: past (who we were), present (who we are now), and future (who we hope to become). This correlates with the *self*, a warm feeling and sense of authenticity when our psyche reflects our actions and behaviors within the social environment. Yet identity is not always congruent with the self. The internal process that mediates the exchange between social and cognitive forces to describe who we are is *self-identity*: a collection of beliefs and perceptions that codes our being by asking, "Who am I?" (Azmitia & Thomas, 2015; Oyserman et al., 2011).

Self-Worth Through Self-Compassion

Self-identity defines who we are objectively and is directly shaped by the similar concept of *self-worth*, a subjective perception of ourselves that acts as a motivator for actions and behaviors in the present. Depending on our interpretations of experiences, self-worth may obscure the internal examination of our interconnected identities that define us. It can be constructed in two ways: 1) *self-esteem*: a degree to which we evaluate ourselves positively, often based on comparisons with others and 2) *self-compassion*: an ability to relate to ourselves via unconditional self-acceptance (Germer & Neff, 2019).

For NOCs, nurturing self-identity through self-compassion may have long-term benefits that support academic success and the prevention of burnout and compassion fatigue as they transition into clinical practice as newly graduated nurses. *Self-compassion*, a transcultural concept prevalent in the East and West, refers to learning how to treat ourselves as we might naturally treat others when they suffer, fail, or feel inadequate. While mindfulness invites us to open ourselves to suffering with spacious awareness, self-compassion allows us to be kind to ourselves during these bouts of suffering. The three components of self-compassion include self-kindness, common humanity, and mindfulness. When these components work in tandem, self-compassion not only promotes resiliency, motivation, and self-concept, but may also mitigate worry, rumination, and other forms of internal conflict (Germer & Neff, 2019).

This chapter provides perspective on intersectional identities and self-care through my journey of self-compassion during nursing school. It offers a reflexive discourse for NOCs to draw parallels to their own lives and experiences and help them craft individualized self-care plans. Starting now, as a NOC myself, I will use "we" to refer to myself as a member of this group identity. The outline of the chapter is broken into sections that contextualize my self-compassionate journey from childhood origins to my current nursing career. Although I focus on the self-care needs of NOCs, this information also extends an opportunity for colleagues to enhance *cultural humility*, the ability to maintain an interpersonal stance that is other-oriented in relation to aspects of cultural identity that are most important to the person (Foronda et al., 2016; Smith & Foronda, 2019). Overall, I hope that this chapter supports the reflexive journeys of readers toward a path of authenticity and kindness and cultivates self-care that feeds the soul (Mills et al., 2015).

A Self-Compassionate Guide to Soul Searching

"If you live the questions, life will move you into the answers."
– Deepak Chopra

As an introvert, I have found myself an avid practitioner of mindfulness, yet my thoughts tend to dangerously border between nostalgia and rumination. For years, I have battled with major depressive disorder, which distorted my self-identity and self-worth to naturally describe and consider myself lesser than everyone else. For most of my life, I defined myself from the expectations and perceptions of others. So, when things went awry in an objective and subjective sense, I would crumble under the pressure. The detachment I had with myself led to my worsening depression. Without acknowledging other dimensions of my identity, I obscured my sight of truly knowing who I am and was bound to repeat the past. To break this pattern, I unknowingly began cultivating self-compassion during a series of misfortunate events during nursing school when I hit one of my lowest points.

Because self-compassion and self-care are analogous to thinking and doing, I use the former to guide the latter. Self-compassion has been essential to my self-care as it has repositioned my thoughts and actions at the center, removed anxieties caused by the outside world, and steeled me for the journey ahead. It has helped me find confidence in who I am and celebrate my predisposition toward open-mindedness, empathy, and childlike curiosity. In fact, my current pursuit of a PhD used to only be a childhood dream that my younger self could only imagine. I feel like I have just found my voice, and I intend to continue learning about myself as I progress through my nursing career and use my knowledge to create positive change and support the introspective journeys of others. This narrative is my meaning-making process of my multiple identities that intertwine with my role as a nurse. I hope it can help serve as a blueprint for self-care by instilling a sense of self-compassion of what came before, what is happening now, and what is planned ahead for your nursing career.

Identity (Mal)formation: Cultural Mismatch

"For someone to develop genuine compassion towards others, first he or she must have a basis upon which to cultivate compassion, and that basis is the ability to connect to one's own feelings and to care for one's own welfare."

–Dalai Lama

During my clinical rotations, I experienced patients who spewed racist remarks based on the incorrect assumption that I was Chinese or Mexican heritage and unit cultures that lacked protocols to handle these events, which is to say that unit leadership (preceptors, charge nurses, and nurse managers) expected me to just brush off these experiences. Once, I broke down into tears days after a preceptor asked if I wanted to apologize to a patient—who was in a manic phase of a psychotic episode and had hurled a racially derogatory term at me on that shift—for finding my demeanor in the room "seemingly rude." I am the type of person that over-apologizes for everything, but this time I felt conflicted. I brewed over this occurrence over and over again; so many thoughts and questions bombarded my mind, particularly, "Am I apologizing for being myself?"

Cultural Tension as a Second-Generation Immigrant

Until my mid-twenties, I felt that I lacked an identity, and thereby any confidence in myself. I meandered through life as my cultural dissonance with Philippine culture continued to grow. This void of identity grew from intercultural and intergenerational conflicts experienced in and outside my home, leading me to identify more with my American identity. Although I grew up surrounded by a large Filipino American family and community, there was always a lack of cultural transmission surrounding Philippine culture and history aside from staple foods and Catholic values.

However, I did learn that homosexuality was taboo early on. During my childhood, "Are you *bakla* [gay]?" served as a derogatory phrase to condition heteronormative behaviors and actions. At seven years old—the age I knew that I was different—my parents enrolled me in Catholic school, where I would occasionally hear that "gay people go to hell." For at least a decade, this traumatized my younger self to suppress perceived aberrations of sexuality and to pray every night for an orthodox marriage and family. I wasted many birthdays wishing to be heterosexual, and eventually, these wishes transitioned into the pursuit of happiness—as I began a downward spiral with clinical depression.

Although my sexual orientation was the straw that broke the camel's back, my depressive symptoms began to take form earlier from the aforementioned culture clash of living in between cultures. Growing up, my first-generation Filipino American parents often took punitive action against me for bad grades, seemingly embarrassing them in public, and accidents like dropping eggs on the floor, which did not help since I was a clumsy kid.

I learned to mute my voice because defending myself would only lead to more punishment. In kindergarten, my teacher sent me to ESL (English as a Second Language) classes despite English being my only known language. I only spoke when spoken to, as my father trained me with military-like obedience to authority figures. As a result, I also developed a sedulous work ethic to compensate for my many perceived flaws and meet my parents' expectations. I also turned to food for solace and went through childhood obesity to deal with the stress of teachers' perceptions of my lackluster social performance and my parents' unattainable standards of filial piety. I was a strange kid, living in my head more than others my age.

The Beginning of Self-Discovery

Specifically, I developed a passion for historical inquiry to make sense of my circumstances and place in the world. I learned to frame my lack of identity within a broader historical context, and this helped me gather the courage to come out when I was 18 years old. I never anticipated my parents would accept my *coming out*—and my gut was right initially. Within my reflexive process, I found a blind spot. My teenage angst refused to empathize with my parents' story—a blatant extension of my own narrative. Yet their overprotectiveness and withholding of Philippine cultural knowledge undoubtedly came from both a place of love to prepare me for the worst but also the fear of losing another loved one. Over the past decade, I asked and listened intently to my parents' narratives and found stories of poverty, death, and struggle: My father, a soldier in the Philippines Marine Corps, lost most of his friends during skirmishes in Mindanao, and my mother, motherless at the age of 14, pursued her dream of becoming a nurse to raise her six younger siblings.

These interconnected dialogues between the past and present provided me with feelings of empowerment and identity that encouraged the accomplishment of shared dreams.

Historicizing (My)Self Across Generations

Before proceeding to my climactic battle with nursing school, now is a good time to impart the usefulness of history as a reflexive tool for self-compassion to fully explore our identities and the baggage they carry. To know ourselves requires an understanding of all the forces that have shaped us—notably, the distant past. Nursing, one of the oldest and most noble professions, often asks us to give much of ourselves to care for others while asking for little to nothing in return. It is a field ripe with intersectionality, intertwining professional status with its largely female presence—a relationship that has resulted in a long history of medicine and hospitals denying autonomous professionalization to the nursing profession (D'Antonio, 2010; Reverby, 1987).

When discussing race in nursing, it complicates the narrative of an already marginalized professional group. *Racialized emotional labor* in nursing is the suppression or inducement of emotions and feelings within one's self across the classroom and clinical environments during interactions with peers, instructors, healthcare staff, and patients and their families (DiCicco-Bloom & DiCicco-Bloom, 2019; Hochschild, 2012). I have often found myself regulating my emotions and behaviors in human service roles, so what were NOCs experiences with racialized emotional labor, particularly Asian American nurses? Until I entered my doctoral program, knowledge about Asian Americans was something almost nonexistent growing up in the South. Outside the often framed Black and White dichotomy, little attention has been paid to the racially ambiguous spaces occupied by Asian American nurses.

Particularly, the identities of my predecessors, Filipino nurses, have been largely influenced by cultural and healthcare environments left by the legacy of Spanish and American colonial regimes in the Philippines. Despite generational gaps, I myself am a postcolonial product of this broader history. After the Spanish-American War, the US acquired various territories, including the Philippines, and imported the US model of nursing into the islands. Since 1911, Filipino nurses have worked and studied at US hospitals and nursing schools, traveling abroad for a number of reasons: educational attainment, socioeconomic and educational opportunities, wanderlust, and financially supporting loved ones back home.

Leading up to the post–Second World War period, the Philippines' overproduction of nurses and inability to create sufficient employment opportunities boded well for the US, which was facing a critical shortage at the mid-century. US policies also supported the migration of internationally educated nurses, which led to the mass migration of Filipino nurses and the associated stereotype of their ubiquitous presence across US hospitals. However, their historicization as a model minority by mainstream media narrates a seamless integration purported by mainstream society. Yet the marginalized voices often recount contrasting stories of identity, belonging, and a renegotiation of color lines.

The following narratives are a part of my research and twenties search for identity. In a similar vein to understanding my parents, reading and listening to their stories empowered not only my perseverance through nursing school but a stronger sense of who I am. Most importantly, they imparted the significance of self-compassion in the face of adversity. The point is not to compare yourselves to them but consider how their lived experiences and emotions relate back to you and your place in the world. See if you can identify or speculate their sources of self-compassion and self-care practices.

Felicidad Nolasco, Paula Nonacido, and Rodolfo Eladio Acena

"That landlady asked the student nurse, 'Are they colored?'
She said, 'No. They are Filipinos.'"

–Felicidad Nolasco reflecting upon her arrival in Cleveland, Ohio in 1926

In 1926, before relocating to Seattle, Felicidad and Paula first arrived at City Hospital in Cleveland, Ohio. Felicidad, a graduate of the Philippine General Hospital School of Nursing, responded to a City Hospital recruitment ad in the Philippines alongside her friend and fellow alumnus, Paula, and together they began their American tale. Despite the protests of her family, Felicidad's wanderlust to see the world ultimately made her decision to board the *Empress of Russia* steamboat and migrate to US proper, scrapbooking her transnational journey along the way. Felicidad and Paula found their time at City Hospital pleasant, forging friendships with their White colleagues, yet the lack of Filipinos in the area, cold climate, and estranged feelings of not belonging directed the pair's movement in 1927 to New York.

While there, Felicidad rekindled a romance with Eladio, her former nursing school classmate who settled in Seattle. On one of his trips to visit Felicidad in New York, the two wed through a civil ceremony in 1928 and then toured the Eastern seaboard. In 1929, a pregnant Felicidad followed Eladio to Seattle. Once there, the Great Depression and increased racism and xenophobia toward Asian Americans on the West Coast prevented her from working in the hospital until the 1940s.

Paula, a faithful friend, followed a year later to provide Felicidad support in raising her newborn. Felicidad became a US citizen in 1949, and although she never returned to the Philippines, she looked back upon her past without any regrets.

Araceli Teodoro Marcial

[In the hospital] I feel that I have two lives. If I am on a 7[a.m.] to 3[p.m.] shift, I eat in the White dining room. If I am working evenings, I eat in the Black dining room. When I go into the community, they [Black people and White people] wouldn't allow us [Filipino nurses] anywhere, so if you go out in the park, you might as well bring your own potty chair.

—Araceli reflecting upon her time in Charleston, South Carolina in 1964

The Exchange Visitor Program (EVP) of 1948 ushered in the initial mass migration of Filipino nurses to the US (Choy, 2003). In 1960, Araceli applied to the EVP for educational attainment and began her journey in New Jersey. However, instead of a student, she felt more like a low-wage laborer. Racial inequity shaped her experience in the program: unequal pay among exchange nurses, shift assignments unwanted by White nurses, assignment tasks normally carried out by student nurses or workers without formal qualifications, and inadequate hospital orientations. During a discussion with a European exchange nurse, Araceli discovered that her stipend was smaller, despite orienting at the same time. After a year, she transferred to a hospital in Pennsylvania. There, she occasionally received prejudiced remarks from White coworkers, like asking if she knew how to use silverware. Although institutional racism was rampant in her work environment, instead of complaining or admitting defeat, she reframed her situation as a learning experience, having said, "I'm a better person than this. I'm here to learn something...I may not know anything at this point in time, but you don't know what I know."

One of the stipulations of the EVP required exchange nurses to return home once they completed the two-year program. Yet Araceli's marriage to a Filipino serviceman in the US Navy stationed in Philadelphia granted her US citizenship. From Philadelphia, she followed wherever her husband was stationed. In 1963, she worked in South Carolina and became more acquainted with racial inequity along the color line, as she noticed the harsher treatment toward her Black nursing colleagues and her own unusual predicament of being neither White nor Black within the Jim Crow South. She navigated her shifting social status across places on her own. Eventually, she settled in Virginia, where she applied the lessons from her experiences with her belief in grassroots change and founded the Philippine Nurses Association of Tidewater and a certified nursing aide school (Capucao, 2019).

Trends of Self-Care Across a Century

Because the Philippines has a predominantly collectivist culture, forming kinship ties among those with shared identities in the US provided a sense of familiarity and comfort and established a base for self-care. For example, during the mass migration of Filipino nurses at the mid-century, many of these nurses arriving together formed sisterhoods to cope with the isolation and foreignness of a new land.

Yet among Filipino Americans of my generation, I have often found estrangement. Many of my peers depict an array of identities across a spectrum of Philippine and American cultures. As of late, I have come to consider that being Asian American, specifically Filipino American, is its own politico-cultural identity that is up to us as a group to define—a collective identity not unlike our self-identity.

The aforementioned Filipino nurses' exploration of the unknown helped them better conceptualize who they were and were not as they learned how to be kind to themselves. I have found myself in awe of these nurses' respect for the past. Their ability to mitigate hardships by reflecting upon past experiences and reframing these experiences as silver linings or necessary obstacles toward a larger goal is a part of my own self-care practice.

While religion, particularly Catholic institutions, provided solace to many Filipino nurses, I have found spirituality and inner strength through other shared activities. For example, I practice photography and scrapbooking as reflexive practices of my ongoing journey. I also share their wanderlust and try to take in new experiences in all the places that I visit for research and conferences. These adventures lead to a constant inquiry of "who am I?" and help bring me closer to my authentic self (Capucao, 2020).

Nursing and Beyond

The beginning and end of stories tend to be the most memorable or celebrated; however, the middle part of my nursing school journey holds the memories that I cherish the most. Under the pressures of school and my own inner turmoil, the middle details my failures as an amorphous blob of disjointed identities and the self-compassion that I managed to nurture when I felt like nothing—breaking a long cycle of malformed identity formation.

As I have come to learn that my mind does not fare well during periods of change, self-compassion is something I wish that I had developed prior to nursing school. During my first semester, I moved into my first apartment living alone. I also stopped taking my prescribed medications for depression due to finally feeling that everything was going right: achieving my academic and professional career goals and being happily in love with my best friend. Yet what resulted was a total disaster. Naturally, a depressive episode overcame me, which led to my inability to focus and failure of an accelerated one-week course. During the meeting with the course professors, I kept apologizing over and over again, being more worried about what my parents, professors, and peers thought about me for being held back a year.

As a hopeless romantic, love was one of the few things keeping my depression at bay and urging me to keep moving forward; I constantly dreamed of finding that one person in the world who would accept me unconditionally and lead me out of the darkness. So, when I found love, I was the happiest that I had ever been but also the saddest. My self-identity would not allow me to be happy especially after failing, which then translated these feelings into other facets of my life, including my relationship.

Five months later, my boyfriend—the first person I have ever loved—and I had parted ways. Both of us struggled with our identities, and we had promised each other we would find ourselves as we went into different directions. There was not only a hole in my heart, but this idea of love that kept my depression at bay had vanished. The state of my mental health was at an all-time low, and suicidal ideation crossed my mind daily—with one attempt at suicide. I could not bear to be with myself and the constant influx of negative thoughts.

To say the least, my first year as a nursing student was a train wreck. Yet I managed to pick up the pieces in the face of depression, failure, and a broken heart by looking deeper into myself and showing myself compassion.

The silver lining about failure is that you can only move upward; these are the moments that make or break you and challenge you to be self-compassionate. After caring for patients and feeling love for someone else—and now living in its absence—I began a massive internal effort to pull myself out of the darkness on my own accord by reminding myself that *this is my* story, which is not a narrative of a tragic hero. I continually played into the trope of the damsel in distress by seeking approval from others and waiting to be saved by the silhouette of Prince Charming. Finally coming to this realization, I recentered myself upon my own design.

First, I addressed the need to improve my mental health and stop blaming myself for things out of my control. I found my drug regiment that best managed my depressive symptoms and underwent transcranial magnetic stimulation therapy. Then, I tried to remember who I was during a point in time when I was still carefree. This reminded me of my childhood dream of becoming a historian of healthcare—a strange dream for a kid, I know. Historical inquiry has always been my primary outlet for reflexivity, yet I never believed I was good enough to receive a doctoral degree. But then, I found a mentor—now my wonderful PhD advisor—who took me under her wing and helped me gain my confidence as a nurse historian.

As I went through my nursing program, I supplemented it with historical coursework addressing my research questions that revolved around identity. The experience was tiresome at times, and I faced naysayers challenging my career pathway, but all that mattered was a growing sense of inner peace within myself. Research for me has become both work and hobby. The perseverance to keep moving forward has been possible by opening myself to self-compassion and lessons from a diverse array of experiences, and more recently, listening to Korean pop band BTS, who provide a reminder to "love yourself." And now, I get to stand proudly next to my mom as a registered nurse and make sense of my identity, profession, and childhood dream as a nurse historian.

In Real Practice

Though complex and sometimes challenging to measure, the interconnected nature of social constructs such as race, ethnicity, gender, and socioeconomic status (to name just a few) are critically important to examine with respect to nursing education. Further, the term, "first-gen" carries two, both distinct and also overlapping meanings—someone who is first-gen might be the first in their family to attend a university, also someone who is first-gen might be the first of their family's generation to be born in the US. Please note that there is no consensus to date in the literature about these definitions of first-gen; thus, it is important to acknowledge first and foremost how an individual self-identifies. All of these factors contribute to an individual's and a community's well-being and thus merit close study.

Walder, Alderson, & Spetz (2020) ask how many of these factors may affect admissions into nursing schools. They find that there remains limited diversity in nursing school applications and that first-gen (first to go to college) students applying to PhD programs were less likely to be accepted. Only 30% of applicants identified as first-gen, and the majority of those applicants were also far more likely to be a student of color, immigrant, or international student. This study reminds us of the pressing need to increase diversity among our student populations and that we must reflect, constantly, on barriers to authentically supporting diversity. Then we should change those barriers to design more equitable schools and admissions processes.

Closing Thoughts

By revealing myself, I intended this chapter to serve as a blueprint for self-compassion among NOCs to address the unique self-care needs of their intersectional identities. Establishing congruency between self and identity has a significant role in developing self-compassion, as it supports self-acceptance amid times of success and failure. We need not agree with our identities, but we must learn to accept them as they permeate our very existence: actions, behaviors, feelings, and dreams.

As you continue on in your nursing journey, you will face structural issues that impose upon your identity, and there will be times you will feel unsettled or be unable to ascertain why you felt discriminated against. Practicing reflexivity through historical inquiry is one approach to explore self-identity and its produced interpretations and perceptions, helping answer the following question: Who am I?

Be kind to yourself and be open to the experiences of others, which will help contextualize your narrative. So, let me end this chapter by asking, "Who are you?"

Key Points

- Because NOCs compose an overwhelming minority within the nursing profession, they experience discrimination within a field made for and dominated by White middle-class women.

- Establishing congruency between self and identity supports unconditional self-acceptance, a shared trait with self-compassion.

- The development of self-worth may come from external (self-esteem) or internal (self-compassion) loci of control.

- Reflexivity, and historical inquiry by extension, nurtures self-compassion by providing a holistic lens of our identity to make sense of experiences surrounding it.

- Self-compassion can support the individualized self-care of intersectional identities of NOCs in environments filled with adversity.

References

Azmitia, M., & Thomas, V. (2015). Intersectionality and the development of self and identity. *Emerging Trends in the Social and Behavioral Sciences*. R. Scott & S. Kosslyn (Eds.). https://doi.org/10.1002/9781118900772.etrds0193

Capucao, R. Jr. (2019). Filipino nurses and the US Navy at Hampton Roads, Virginia: The importance of place. *Nursing History Review, 28*(1), 158–169. http://dx.doi.org/10.1891/1062-8061.28.158

Capucao, R. Jr. (2020, February 14). For the love of family: The Filipina/o nurse diaspora. *Routed Migration & (Im)mobility Magazine, 8*. https://www.routedmagazine.com/filipino-nurse-diaspora

Crenshaw, K. (1989). Demarginalizing the intersection of race and sex: A Black feminist critique of antidiscrimination doctrine, feminist theory and antiracist politics. *University of Chicago Legal Forum, Vol. 1989*(8). https://chicagounbound.uchicago.edu/uclf/vol1989/iss1/8

D'Antonio, P. (2010). *American nursing: A history of knowledge, authority, and the meaning of work.* Johns Hopkins University Press.

DiCicco-Bloom, B., & DiCicco-Bloom, B. (2019). Secondary emotional labor: Supervisors withholding support and guidance in interdisciplinary group meetings in a community hospice program. *Work and Occupations, 46*(3), 339–368. http://dx.doi.org/10.1177/0730888419848042

Foronda, C., MacWilliams, B., & McArthur, E. (2016). Interprofessional communication in healthcare: An integrative review. *Nurse Education in Practice, 19,* 36–40. http://dx.doi.org/10.1016/j.nepr.2016.04.005

Frey, W. H. (2018). The US will become 'minority White' in 2045, Census projects: Youthful minorities are the engine of future growth. *Brookings.* https://www.brookings.edu/blog/the-avenue/2018/03/14/the-us-will-become-minority-White-in-2045-census-projects/

Germer, C., & Neff, K. (2019). *Teaching the mindful self-compassion program: A guide for professionals* (1st ed.). The Guilford Press.

Graham, C. L., Phillips, S. M., Newman, S. D., & Atz, T. W. (2016). Baccalaureate Minority Nursing Students Perceived Barriers and Facilitators to Clinical Education Practices. *Nursing Education Perspectives, 37*(3): 130–137. doi:10.1097/01.NEP.0000000000000003

Hochschild, A. R. (2012). *The managed heart: Commercialization of human feeling* (3rd ed.). University of California Press.

Loftin, C., Newman, S. D., Dumas, B. P., Gilden, G., & Bond, M. L. (2012). *International Scholarly Research Network, 1*(19): 1–9. doi:10.5402/2012/806543

Mills, J., Wand, T., & Fraser, J. A. (2015). On self-compassion and self-care in nursing: Selfish or essential compassionate care? *International Journal of Nursing Studies, 52*(4), 791–793. http://dx.doi.org/10.1016/j.ijnurstu.2014.10.009

Oyserman, D., Elmore, K., & Smith, G. (2011). Self, self-concept, and identity. In Leary, M. R., & Tangney, J. P. (Eds.). *Handbook of self and identity* (2nd ed.). ProQuest Ebook Central. https://ebookcentral-proquest-com.proxy01.its.virginia.edu

Reverby, S. M. (1987). *Ordered to care: The dilemma of American nursing, 1850–1945.* University of Cambridge Press.

Smith, A., & Foronda, C. (2019). Promoting cultural humility in nursing education through the use of ground rules. *Nursing Education Perspectives.* Advance online publication. https://doi.org/10.1097/01.NEP.0000000000000594

U.S. Department of Health and Human Services, Health Resources and Services Administration. (1992). *The registered nurse population: Findings from the 1992 national sample survey of registered nurses.*

U.S. Department of Health and Human Services, Health Resources and Services Administration. (2010). *The registered nurse population: Findings from the 2008 national sample survey of registered nurses.* https://bhw.hrsa.gov/sites/default/files/bhw/nchwa/rnsurveyfinal.pdf

U.S. Department of Health and Human Services, Health Resources and Services Administration. (2020). *The registered nurse population: Findings from the 2018 national sample survey of registered nurses.*

Wagner, L. M., Alderson, A., & Spetz, J. (2020). Admission of first generation to college pre-licensure master's entry and graduate nursing students. *Journal of Professional Nursing. 36*(5), 343–347. https://doi.org/10.1016/j.profnurs.2020.02.001

8
Narrative Practices

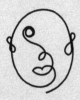

Tim Cunningham
pronouns: He/Him

Tim Cunningham began his professional career as an actor, then a hospital clown. He began doing international humanitarian work with Clowns Without Borders. While a clown, he fell in love with nurses' ability to connect with patients and families, even in times of terrible suffering—so he became an emergency nurse. The rest is history.

"Take no one's word for anything, including mine—but trust your experience. Know whence you came. If you know whence you came, there is really no limit to where you can go."

—James Baldwin

This chapter explores narrative practices and how they can be critical to not only self-care, but also in fostering compassion.

Narrative practices, reflective writing, and intellectual discourse have a common thread—one that is common throughout this text—the necessity of paying close attention. Research on narrative medicine for nurses and physicians suggests that engaging closely with the arts or literature (e.g., if you're examining a piece of literature, spending time looking deeply into writing style, theme, tone, and voice) can, over time, increase empathy scores and attention scores on various scales (Mangione et al., 2018; Ward et al., 2012). One study found that surgical residents were able to sharpen their attention skills through close involvement with the arts (Naghshineh et al., 2008). If you were about to undergo a surgical procedure, wouldn't you want the surgeon to have sharp attention skills? In your role as a nurse, don't you want to know that you won't miss a subtle change in your patient's status, a critical diagnosis, or some other telltale event that could cause injury or a decline in health?

Here, we begin with narrative medicine, a concept that is wholly interprofessional and that emphasizes ways by which we, as health professionals, can pay closer attention to the nuance and needs of the patients we care for. Narrative medicine provides us with a series of practices through which we can hone our attention skills and find stress reduction (Charon, 2016; Frank, 2017). By using narrative practices, we notice self-care occurring when nurses experience a sense of ease while growing as stronger, more attentive clinicians.

Dr. Rita Charon, a pioneer in narrative medicine, suggests:

> The effective practice of [healthcare] requires narrative competence, that is, the ability to acknowledge, absorb, interpret, and act on the stories and plights of others...Adopting methods such as close reading of literature and reflective writing allows narrative medicine to examine 4 of [healthcare's] central narrative situations: [caregiver] and patient, [caregiver] and self, [caregiver] and colleagues, and [caregivers] and society. With narrative competence, [healthcare professionals] can reach and join their patients in illness, recognize

> their own personal journeys through [healthcare], acknowledge
> kinship with and duties toward other healthcare professionals, and
> inaugurate consequential discourse with the public about health
> care. (Charon, 2001, abstract)

In the citation above, I have changed all terms in brackets from terms like "medicine" or "physician" to represent more inclusivity in healthcare.

Narrative medicine, by nature, is inclusive of all who provide care, but because it was originated by physicians, much of the early literature about narrative medicine is written from the physician point of view. This should not dissuade the reader, as you will soon see in this chapter that narrative medicine and narrative practices are necessarily interprofessional.

Let's begin by practicing: Alone, or with a small group of classmates or colleagues, choose one of the following websites for one of these world-renowned art museums.

- The Tate Modern: https://www.tate.org.uk
- The Metropolitan Museum of Art: https://www.metmuseum.org
- Museo Botero: https://www.banrepcultural.org/bogota/museo-botero
- The National Bardo Museum: http://www.bardomuseum.tn
- Tokyo National Museum: https://www.tnm.jp/?lang=en
- National Museum Australia: https://www.nma.gov.au

After you choose a museum website, scroll through and find a painting, sculpture, or other piece of art. Then, as a group, take a close look at that piece of art. Examine every little detail (and take your time doing this)—the lines, the hues, the brushstrokes, and the tone. Try to imagine what the artist was thinking when they made this piece, and then imagine what they were trying to convey with this art.

As a group, discuss in detail all the aspects mentioned above. Finally, converse with each other about how this work, this conversation, this exploration, made you feel. There are no right or wrong answers here. The key to this exercise and all the exercises within narrative medicine focus on close viewing, close listening, close reading, and concentrated, detailed discussion about the effects that the art, literature, or music has on you.

Think about your experiences with another art form: music. Have you ever found yourself so enraptured by a piece of music that tears well up in your eyes? A colleague and friend of mine, Dr. Chuck Callahan, once taught me that when he practiced as a pediatric intensivist and he would witness the death of a sick child, or when he had to give bad news to a child's family about the onset of a terminal illness, he would always take a few minutes—even during the busiest of shifts—to find a quiet place and listen to "Largo from Xerxes: Ombra mai fu" by Handel. He and I both listened to that song frequently in 2015 when we worked together treating Ebola patients during the West Africa Ebola outbreak. With what seemed to be endless suffering of all our Ebola patients, we found respite when listening to this song.

Books like *Violation*, by nurse Sallie Tisdale (2016); *When Breath Becomes Air* by physician Paul Kalanithi (2016); and *The Empathy Exams*, by standardized patient (or medical actor) Leslie Jamison (2014) can bring a sense of relaxation or elevated emotion when read. In fact, many nurses, physicians, and members of the allied health practices read these authors and many others, like Abraham Verghese or Atul Gawande, to reflect on their own experiences in healthcare and to sometimes make sense of the pain, suffering, *and* healing that we witness every day as care providers. Reading can bring relaxation; so too—for some—can writing.

This chapter will explore the benefits of narrative practices as forms of self-care. Inspired by the innovative narrative medicine work developed at Columbia University (Charon, 2017), this chapter will provide insights on how to use narrative practices to practice self-care. It will then set the stage for the two following chapters, which model self-care via narrative practice as shared by physician Mick Krasner.

Lived Experience

Neither classroom, nor course syllabus, nor any standardized exam will ever fully prepare you to truly, holistically care for another human being in the clinical setting. Consider what brought you into this profession. There is a common humanity among nurses and caregivers, a calling. That is a calling toward bringing health and healing. That is a calling that is not measured by Press Ganey patient satisfaction scores, Hospital Consumer Assessment of Healthcare Providers and Systems (HCAHPS) surveys, or board examinations—that is a calling that is experienced in the day-to-day engagements with other patients and their families. And it is that calling that narrative medicine and other narrative practices can help you understand. That calling is at the core of our lived experience. Uniquely ours, lived experience is an important aspect of our lives to examine because, from it, we will know ourselves better. In knowing ourselves better, we'll better understand our own, individual and critical self-care needs.

Lived experience is clearly subjective. It is the cumulation of your life experiences, to date, mixed in with the way you make plans, envision your future, and create your life goals. Lived experience is very challenging to measure or put in a concise box. Rather, it is abstract and even, in some opinions, subconscious. Max van Manen (2016) suggests that lived experience is *temporal*, meaning it blends periods of your life that are reliant on time—how your present is affected by your past and how your past helps to determine your future choices. In his scholarly book on poetry, Wilhem Dilthey includes an early definition of lived experience that helps explain the abstract nature of this term:

> A lived experience does not confront me as something perceived or represented; it is not given to me, but the reality of lived experience is there-for-me because I have a reflexive awareness of it, because I possess it immediately as belonging to me in some sense. Only in thought does it become objective. (Dilthey, 1985, p. 223)

This quotation may be confusing about lived experience. For example, how is a thought ever "objective" as mentioned in the last sentence? A thought cannot be objective, as thoughts only occur within the self; meaning that thoughts are subjective by nature. Further, Dilthey suggests that a lived experience is something that is not given to you, but a culmination of an experience in your life and how you interpret it. As you think about your cumulative lived experience, consider how you can use it to design your own self-care practices addressing your unique needs.

Self-reflection is another way to think about how you interpret your life and your experiences. There is a whole series of research methods designed to understand self-reflection; it is called *qualitative research*. Like lived experience, qualitative research, by nature, is also not objective. It collects data about the lived experiences of other people—their subjective experiences—and uses robust methods in order to understand that subjectivity. This kind of research validates aspects of human life that are not measurable by numbers, or with quantitative approaches. Qualitative data, therefore, are rich with nuance, as is lived experience.

By practicing various ways to reflect upon and understand your own lived experience, you can practice self-care. It is in better understanding yourself, the reasons why you are drawn to other people or not, the reasons why you make the choices that you do, that can also help you determine the best ways to care for yourself. Lived experience requires paying attention. It requires keen reflection. It can be challenging and also inspirational. To understand your own lived experience as well as that of others, you must begin with practices that resonate with mindfulness.

Using Poetry as a Tool for Reflection

−Irène P. Mathieu, MD (she/her)

Shortly after my grandfather died, a patient I had been caring for in the pediatric intensive care unit during residency passed away. It was a particularly tough situation for our entire team. A big part of self-care for me is about listening to what my body needs, and what I needed in that moment, physically, was yoga. I felt unmoored by my anguish, numb, and guilty for being alive. I needed to "be as inside of myself as possible." I also needed to process the disembodied feeling I had in that moment of compound grief, so after an hour of yoga practice I opened my laptop and started to write this poem.

I process things verbally—either out loud or on the page—so writing has always been a big part of my life. I don't ordinarily write about patients, but when I do I am careful to make sure that anything I share publicly is completely de-identified. But I still worried about voyeurism, as if I did not have a right to feel this grief for my patient. I shared the poem with my (nonmedical) writing group, and they gave me the space and permission to feel everything and to share what I felt. This poem illustrates the cornerstones of self-care that got me through residency—listening to my body, processing out loud, and surrounding myself with supportive loved ones.

---

having seen a child die I crave embodiment

I want to be as inside of myself as possible.
I am so swollen at times with my own blood & bones
it feels like a sin.

I stretch my hips & stand on my head for as long as I can stand it
and feel my stomach pitch with
someone else's grief.

I am as fit to bursting as the nectarines on my counter,
juicy suns wrapped in taut skin, sweet lucky tree babies—
hush a while, I want to say, to myself I mean, be the stillest thing
in the room for once.

my songbird hands don't get the message,
so once again I'm somewhere in the rafters
watching a platoon of words drumbeat for more. they know nothing
if not how to fight, and I've taught myself a mind is for nothing
but to make everything right. I've half a mind
to wrestle this down to the floor.

and then I think of when a plum-sized heart quiets,
the moment I watched
numbers drop
& drop

until it seemed they
would fall through
the earth,

and
they did.

they broke
the ground and through the hole
a fruit / a child slipped.

imagine being tucked
into the pocket of the earth,
how dark & warm
how nothing moves
how the body runs out.

the moment just before:
all that fight evaporating,
all the lightness
I would feel—
how blinding.

What Is Mindfulness?

Mindfulness is the act of paying attention. That's it.

When you sum it up and reflect upon this frequently, if not overly, used term, "mindfulness," it's all about paying attention. There are myriad definitions of mindfulness (Ludwig & Kabat-Zinn, 2008; Nilsson & Kazemi, 2016; Reibel & McCown, 2019; Young, 2016), but they all tend toward the simple adage of "pay attention." Paying attention; however, is not that easy to do. And to what degree should you pay attention? What are ways that you can practice paying attention?

The art of paying attention is discussed throughout this book, although we have tried to be intentional about placing mindfulness within contexts that connect the practice to real-life, in-the-moment situations. If you are interested in learning more about the practice of mindfulness, there are ample publications in the literature (nursing literature and beyond) about this practice. We are also aware that the term "mindfulness" has been used so frequently and in so many different aspects, it has become confusing. There can be a sense of elitism that is associated with mindfulness. Magazines about this practice often feature very affluent people in expensive, nonaccessible settings (for most people), thus subtly suggesting that one must have a certain and elevated socioeconomic status to be able to learn about and practice mindfulness. We do not want to promote that in this book.

Take a moment to look again at the image or piece of art that your group chose at the beginning of this chapter from a museum website. What new things do you notice about it? Do you feel the same about it now? To pay attention requires reflection, and as we reflect we may notice new differences or similarities. We may notice new tones or colors. The art of paying attention is the art of noticing how things change. Further, the art of paying attention helps us become more open to these changes as they occur.

Reflection, Refraction, Deflection, and Awareness

While you practice reflecting on an experience, a piece of art, the words said to you by a teacher, colleague, family member, or friend, have you ever noticed how others might be affected by that experience, too?

Reflection and paying attention, in this sense, is not just about you. Your own experience, whether it's tears during the sweet scene of a movie or laughter shared at a comedy show, affects others around you, whether you are aware of it or not. Think of the adage, "laughter is contagious." People around you may cry or laugh with you; they may do the opposite; they may have some other unpredictable reaction as they witness you reflecting on an occurrence.

As you reflect on an experience, *refraction*—the change in direction of a wave passing through one medium to another—can occur when others experience a piece of art, a patient interaction, a good book, through you. Some people might see you having an emotional response to an experience and they may, for their own defensive well-being, shut down emotionally or develop a flat affect while you are feeling intense emotions. This is a form of deflection.

What skills can you build to notice what happens when you or someone else reflects upon a thing or experience? How do you, or they, refract or deflect that experience? Awareness develops over time, with focus and intention. Your evolving awareness of how others experience events in their lives will help you develop a sense of connection to others, camaraderie with those you care for, and ultimately a sense of community, which is a form of shared self-care. This process of seeing how you affect others and are affected by others begins with reflection, and it provides a lens through which you can experience a phenomenon called "the space in between."

Personal Perspective

The Narrative Power of Music for Self-Care

-Lerner L. Edison, MSN, MA, RN, CNL (he/him)

Let's define self-care as a multifaceted practice. To me, music therapy is the key to the soul. I grew up in the arts as a French horn player and a mass choir singer. It was a time of joy and calmness with a renewal of passion for life itself. However, most of my days as a critical care nurse consist of death, grief, pain, and sorrows with minor celebrations. You have the power of life and death within your hands, while each intervention you do for your patient requires accountability. You must fight for the vulnerable, advocate for change, and think of others over self. These are some of the untold pressures as a nurse, especially a new graduate.

Self-care is a process to detach from others and create a safe space to reflect, meditate, and listen. Music therapy is an opportunity to self-isolate with a sense of protection from the outside world. It is a reminder of good health, financial stability, great relationships, and most importantly, the renewal of passion for nursing. This renewal allows countless opportunities to meet each patient, family member, and team member where they are. A simple touch, gesture, or word can change the patients' perspective or calm the environment. The music echoes are a reminder that nursing is a calling to lead, to care, to prevent, to change, and to show nonjudgmental compassion. We not only need self-care to heal self, but to heal others.

Sympathetic Resonance: The Space in Between

"The space in between," is a rather abstract concept. To help understand it, let's explore an idea called sympathetic resonance.

In its essence, *sympathetic resonance* shows how objects that are capable of vibrating will in fact begin to vibrate if they are in a space near another object that is vibrating (Von Helmholtz, 1912). If you are a musician, you can actually hear it sometimes.

Envision Sympathetic Resonance as a Symphony Orchestra

Imagine, for a moment, a symphony orchestra. You are an audience member in a full concert hall. On the stage, you see artists sitting with their violins, violas, cellos, double basses, percussion, and other brass and woodwind instruments. There is a piano on stage, too. If you've ever been to such a symphony, close your eyes and reflect upon the experience you had there.

Now, imagine in this specific symphony that there are suddenly no musicians on the stage. There is still a full audience of spectators and all the instruments are still there, laying on stage—perhaps they are in the musicians' chairs or in an instrument stand. The stage remains full, but with only instruments and no people. Once you have that image in your head, now imagine an individual person walking out into the middle of the stage. Just one person, and they're carrying a violin. That person stands on the platform where the conductor would normally stand, they lift the violin to their left shoulder and with their right left arm, bow in hand, they play an "A," the open position on the violin's A string. So, what happens next? Remember, the only person on the stage full of stringed instruments is that person who is playing just one note.

Every other A-string on that stage, on any instrument that has one (cello, double bass, violin, viola, harp, piano), begins to vibrate. You can measure this. The sound waves generated by the A string on the violin being played by a human resonate with all the other A strings on the stage. This phenomenon is called "sympathetic resonance."

The vibrations of one body can serve as the set of weak impulses that can set another nearby body into vibration. For example, if one strikes a tuning fork, its vibrations will cause vibrations in a nearby, similarly tuned tuning fork. This latter phenomenon—in which the vibrations in one object produce vibrations in another—is called sympathetic resonance.

Sympathetic resonance is an example of physical entrainment, in which periodic behavior of one object can be communicated to another, even when there are no direct physical connections between the two. (Dawson & Meddler, n.d.)

Let's take this a step deeper now: Think about a time when you experienced a piece of art or literature that moved you so much that you felt an emotion of joy or sadness. If this has never happened to you, consider a song that you've heard that resonates with you by stirring up a memory of the first time you heard that song. Another way to consider this is to think about a time when someone did something nice for you, gave you a gift, or simply said the words, "I love you." Did you feel those experiences in your body?

Think about a time when you encountered a patient, friend, or family member who was sick and being treated in a hospital. Did you feel emotions or a different kind of energy when you walked into the room? Did you, in some ways, feel their pain and connect with their emotional state? These feelings that you noticed align with the concept of sympathetic resonance. But remember that sympathetic resonance is physics, measurable science (Von Helmholtz, 1912). At this point, we're now experiencing emotional resonance, so let's change the term and take this concept to the next level: empathetic resonance.

Empathetic Resonance

Empathetic resonance is essentially connecting with—or vibrating with (if that's a phrase you can relate to)—another person's emotional state. Empathetic resonance is absolutely crucial when it comes to the healing arts, regardless of your profession within healthcare (Richards, 2018). As nurses, we experience empathetic resonance when we encounter a patient who is suffering. Through narrative practices that we'll explore in this chapter, you can practice your skills at empathetic resonance and reading "the space in between." And it is in this "space in between" where the empathetic resonance passes and occurs.

Compassionate Resonance

Let's next examine one final stage of the resonance process, which is called *compassionate resonance* (see Figure 8.1). As we resonate with one another, we can experience sympathy (knowing that someone is suffering); empathy (feeling someone else's suffering) and, if we choose, compassion (**doing** something about someone else's suffering).

As nurses, we may not always feel like we are stepping into compassionate resonance, the third and highest level of caring; alternatively, we may not even realize that we are doing it. Often, when there may not be enough supplies, or enough staffing on a unit, we must be creative in order to provide the safest, highest-quality and most compassionate care.

So how do we build creativity? Narrative practices are not only methods by which to practice self-care, but robust means through which to build creativity. In the next section I'll provide some ways to practice.

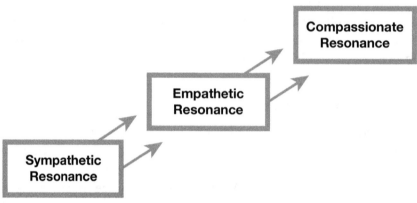

FIGURE 8.1   The resonance process.

Where are some places that you could practice narrative skills, or close viewing? In the next section, we'll practice this together.

Narratives of Health and Healing

To examine narrative medicine and narrative practices, you do not have to look just at nursing or medicine literature. In fact, you can and should expand your thinking far beyond these fields and look at how much of what is written or created artistically in this world has been inspired by health.

Music: Beethoven's immaculate *Missa Solemnis in D Major, Op 123* (1823), was written at a time when the composer was rapidly losing his hearing and literally shouting out into the universe as he mourned the loss of the skill that made him a virtuoso in symphonic music (Drabkin, 1991).

Graphic Autobiography: The graphic narrative turned musical, *Fun Home*, by Alison Bechdel (2007), encompasses themes of mental health and strained family relationships all the while layering its narrative arc within that of James Joyce's *Ulysses*, first published in 1922 (1993). Health drives our creativity, and ultimately our lived experiences.

Nonfiction: Let's consider the following excerpt from *The Autobiography of Malcom X*, where El-Hajj Malik El-Shabazz (Malcom X) describes his personal experience of witnessing his mother's care, and her state of health, in a mental health hospital. Read the passage below and then consider the following prompts as you practice close reading and reflection.

Applying Narrative Medicine Practice

It was so much worse than if it had been a physical sickness, for which a cause might be known, medicine given, a cure effected. Every time I visited her...I felt worse...

I can't describe how I felt. The woman who had brought me into the world, and nursed me, and advised me, and chastised me, and loved me, didn't know me. It was as if I was trying to walk up the side of a hill of feathers...But there was nothing I could do.

(X & Haley, 1993, pp. 22–23)

First, you should consider the monumental value of El-Shabazz's autobiography as a whole. His life, advocacy, and struggle has transformed the lens through which the US examines racial justice and equity.

Then looking more closely into this excerpt, you may notice El-Shabazz's concern that his mother is considered nothing more than "a case, a number" by the staff at the hospital where she is being treated. How does that resonate with your experience so far as a new nurse or student?

As his mother succumbs to her dementia, she no longer recognizes her son, Malcom, while in the hospital. El-Shabazz goes on to say, "I can't describe how I felt." We can look into this line and experience, for a moment, empathetic resonance, for those of us who have experienced a loss of words at the sight of a suffering family member.

As you continue your exploration into this narrative, it should not be taken lightly that Malcolm X, as brilliant an orator and leader that he was, was at a loss for words. You can imagine how this moment must have caused so much pain for him. Finally, to wrap up this brief examination, take the line, "It was as if I was trying to walk up the side of a hill of feathers." What kind of imagery does that evoke to you?

You could take hours to examine just a short sample of text like what we've done here. If you find joy in this kind of analysis, I'd encourage you to find more opportunities to practice it. Examine what the arts mean to you and the space in between—that is between you, the art, and others—and the many ways you are affected and how you affect others. Ultimately, this work will build your attention skills.

Narrative Practice in Action

From my experience as an assistant professor at a large nursing school in an even larger university, I have learned that narrative practices do not bring joy to all students. Please remember that self-care is not a one-size-fits-all model, thus if close readings, close engagement with the arts, or writing your own reflections do not feel like self-care to you, you do not need to push it.

If, on the other hand, you find inspiration in work like this, I'd encourage you to look deeper into it. By building your own narrative practice, you will see the world through different and variegated lenses, which could, over time, help you build your own clinical practice—one that is full of resilience and compassion.

The next chapter in this book is an example of how a clinician has incorporated narrative and mindfulness practices into his life's work as a physician, teacher, and scholar. As you read the chapter, consider how the many aspects discussed in this chapter are interconnected.

In Real Practice

Nurse researcher Dr. Carolyn Phillips and colleagues (2020) aptly combine the practices of storytelling, songwriting, and compassion to understand innovative methods by which to support the well-being of oncology nurses. In recognition of the suffering witnessed by oncology nurses, in particular, Phillips designed and then tests a intervention called "Storytelling Through Music." To test this intervention, which includes focus groups, narrative reflection, and songwriting with a professional musician, Phillips implements a quasi-experimental study—two-groups, intervention and control. The research team learns from their 43 nurse participants that through group reflection of their own suffering and then applying the performing arts to their experiences, this music intervention supports a sense of camaraderie. Further, it is shown to increase a sense of self-compassion and decrease a sense of loneliness.

In the next chapter, and our corresponding workbook, you will have opportunities to examine, experience, and practice empathetic resonance. Key to self-care is recognizing—paying attention to—the interconnectivity and *intra*connectivity of ourselves and our lives as professionals and human beings, friends and colleagues.

Closing Thoughts

Narrative practices, like narrative medicine, are evidence-based methods that not only can support self-care (if these are practices that resonate with you), but increase empathy and sharpen attention skills. Paying attention is key to these practices, as it is to the many ideas shared in this book, and it is also key to mindfulness. The arts remind us about the interconnectivity of health, well-being, and what it means to be human. By reflecting on experiences or art, then learning to build awareness about how your experience may be refracted or deflected by others, you can learn over time how to understand "the space in between," which is the space of lived experience and how it is shared between people.

Key Points

- Reflective practices can reduce stress, support self-care, and increase your ability to pay attention and build awareness.

- Health is often the root of many artistic expressions, and it binds us all in common humanity.

- As a nurse, recognizing how people respond to or detract from lived experiences can help you learn to acknowledge the wholeness of your patients and of yourself.

- Creativity is key when you practice narrative or reflective practices.

References

Bechdel, A. (2007). *Fun home: A family tragicomic.* Houghton Mifflin Harcourt.

Carroll, L. (2004). *Through the looking-glass.* Dover Thrift Edition. Digireads.com. (Originally published 1871). p. 14–15.

Charon, R. (2001). Narrative medicine: A model for empathy, reflection, profession, and trust. *JAMA, 286*(15), 1897–1902.

Charon, R. (2016). The shock of attention. *Enthymema, 16,* 6–17.

Charon, R. (2017). *The principles and practice of narrative medicine.* Oxford University Press.

Dawson, M., & Meddler, D. (n.d.). *Dictionary of cognitive science.* University of Alberta. http://www.bcp.psych.ualberta.ca/~mike/Pearl_Street/Dictionary/contents/S/sympres.html

Dilthey, W. (1985). *Poetry and experience* (Vol. 5). Princeton University Press.

Drabkin, W. (1991). *Beethoven: Missa Solemnis.* Cambridge University Press.

Frank, A. W. (2017). What is narrative medicine? *Journal of Medical Humanities, 38*(3), 339–343. https://doi.org/10.1007/s10912-017-9464-2

Jamison, L. (2014). *The empathy exams: Essays.* Graywolf Press.

Joyce, J. (1993). *Ulysses: The 1922 text.* Oxford University Press.

Kalanithi, P. (2016). *When breath becomes air.* Random House.

Ludwig, D. S., & Kabat-Zinn, J. (2008). Mindfulness in medicine. *JAMA, 300*(11), 1350–1352. 10.1001/jama.300.11.1350

Mangione, S., Chakraborti, C., Staltari, G., Harrison, R., Tunkel, A. R., Liou, K. T., Cerceo, E., Voeller, M., Bedwell, W. L., Fletcher, K., & Kahn, M. J. (2018). Medical students' exposure to the humanities correlates with positive personal qualities and reduced burnout: A multi-institutional U.S. survey. *Journal of General Internal Medicine, 33*(5), 628–634. https://doi.org/10.1007/s11606-017-4275-8

Mathieu, I. (2019). *Grand marronage.* Switchback Books.

McPhail, S. (2016). Multimorbidity in chronic disease: impact on healthcare resources and costs. *Risk Management and Healthcare Policy.* 9, 143–156. https://doi.org/10.2147/RMHP.S97248

Naghshineh, S., Hafler, J. P., Miller, A. R., Blanco, M. A., Lipsitz, S. R., Dubroff, R. P., Khoshbin, S., & Katz, J. T. (2008). Formal art observation training improves medical students' visual diagnostic skills. *Journal of General Internal Medicine, 23*(7), 991–997. https://doi.org/10.1007/s11606-008-0667-0

Nilsson, H., & Kazemi, A. (2016). Reconciling and thematizing definitions of mindfulness: The big five of mindfulness. *Review of General Psychology, 20*(2), 183–193. https://doi.org/10.1037/gpr0000074

Peterson Foundation. (2020, July 14). *How does the U.S. healthcare system compare to other countries?* Peter G. Peterson Foundation. https://www.pgpf.org/blog/2020/07/how-does-the-us-healthcare-system-compare-to-other-countries

Phillips, C. S., Volker, D. L., Davidson, K. L., & Becker, H. (2020). Storytelling through music: A multidimensional expressive arts intervention to improve emotional well-being of oncology nurses. *JCO Oncology Practice, 16*(4), e405-e414. doi:10.1200/JOP.19.00748

Reibel, D., & McCown, D. (2019). Mindfulness-based stress reduction. In I. Ivtzan (Ed.), *Handbook of mindfulness-based programmes: Mindfulness interventions from education to health and therapy*. Springer.

Richards, R. (2018). Empathy and relational creativity. In R. Richards (Ed.), *Everyday creativity and the healthy mind* (pp. 243–265). Palgrave Macmillan.

Rosenbaum, L. (2020). The untold toll—The pandemic's effects on patients without Covid-19. *The New England Journal of Medicine*. 382. 2368–2371. https://www.nejm.org/doi/full/10.1056/NEJMms2009984

Tisdale, S. (2016). *Violation: Collected essays*. Hawthorne Books and Literary Arts.

van Manen, M. (2016). *Researching lived experience: Human science for an action sensitive pedagogy*. Routledge.

Von Helmholtz, H. (1912). *On the Sensations of Tone as a Physiological Basis for the Theory of Music*. Longmans, Green.

Young, S. (2016). What is mindfulness? A contemplative perspective. In K. A. Schonert-Reichl & R. W. Roeser (Eds.), *Handbook of mindfulness in education* (pp. 29–45). Springer.

Ward, J., Cody, J., Schaal, M., & Hojat, M. (2012). The empathy enigma: An empirical study of decline in empathy among undergraduate nursing students. *Journal of Professional Nursing, 28*(1), 34–40. https://doi.org/10.1016/j.profnurs.2011.10.007

X, M., & Haley, A. (1993). *The autobiography of Malcolm X: As told to Alex Haley*. Ballantine.

Presence With COVID: A Day in the Life of an ICU Nurse

In his book, *Through the Looking-Glass,* Lewis Carroll provides a timely reflection. A young girl named Alice drifts off to sleep and dreams herself wandering through a backward world. At one point, she is standing at an enormous chessboard with a game in progress. She joins in, starting as a pawn yet hoping to become queen. After a while, Alice meets an actual queen and then finds herself sprinting as fast as she can after her. Alice runs so fast it's all she can do to keep up, but the queen keeps yelling, "Faster! Faster!" Eventually the queen allows Alice some time to rest and props the girl against a tree.

Alice realizes that, despite all the running, nothing around her has changed, as if she'd been on a treadmill the whole time.

For me, without being intentional about practicing self-care, I become Alice, exhausted and bewildered, running in place. My tendency is to run hard, work through lunch, and check email on my days off. There is certainly a time and place for hard work, but leaving these things un-checked, I become consumed by depression, anxiety, and hopelessness. Why am I doing all of this? What's it all for?

As I write this, it's been nearly seven months since the COVID-19 pandemic began. These months have been a blur. Making it through the first wave of this disease has highlighted how cumulative self-care is for me. Caring for myself—or not—adds up.

This pandemic is the most significant of any in our lifetime. As nurses, we find ourselves, as Alice did, running faster and faster, oblivious to the world around us, with barely time to catch our breath.

Amid this chaos, we must stop, slow down, and fiercely care for ourselves.

This day-in-the-life account affords me the chance to share some of my life as an ICU nurse during COVID-19 juxtaposed with the self-care habits I strive to practice. I hope it will give insight into how self-care can be woven into a typical, or not-so-typical, day. Self-care, thankfully, doesn't really take a lot of investment. What it does take is persistence—tenacity even—because doing small things for myself everyday—whether it be preparing a home-cooked meal, going for a 20-minute run, or taking 10 minutes to meditate—is what fortifies my ability to serve a purpose greater than myself.

Morning

The birds are chirping again, bringing me a sense of comfort. That's the first thing I notice, even before I'm aware of whether it's light or dark outside. The sounds of the morning contrast sharply against the noise of the intensive care unit where I work, where I'll soon be headed.

The ICU is full of bells, dings, beeps, whirrs, and the occasional screaming patient. The commotion is exhausting day after day, and we've added even more noisy equipment, loud humming fans called air scrubbers, to protect everyone from airborne contagion. While it looks like COVID-19 is only transmitted through the air under certain conditions, that we might be exposed to contaminated air is unsettling.

I've seen COVID-19 kill a lot of people, yet it's not a death sentence for most victims. The unknowns, public hysteria, lack of personal protective equipment—it all piles stress on top of stress. I no longer take my self-care for granted. To get through this first wave of the pandemic, I will revert to my healthy habits and hang on for dear life.

But now, I am lying in bed, listening to birds chirp. They invite me to wake up, to enjoy the morning.

My girlfriend Bharvi wakes up every time I try to leave, my anchor to the bed.

"Stay," she says, brushing my arm.

For a moment, I move closer to her and breathe her in. I feel a pleasant sense of gratitude. Pandemics strain relationships, but our relationship has deepened, and we have persisted in spite of, or because of, the crisis.

"Be present in this moment," I tell myself. I take a deep breath and feel the air moving through my nostrils, inflating my lungs. These small doses of mindfulness are a well that refills every time I draw from it.

I roll out of bed and chug a glass of water. I feel more energized and alert when I drink enough water during the day. Plus, the extra trips to the bathroom force me to take little breaks to clear my mind. I go through my morning routine, and in the quiet, I meditate for a few minutes with instruction from an app on my phone. My mind wanders and then returns to the present moment.

In through your nose, out through your mouth.

I assemble my lunch and grab something to eat on the way into work.

The Ebb and Flow of Self-Care

I do self-care in cycles. I can be nearly "flawless" for a while, saying no to the right things, eating well, exercising regularly, and meditating daily. Then life happens and knocks me off the self-care wagon. Being tenacious about self-care to arrive at the coveted destination of "healthyness" isn't how it works though. My mentor, Patrick, told me, "These are tools in a toolbox. Just because you have a hammer doesn't mean you need to go around banging on shit all the time." Moderation in all things.

I'm psychologically trying to stack the deck in my favor.

With COVID-19, my commute to work includes some dread about the day to come. Yesterday was hard. I know I'll have the same patients I had yesterday, although one patient may have died overnight. My other patient has a demanding family with frustrating and difficult personalities to contend with. I need to stay in the moment. Worrying doesn't help.

I've grown a lot as a nurse over the past four years. I continue to grapple with the uncomfortable parts of my work and my life. It's okay to be uncomfortable, and sometimes discomfort is necessary. I often tell my patients, "Part of my job is to push your comfort zone. You won't get stronger if you don't keep pushing."

The Shift Begins

I clock in, attend huddle, and get report from the night shift nurse for my patients today. Then I tidy up my workstation and patient rooms. Even though I know it will be trashed by the end of the shift, beginning with a clean workspace helps me think clearly. It makes it easier to notice when something is out of place, when supplies need to be refilled, or when my patient needs a closer look. It gives me a fleeting sense of control over my environment. I just have to avoid the temptation to keep straightening when it's time to care for my patients, to chart, or focus on quality improvement projects around the unit.

I call self-care a *practice* because it's largely about developing habits that condition my brain for when the game is on. I "practice" self-care on my downtime so that healthy thoughts and behaviors are more likely to bubble to the surface during and after times of stress.

It's like learning to put on PPE for patients with COVID-19. It took a lot of focus at first, intentionally thinking through each step: sanitize hands, put on gloves, sanitize gloves, put on gown, sanitize gloves again, put on another set of gloves, sanitize those gloves, put on mask, sanitize gloves, put on face shield, sanitize again, enter the room, and one more time, sanitize gloves. This process seemed painfully redundant in the beginning, but now I've done it so much I barely think about each step. The practice has been ingrained into my muscle memory, so that even during an emergency, I know I've placed my PPE safely. I know I'm protected.

One of my patients (I'll call him Mr. Jones) isn't doing well, so it will be a busy shift. When hearts stop beating, when we have to code patients , those are the days that stand out the most. The feeling of ribs popping and cracking beneath my palms is not a thought soon forgotten. Equally memorable are the days we counsel families as their loved one transitions through the end of life. But days where I care for patients like Mr. Jones are what really wear me out. He is very sick with a long road ahead of him, and our team is doing everything we can to give him that chance to recover, or at least a little more time for his family to find closure.

Mr. Jones is in his late 50s, in generally good health, but COVID-19 has been especially hard on him. His fingertips have turned a dusky black color with a purple hue, the cells dying right before our eyes. I feel stress build as I toil to keep him alive.

Small releases foster my own well-being. One way I do that is by verbalizing to folks around me how I'm feeling. I don't get too deep, but I at least acknowledge it and move on. This is another way meditation has helped me become a more resilient nurse. It has helped me identify and name what I am feeling.

Talking about feelings can be a challenge, especially in an ICU where colleagues talk tough. I get it, that their nonchalance about life and death is protective. Sometimes we have to make light of the daily traumas with humor, and I do that too, at times. It's not helpful to dwell.

Taking a full 30-minute lunch break is another cornerstone of my self-care at work. But it's easier said than done.

The third cornerstone is simply doing the work that needs to be done throughout the day. Being able to leave work with a clear mind demands that I put everything I can into the health and safety of my patients and my team. Some days I do better at that than others.

In addition to caring for some of the sickest patients our unit sees, I'm heavily involved in quality improvement projects and other shared-governance initiatives. These projects, while I often feel very energized by them, also pose a risk for further burnout because they distract me from my own health.

I'm proud and grateful that I feel so passionate about this work, yet without boundaries my passion can set me up for despair. I remind my supervisors of this sometimes, even though I fear coming off as needy, weak, or incapable. When my boss approaches me with a new project and I'm feeling overwhelmed, I'm honest about it. "I've been feeling pretty burnt out, and I need to take some time to address that." Saying "no" to new projects is a form of self-care.

Nearing the end of my 12-hour shift, I'm able to breathe easier. Mr. Jones has stabilized for the time being. My other patient passed. Despite the day's challenges, I believe I've offered some degree of relief to their families. As I get ready to hand off care to my night-shift colleague, it occurs to me that for all the fanfare about healthcare workers fighting COVID-19, not much has fundamentally changed in what we actually do.

While community members clap from balconies and fill our breakrooms with food, it does feel good to know folks are taking notice of nurses, but that doesn't relieve pressure from one of our most persistent challenges in healthcare: exceedingly limited resources (McPhail, 2016). Despite spending more on healthcare than any other developed country in the world, many of our health outcomes still rank as some of the poorest (Peterson Foundation, 2020). COVID-19 has magnified problems that already existed. I would feel less stress if we could treat these people better, if our workers felt safer, and if we had the staff and equipment to match our communities' needs.

Therein lies the importance of wise and prudent leadership within us and among others. Whether we can practice self-care as frontline workers during a pandemic isn't really the question. For most of us, self-care probably doesn't look that different than it did prior to COVID-19. What does strike me after this shift is that the most helpful kind of self-care should start long before disaster strikes. I hope more people are waking up to this reality.

Letting Go

After my shift, I walk to the car and start to decompress. I check in with how I feel and give myself space to talk about my day with Bharvi. I really don't want to explore my feelings, but I need to. They deserve attention and shouldn't be left in my head unchecked. Taking my eyes off the mental landscape would be like having a boss who neglects their responsibilities.

Today is hard because I'm angry. And I'm sad. There were the usual irritations: complaining co-workers, limited resources, too much work for one person. There were also the familiar moments where I caught myself in a negative headspace, imagining arguments with people that have never actually happened. But today felt heavier than usual. I wish more than anything that people would leave me alone.

"Sorry for being a grump earlier," I tell Bharvi, still steaming, still hurting from the day's events, from the exhaustion of COVID-19.

"You're a cute grump though," she replies, hugging me as we walk to the car. The nice thing about dating another nurse is that they generally "get it" without much explanation.

There's been a lot of death on our unit lately, and it's different now because family visitation has been suspended. Now the muscles in my arms burn as I hold a video phone, leaning over dying patients, with crying loved ones on the other end of the line.

Not only has COVID-19 itself presented us with sicker people, the uncertainties of the disease have further complicated treatment of more familiar ailments. Some folks are afraid to come to the hospital, so they're even sicker when they do finally show up (Rosenbaum, 2020).

As Bharvi and I gently unpack our workday together, I realize there's a silver lining amid all this negativity. Sometimes I just need to be angry and sit with this sadness. Sometimes I need to stew over the fact that the world's not perfect. I can be angry without treating others poorly. Anger can be scary, but it's only harmful if we approach it without respect.

At home, I do simple hobbies, and that helps. I always have a paint-by-numbers project I'm working on, or a few simple guitar chords I strum into a rhythm. Lately, Bharvi and I have been chipping away at puzzles. There's gardening, too. We only have a 10- by 3-foot balcony at our third-floor condo, but I enjoy the challenge of bringing nature home. These outlets, along with pure, unapologetic rest, reinvigorate me the most.

My self-care during COVID-19 is less about the tools I use to weather the storm, and more about forming healthier habits before the next crisis comes. The main tenets I return to involve practic-ing mindfulness, eating well, getting exercise, exploring hobbies, and embracing rest. My hope is these reflections will give you more confidence to practice and commit to self-care before whatever storm you face arrives.

As I wrap this up, writing this record of my day, there are indications of a second COVID-19 surge in the city of Atlanta where I work. I think of Alice, running so hard yet going nowhere. All kinds of thoughts are flying through my head about ways I can try to add value to the work we do, but for now that must wait. Like Alice, I may end up where I started, but perhaps it is *how* we run that matters.

9
Mindful Compassion:
A Life in Practice

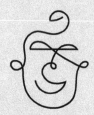

Mick Krasner
pronouns: He/Him

As the fifth of six children whose father was the seventh of seven children, Mick Krasner used his chaotic extended-family upbringing as his motivation to make sense of human flourishing. He attends to a busy primary care practice in internal medicine and also directs mindful practice workshops to help colleagues flourish in the chaotic and uncertain social networks within medicine. For fun, he enjoys walking—to nowhere in particular.

"In a world myriad as ours, the gaze is a singular act: to look at something is to fill your whole life with it, if only briefly."

—Ocean Vuong

As I contemplate what it means to bring compassion into the center of a life in healthcare, I cannot separate life into isolated parts—a life in medicine and another life outside of medicine. Compassion lives within all of life, unseparated, and is a potent and reinforced biological imperative that has not only survival implications for an individual and a community, but no less important repercussions for living a life of purpose, meaning, and joy. And this truth includes not only being with and acting toward the suffering of others, but equally and importantly doing the same for oneself. The two are facets that require one another.

So how do I write about this in a way that a reader of this chapter will be touched and perhaps transformed by the moments spent sharing the words on these pages? What strikes a strong chord within me has to do with intention and impact, using both narrative practices and my own experiences in exploring mindfulness. What are my intentions in sharing thoughts and ideas for something as important and fundamental to healthcare and to life as compassion? What impact might sharing thoughts and stories about compassion from my work in healthcare have? And, how do I craft a chapter that will have a positive impact and inspire the reader to cultivate the parts themselves that can enact compassion toward oneself and toward others?

What follows is not the usual chapter one would find in an edited scholarly edition on this topic, but a series of narratives and reflections illustrating how compassion and healthcare are inseparable, have always been inseparable, and are at the heart of not only a life in medicine but a life of meaning and the flourishing of humankind.

Mindfulness and the Beginner's Mind

"The only true voyage of discovery…would be not to visit strange lands but to possess other eyes."

–Marcel Proust (Proust, 1981, p. 260)

One of the things that has been important to me in my medical career has been integrating, teaching, and investigating mindfulness, and developing ways to share its promise with health professionals for improving quality of care, quality of caring, and personal well-being. My colleagues and I have created an intervention we call *Mindful Practice* (Krasner et al., 2009; University of Rochester Medical Center, n.d.), and among the qualities cultivated through this program is the well-known attribute of "beginner's mind." This capacity to see things, no matter how mundane or common, as new and emerging *in the now* sounds simple but is one of the most challenging qualities to bring forth in our clinical work.

Beginner's mind is a quality of *compassion*, of *suffering with*. Beginner's mind asks us to have an open and receptive orientation toward any experience, however difficult or easy, however rare or common, however complex or simple. It is a challenging quality to maintain, as there are so very many things that pull our attention and focus away from the present moment mindset, even if we have consciously and intentionally set our mind to see things freshly and experience moments as if they have never occurred before.

Barriers to Beginner's Mind

There are the regular distractions in work—from the "outside," such as telephone calls, staff interruptions, computer screen prompts, and from the "inside," such as the awareness of time pressures, the multiple tasks that need to be completed, the striving not to miss "big" or "risky-if-missed" diagnoses. At times, for myself I must admit, there are also the moments of such complete and rapid certainty that I close myself off to possibly being mistaken. We say things to ourselves like "it is textbook" or "we see this all the time." Honestly, there are times when I see another's suffering as one that I can understand fully, a suffering that is expected, and a suffering that just requires intervention x, y, or z to manage and fix. But the truth is that I have not actually lived within that person's experience, never, even though I do empathically resonate and feel something very real in relationship to it. No matter how much experience I have, no matter how deep my relationship with the other, it is impossible for me to fully know that person's experience.

But once in a while, even without our conscious and intentional efforts to return mindfully to the quality of beginner's mind, we experience events that do the work for us, that reframe our habitual views into panoramas that are more spacious than we thought possible. Moments like these remind me of the mystery of our work in medicine and deepen the meaning derived from that work. They are further reinforcements for the compassion that evolution has preserved so assiduously and for so many eons.

Personal Perspective

Designed for Compassion: A Story
−Elgin Cleckley, Assoc. AIA, NOMA (he/him)

It's been almost 10 years since a close friend of mine, who I will call S out of respect for his memory, passed away in a hospital room in a large North American city's main hospital. As his organs failed, creating swelling in the bottom half of his body in ways I had never seen, I remember S staring up through a morphine haze at the dilapidated, water-stained ceiling punctured with the usual array of flickering fluorescent lights from your average horror movie. The room, and the entire palliative care wing of this immense hospital, was grim. Concrete masonry unit walls cast eerie shadows through chipped beige paint, seeming to melt your thoughts in the un-air-conditioned hallways spotted with window fans struggling to create a breeze.

Cut to the hallway—our de facto conference room for consoling my friend's mother and relatives among more beige concrete masonry units. This became our space to have a good cry to not upset S. After one of these good cries during the last week of S's life, I realized that most of the lights were turned off to reduce heat from the blistering July day outside. The shadows onto the drab hallway seemed to intensify our pain—especially one day as we waited for a doctor to meet with us. We later chased him down in the parking lot, urgently wanting to know if test results from another hospital showed any hope. They did not.

I often think back to this scene, moving through thoughts of S's life and legacy, but also thinking about the six design elements (I call them 6D in my work) surrounding his last month. 6D are the spaces within the hospital, the systems of care, the objects and products utilized, the graphics throughout the facility, and the experiences of S, and us, in the palliative wing. 6D includes the organization and communication of doctors and nurses, the lighting and colors of his room, the fading signs of the wing, and the aged plastic pitcher holding ice shavings for S's forehead. What if these 6D were designed with compassion? S was quite particular of the artifacts around him in his short life, mentioning the drab space during one of his semi-lucid moments, saying to us, "This is a glamorous space to be in, eh?" I had no response to S, just quiet, agreeable silence.

Sometimes a Patient Makes Us Feel Seen

Recently I saw a patient I have cared for over 20 years, through challenges of the loss of her husband, family difficulties, complex medical problems and debilities, whom I was following up with after I received a call from her cardiologist suggesting that she enter into palliative care. We have a good relationship, and she is straightforward in her demeanor and does not hide her discouragement or her irritations. So, when I opened the conversation about her rapidly failing health, including the extreme unlikelihood of any recovery or even a plateau in her status, I expected to meet resistance or irritation or deep discouragement. Instead, I was taken aback when her response was one of relief. She shared with me how tired she has been of the struggle. She talked about the new opportunity in not proceeding in quite the same way as she had until now. She wanted to talk about what mattered most to her—how to simply sit comfortably, how to be a bit less breathless, how to comfortably allow others to assist and support her as her life draws to an end.

And then, quite surprising to me, she thanked me for helping her through all that she had been through. She did this in a way that seemed to understand the challenges I face as a clinician. As I felt compassion for her, this desire and need as a physician or any caring health professional to be with her suffering in an active way, a way that could lift her up even as she was falling and a way that could allow her to have a new view of her life, in that moment she was also engaging in a reciprocal process of compassion toward me. She could be with the suffering of her physician, the acknowledgement of the uncertainties and challenges I face of not only recommending the right care to the best of my capacity among the many choices available, but also being present with the inevitability of her own death. It felt as if she was standing in my shoes and seeing my world, at least imagining what it might be like.

And not only that, it felt as if she wanted to lighten my burden through her own compassionate action, if only just a bit. In that moment, I could not only extend and enact compassion toward her, but toward myself and direct self-compassion. There was mutual transformation in this exchange, and this is some of what the compassion imperative infuses within me, within us. Experiencing this mutual transformation through compassion, I understood the world slightly differently than I did previously. Facing this, I now see the work I do in a different light. Feeling this, I know now that my gaze has changed, and my vision can see more clearly and more deeply, as if I had new eyes.

"In difficult times carry something beautiful in your heart." –Blaise Pascal (Goodreads, n.d.)

The Mindful Practice program's objective is to enhance quality of care, cultivate relationship-centered qualities and thereby improve the quality of caring received, and improve well-being for the health professional. The contemplative practices, narrative exercises, and appreciative inquiry that are the building blocks of Mindful Practice work together to enhance the interpersonal and intrapersonal awareness that can influence the enactment of compassion within the clinical encounter. These qualities of awareness (which have the potential to interrupt habitual patterns of reactivity) are rarely more important than when encounters with suffering are complicated by the unexamined and habitual reactions to the empathic resonance they stimulate.

Empathic resonance, an evolutionarily developed and preserved feature of our humanity, occurs instantaneously without cognitive modification. It is a mirroring intrapersonally of what the other is experiencing (Ekman & Krasner, 2017). It is the first step in a sequence of events that leads then to a cognitive appraisal resulting in a choice of how to respond and whether to initiate a compassionate response. One of the challenges occurs when faced with human situations where either the suffering seems too much for us to be with or the darker aspects of humanity invoke fear or disgust. In such situations, our cognitive appraisals may lead us to distancing or blaming the other or turning that dissonance into personal distress, invoking a cycle of self-criticism or a lowered sense of self-worth. These reactions render compassionate responses much more challenging.

I currently see a patient I have been caring for a number of years who is now suffering from the ravages of alcoholic liver disease. There are times when it seems, despite severe illness requiring hospitalization for gastrointestinal bleeding or peritonitis, that he won't make the changes necessary to decrease his risk for further complications or for, dare I say, saving his life. And I have noticed moments of awareness when I feel within me anger, disgust, and disbelief arising. Yet, there are also moments when I can not only imagine but also feel and see the fear he lives with, the dread that his wife holds, and even the beauty of two people doing the best they can or being the best they can be in that moment. And I find that there is almost always a choice in how I want to hold his situation and his illness in my awareness. That holding can be described in no other way than compassion, simply being with the suffering. Part of that is also having compassion for my own sense of helplessness and for the human part of me that experiences those sensations of frustration, anger, and disgust. Sometimes it is helpful to me to simply acknowledge the presence of suffering of the patient. When I can and when I do, there is an inclination toward compassion.

I find it helpful to carry within my imagination images of beauty that deal with the truth of suffering, some of these by our greatest artists, who through their genius allow us to see and feel, to empathize and have compassion. In this way the world of art creates a laboratory for us to experiment with empathy—the feeling that arises when we can identify suffering, and compassion—the desire to be with that suffering and take some action. I am thinking of Van Gogh's *Sorrowing Old Man (At Eternity's Gate)*, Leo Twiggs' *Hooded*, Goya's *Self Portrait with Dr. Arrieta*, and Sir Luke Fildes's *The Doctor*. Not only do these images add elements of color, history, context, and diversity to the suffering witnessed in our work in medicine, but they add the truth of the universality of suffering and its centrality as a human experience in medicine and in life.

I urge you to search the internet for these paintings, or any other paintings that depict human suffering. Take a few moments to look at each painting, allowing yourself to empathically resonate and allowing compassion to arise. Notice what you observe in the paintings. Notice what you observe in yourself. Notice what you would say or do if you met the people depicted as they are depicted in these photographs.

> **"We've all heard that we have to learn from our mistakes, but I think it's more important to learn from successes. If you learn only from your mistakes, you are inclined to learn only errors."**
> –Norman Vincent Peale (Decision Innovations, n.d.)

Among the most challenging experiences for health professionals are the inevitable encounters with errors, our own and others, in our medical work. Even though it is understood that not all errors result in bad outcomes, and not all bad outcomes are the result of error (Blendon et al., 2002), the experience of errors in medicine challenges the health professional's sense of competence and self-worth (Wu, 2000). As a result, quality of life, depression, burnout, isolation, and future errors loom as downstream effects.

One particular quality of compassion—self-compassion—directs our capacity for being with the suffering of ourselves. Self-compassion can help mitigate some of the negative, self-perpetuating, and potentially harmful effects of errors experienced in medicine. Instead of focusing on self-criticism or denying and ignoring the internal experiences of suffering and pain, Mindful Self-Compassion—which is composed of self-kindness, mindfulness, and the recognition of our common humanity—can both soothe our emotional distress as well as open us to the pain of the suffering experienced, giving it space to transform and heal (Neff, 2011).

Working Through a Medical Error

The Mindful Practice program likewise contains an approach that helps health professionals explore errors and their effects on the individual practitioner and healthcare teams through sharing personal narratives about errors. This helps participants discover capacities to heal, grow stronger, and improve future quality of care. At its foundation, the intentional act of sharing stories about errors in medicine engages the bidirectional nature of compassion discussed previously. The storyteller, through contemplating and speaking aloud about the experience, and through examining personal attributes that help one to work through the episode, engages in a self-compassion process. The listener, by providing a nonjudgmental ear and by understanding as a fellow health professional what the experience of an error in medicine may be like for the storyteller, enacts compassion by being with their colleague, face-to-face with expressive human eyes behind them (Walker, 1998).

Early in my career, I took care of an elderly patient with multiple medical morbidities who presented with malaise and nonspecific symptoms. He appeared ill, but my exam revealed no particular focus. Lab evaluation did show evidence of something seriously amiss, however. Before I had a chance to review the labs, this patient had deteriorated and was admitted to the hospital ICU for sepsis from Fournier's gangrene. I had not examined the pertinent body part that would have helped me recognize this rare and serious acute infection. Needless to say, I was devastated, felt fully responsible, assumed the worst about my knowledge and skills, and questioned my commitment to my work, even my suitability for a life in medicine.

Shaken, I did turn toward the difficulty; I remained engaged in this patient's care and the long recovery process after the hospitalization. This included a series of home visits through the slow recuperation, a time where I was not only exposed to the intimacies of another person's life, but also began to develop a deeper sense of empathic resonance and potential for compassionate action. The lessons I learned from this formative experience have remained with me over the ensuing decades of primary care practice. Embedded within the error have been successes, capacities that I have been able to generalize in my work and in my life going forward. These faculties include the capacity to turn toward the dissonance, to be aware of the empathic resonance even when it is unpleasant, to engage in self-compassion, and to remain connected and in relationship despite complex challenges.

> **"Self-transformation is precisely what life is, and human relationships, which are an extract of life, are the most changeable of all, rising and falling from minute to minute."–Rainer Maria Rilke (Rilke, 1945, p. 151)**

COVID-19: The Greatest Healthcare Challenge of an Era

I am completing the writing of this chapter in the middle of one of the most challenging periods for healthcare professionals worldwide. The COVID-19 pandemic has presented challenges for patients, their families, healthcare professionals, and all their communities. One need only reflect on the realization of compassion as individuals and groups of health professionals selflessly place themselves face-to-face with the immense suffering at hand at great personal risk. Why do they do this?

Health professionals have the opportunity to live a life of meaning, satisfaction, and personal and professional flourishing through the transformative nature of human relationships. The biological drive to care for each other, and the sociological structures that make it possible to engage in a work where lives are transformed, supports individuals and groups of health professionals to be changed themselves. The changes they experience are reinforced at the individual one-on-one level, collegially, and communally.

We are all embedded in a complex web of interdependence, and human survival as well as human flourishing depends now and has always depended on our cooperation and connection. Compassion, which includes the triad of recognizing suffering, emotionally resonating with it, and taking action to relieve it, is a prosocial imperative for humankind. Health professionals, through the intimacy of

In Real Practice

It begins with paying attention. For many of us, we need coaching and support on how to do that in a healthcare context. Slatyer and colleagues (2017) present a controlled trial in which they try to measure the effectiveness of a mindfulness/resilience intervention. This study has no randomization to groups, which technically weakens the robust nature of the study, but, nonetheless it provides inspiring findings that should encourage future researchers to continue this kind of work.

In this study, participants in the intervention group were exposed to a day-long mindfulness retreat. After the retreat they received resilience coaching on a regular basis. Ninety-one nurses participated in this work, and although there were no statistically significant findings, a cursory (or anecdotal) analysis found that participants reported improvements in self-compassion and compassion satisfaction. The authors here suggest that there can be positive benefits from engaging in mindfulness and resilience coaching.

their encounters with suffering and their capacity to provide real, tangible healthcare, are the human embodiment of society's capacity to express concern, provide care, and enact compassion. Self-compassion cannot be separated from this because they must coexist. Compassion that embraces attentiveness, awareness, and love of humanity—philanthropy—in the end is as much a giving as it is a receiving and remains a moral beacon for all health professionals.

Closing Thoughts

Compassion and self-compassion are biological imperatives for humankind, and central drives that not only bring individuals into the practice of medicine, but also provide support for the complex and challenging experiences of health professionals. Through the lens of Mindful Practice, narrative reflections on professional experiences help cultivate some of the qualities of compassion. Within these narratives can be discovered qualities of curiosity, beginner's mind, recognizing the beauty within difficult human conditions, and even the ability to examine our own imperfections. The health professional, through intimacy with suffering, can enact compassion toward others and toward oneself and by doing so foster a life of meaning and purpose. To move forward into self-compassion and compassion for other, the healthcare professional must begin this journey with self-care.

Key Points

- Healthcare and compassion are inseparable.
- Compassion and self-compassion are mutually transforming.
- Beauty may be found within even the most challenging life experiences.
- Turning toward dissonance is an act of compassion.
- Philanthropy—love of humanity—involves giving as well as receiving.

References

Blendon, R., DesRoches, C. M., Brodie, M., Benson, J. M., Rosen, A. B., Schneider, E., Altman, D. E., Zapert, K., Herrmann, M. J., & Steffenson, A. E. (2002). Views of practicing physicians and the public on medical errors. *New England Journal of Medicine, 37*(24), 1933–1940. https://doi.org/10.1056/NEJMsa022151

Decision Innovations. (n.d.). *Quotes about mistakes in decision making.* Retrieved May 2020 from https://www.decision-making-solutions.com/quotes_about_mistakes.html

Ekman, E., & Krasner, M. (2017). Empathy in medicine: Neurscience, education and challenges. *Medical Teacher, 39*(2), 164–173. https://doi.org/10.1080/0142159X.2016.1248925

Goodreads. (n.d.). *Blaise Pascal quotes.* https://www.goodreads.com/quotes/410084-in-difficult-times-carry-something-beautiful-in-your-heart

Krasner, M. S., Epstein, R. M., Beckman, H., Suchman, A. L., Chapman, B., Mooney, C. J., & Quill, T. E. (2009). Association of an educational program in mindful communication with burnout, empathy, and attitudes among primary care physicians. *Journal of the American Medical Association, 302*(12), 1284–1293. https://doi.org/10.1001/jama.2009.1384

Neff, K. (2011). *Self-compassion: The proven power of being kind to yourself.* William Morrow.

Proust, M. (1981). *Remembrance of things past, The captive.* Random House.

Rilke, R. (1945). *Letters of Rainer Maria Rilke, 1892–1910* (J. Greene, & M. Herter Norton, Trans.). W.W. Norton and Company.

Slatyer, S., Craigie, M., Heritage, B., Davis, S., & Rees, C. (2017). Evaluating the effectiveness of a brief mindful self-care and resiliency (MSCR) intervention for nurses: A controlled trial. *Mindfulness, 9*(2), 534–546. https://doi.org/10.1007/s12671-017-0795-x

University of Rochester Medical Center. (n.d.). *Mindful practice programs.* www.mindfulpractice.urmc.edu

Walker, A. (1998). *Anything we love can be saved.* Ballantine Books.

Wu, A. (2000). Medical error: The second victim. The doctor who makes the mistake needs help too. *British Medical Journal, 320*(7237), 726–727. https://doi.org/10.1136/bmj.320.7237.726

10

Self-Care and Systemic Change: What You Need to Know

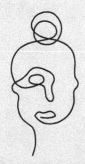

Ashley R. Hurst
pronouns: She/Her

After her legal career, Ashley R. Hurst became a clinical ethicist for an academic hospital. She quickly learned that nurses play a pivotal role in preventing and addressing ethical dilemmas in the clinical setting. She now teaches nursing students how to advocate for patients and changes to healthcare systems to promote the well-being of all.

"The moment I found myself envious of the man lying down on the operating room table was a startling and dark admission of the effects of my fatigue. I think of that time when I realize I have again ignored my own well-being."

—Rishi Doshi, MD

Note to reader:

This chapter presents a perspective that you might not expect to find in a self-care book, but we felt we would be remiss if we did not directly address the issue of institutional responsibility for staff well-being. We weave this issue throughout this book, beginning with the myth that individual self-care practices let organizations off the hook, and a chapter on the importance of finding a healthy work environment for your first nursing position.

The inclusion of this chapter became even more urgent with the onset of COVID-19. As it did with so many things, the pandemic starkly revealed many of this nation's (and other countries') strengths, as well as its weaknesses. At our own institutions and beyond, we saw frontline nurses (as well as physicians and other staff) suffering in unimaginable ways. The unrelenting stream of patients, death, and isolation seemed more than anyone should have to bear, especially those working so hard to comfort the sick and dying. To our regret, much of nurse suffering could have been alleviated by the hospitals where they work. Many institutions failed to adequately offer care and compassion to their own staff. It is not a stretch to suggest that much clinician distress can be addressed by the institutions where it occurs, and that individual self-care practices alone do not preclude suffering due to unhealthy work environments. This tension between self-care and institutional responsibility is the focus of this chapter.

Are self-care practices enough? You may have met or heard about nurses who regularly practice self-care but who still struggle with the stressors in their work environments. Unfortunately, this can sometimes be the case, and one reason may be factors that you cannot control. The power of self-care practices to help you handle stressful situations in your nursing practice is backed by years of research. But these practices can't fix many of the systemic problems nurses face. Thus, self-care practices come with a caveat: Self-care practices play an important role in your well-being and professional satisfaction, but they can't fix everything, nor should they.

Causes of Burnout in Nursing

One of the many reasons to incorporate self-care practices into your routine is to cope with the stresses of the nursing profession. Some work stress is to be expected in the demanding nature of nursing practice and modern healthcare. Yet, work stress can rise to abnormal levels, leading to burnout. Burnout is a leading cause of nurses leaving their professional practice (Brown et al., 2018; National Academies of Sciences, Engineering, and Medicine [NASEM], 2019). There are also multiple negative consequences for nurses, patients, and the healthcare community from burnout, such as substance abuse, depression and anxiety, disengagement, higher mortality rates for patients, and nursing shortages (Halm, 2019; NASEM, 2019). The top causes of nursing burnout are excessive workload; moral distress; and lack of resources, professional autonomy, and decision-making authority (Mudallal et al., 2017). A regular self-care practice is one way to reduce burnout. But there is more to the story.

Consider some concerning facts about nursing burnout:

- 35–45% of nurses experience burnout
- Nurses in hospitals and nursing homes have the highest rates of burnout
- Younger nurses have higher rates of burnout
- Women have increased rates of burnout relative to male colleagues

  (NASEM, 2019; Rees et al., 2016)

One unintended consequence of promoting self-care practices as a way to reduce burnout is the focus on the individual practitioner in isolation, rather than as a professional member of a team and complex system.

Pause for a moment and consider this poem by Dr. Rishi Doshi (Figure 10.1). The image that it is cast on came from a collaboration between Doshi and the artist, Nikeeta Shah.

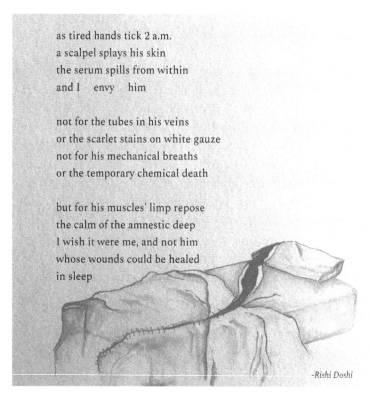

as tired hands tick 2 a.m.
a scalpel splays his skin
the serum spills from within
and I   envy   him

not for the tubes in his veins
or the scarlet stains on white gauze
not for his mechanical breaths
or the temporary chemical death

but for his muscles' limp repose
the calm of the amnestic deep
I wish it were me, and not him
whose wounds could be healed
in sleep

-*Rishi Doshi*

FIGURE 10.1   "Night in OR #5," Rishi Doshi, MD (@rishipoetry).

After writing this poem, Dr. Doshi reflected on what inspired him to create this work that revealed his own burnout in a haunting and meaningful way. You can read his thoughts in the epigraph to this chapter, when he states: "The moment I found myself envious of the man lying down on the operating room table was a startling and dark admission of the effects of my fatigue. I think of that time when I realize I have again ignored my own well-being" (NAM, n.d.b).

Clearly, burnout affects us all, and it should never be put on us as individuals to solve on our own. In fact, one unintended consequence of promoting self-care practices as a way to reduce burnout is the focus on the individual practitioner as the problem to be fixed and not the systems causing the stressful work environment. Many hospitals and clinical practices offer programs that focus on the individual

clinician, such as mindfulness-focused workshops and incentivized exercise programs. It follows, however, that if work stress is the result of inadequate staffing,
lack of practice autonomy, and interprofessional collaboration, for example, then
self-care alone will not remedy these issues. Organizational leadership must focus on solving these complex issues with more than clinician-focused programs
(NASEM, 2019; Shanafelt & Noseworthy, 2017). Instituting clinician-focused
programs without institution-wide efforts to address systems issues sends the message that individual clinicians are on their own when it comes to their well-being.
Healthy work environments with supportive administrations are keys to reducing
burnout; but organizational programs that focus solely on a provider's individual
practices inadvertently blame the provider for their own burnout.

Nurse and artist Julie Shinn brings to life the challenges nurses face, acutely so
during the COVID-19 pandemic (Figure 10.2).

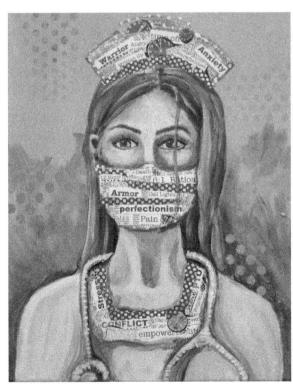

FIGURE 10.2   *Isolation Mask* by
Julie Shinn.

Shimm describes her own work of art saying:

"Health care is physically, emotionally, and mentally draining, and while great strides have been instituted to protect patients, more needs to be done to protect clinicians. Adequate staffing is a must, as is a less punitive work environment" (NAM, n.d.a).

As a nursing student or early career nurse, it is important to recognize that no self-care practice can fix the system you work in. When you valiantly try to breathe, meditate, walk in the woods, or exercise and you aren't feeling relief, this is a sign that something in the system needs to change.

Moral Distress and You

A leading cause of burnout in nurses is moral distress (Epstein et al., 2019). *Moral distress* is generally defined as the belief that you know the morally right thing to do but cannot do it because of external or internal barriers. It has been studied in nurses for decades and is the result of systems issues that prevent nurses and other healthcare providers from engaging in morally correct actions. The root causes of moral distress are institutional causes, not personal ones.

Common causes of moral distress include continuing aggressive care not in the best interests of the patient; watching patient care suffer from lack of provider continuity; staffing shortages that endanger patient care; and poor team communication (Whitehead et al., 2015). However, moral distress is *experienced by* the individual nurse, physician, or other clinician. In other words, you experience moral distress, but its cause is rooted in the work environment.

Resiliency training and other self-care related practices have been encouraged as ways for nurses to address moral distress and the related burnout (Brown et al., 2018). However, as noted with burnout, because you are not the root cause of the moral distress, you cannot change something about yourself to fix the root causes of moral distress. Instead, organizational leadership (e.g., unit managers, medical directors, hospital administrators) must address the causes through policy changes, resource support, and empowered decision-making.

Moral Distress, Empowerment, and Advocacy

Nurses in a medical ICU experienced moral distress due to high nurse-to-patient ratios. The unit's high nurse turnover resulted in the high ratios, as did the recent decision by leadership to eliminate all part-time nursing positions. The ICU nurses believed they were unable to provide safe, high-quality care to all their patients due to the staffing ratios. However, many nurses did not speak up for fear they would be seen as not a team player and not a hard worker. Other nurses did speak up to their unit manager but were told budget cuts required this level of staffing.

After a near-fatal patient event, nurses asked to debrief the event with a non-unit-based ethicist. In the discussion, the nurses identified the staffing shortage and attendant stress as a contributing factor to the patient event. The nurses also validated each other's fear of being seen as weak or not a team player and feeling like nothing could be done about staffing because it was an administration decision.

However, hearing and affirming each other's concerns empowered the nurses to speak to unit leadership as a group. As a result of their advocacy, hospital management authorized the closing of ICU beds when staffing was low. By debriefing and then acting collectively in response to their moral distress, the nurses affected system changes to support their patients and themselves.

You play a critical role in bringing morally distressing events to the attention of leadership, as well as playing an active part in solving systems issues that cause or enable moral distress. Although upsetting, your experience of moral distress can serve as a catalyst to meaningful, systemic change. Thus, if self-care practices are viewed as a way to fix your moral distress, they won't help. But they can support you through morally distressing events so you can advocate for change.

The Resiliency Dilemma

Some would argue that healthcare organizations and educators are promoting a more resilient nursing workforce as the answer to nursing shortages, high turnover rates, and other challenges facing the nursing profession. But what are the benefits of resiliency for nurses and healthcare in general, and is the goal of more resilient nurses a good one?

Resiliency means the ability to adapt to or bounce back from distressing situations (Rushton et al., 2015). Given the high demands on nurses and other clinicians, the ability to bounce back from distressing situations is an important skill for well-being. The ability to return to a demanding environment shift after shift—whether in the ICU, emergency department, or an understaffed floor or clinic—is considered the hallmark of a resilient nurse. But should our goal be for nurses to increase their individual capacities to bounce back from traumatic, distressing events so that they can continue to face more of them? Does the call for resilient nursing allow healthcare administrators, systems, and society at large to ask more from nurses than is just?

The origins of the nursing profession in the Western world were steeped in a mythology of heroic, self-sacrificing women who cared for the sick and injured out of a sense of divine calling and innate ability (Gordon & Nelson, 2005). The legend of Florence Nightingale became the archetype of the "good nurse." We clearly saw the echoes of this origin myth during Hurricane Katrina in New Orleans in 2005 and more recently during the COVID-19 pandemic.

On one hand, nursing is consistently voted the most trusted profession in America (Reinhart, 2020). On the other hand, nurses face the most workplace violence of any profession, with very little public awareness (Occupational Safety and Health Administration, n.d.). And, as we saw during the COVID-19 pandemic, while nurses were being hailed as heroes, they also faced increased exposure risks, particularly in settings with inadequate PPE and other resource supports. Many nurses were then flexed or furloughed from their jobs due to hospital financial instability when the COVID-19 caseload decreased.

We trust nurses to care for us and our loved ones, but it seems that we also trust them to bounce back from whatever adversity comes their way. Is this a fair and just expectation? Do we need nurses to be even more resilient so they can face even more trauma and distress? Or do we owe nurses meaningful change that reduces the traumatic and distressing situations they face in practice? Building nurses' personal resilience is certainly important. However, if the primary goal is their well-being, we must not ignore the underlying systemic issues that, if addressed, will reduce the distress and traumatic experiences nurses routinely face.

Working for Change

As noted above, self-care practices often focus on helping nurses be more resilient and avoid burnout. Our society and all healthcare systems depend on nurses to provide safe and effective care. But we also need nurses who can advocate for changes in systems that fail to promote the health of patients and providers. Speaking up against policies and procedures that don't support patient and provider well-being is an essential role of the nurse.

Self-care practices play an important role in enabling nurses to continue working in the profession and to continue working for change. Pairing self-care practices with advocacy empowers nurses to change systems that are not promoting health for all. As poet and social activist Audre Lorde famously said, "Caring for myself is not self-indulgence, it is self-preservation, and this is an act of political warfare" (Lorde, 2017, p. 130). We need nursing voices in every arena of healthcare to call for change and help implement it. A focus on self-care practices without coupling them with changes in the system undermines the power of self-care.

#selfcare

There is another cultural phenomenon at play here: #selfcare. Self-care concepts have taken social media by storm recently, with posts and pictures of the latest practices and fads. Although entertaining at times, the social media version of self-care is often misleading and needs to be differentiated from the self-care practices in this book.

The #selfcare social media movement is frequently presented as a hyper-feminine form of self-indulgence. From bubble baths to spa days, what is depicted on social media is often a caricature of self-care practices aimed at selling products and competing with one's Instagram followers. The explosion of the #selfcare movement has created a $10 billion industry (Silva, 2017). Even Mattel, a global toy company, is riding the #selfcare wave by introducing a line of self-care Barbies, including Breathe with Me Barbie, Fitness Barbie, and Spa Barbie that come with bath bombs, face masks, and yoga pants (Lampen, 2020). Although there is nothing inherently wrong with relaxing soaks or massages, the #selfcare message echoes unhelpful gender stereotypes of pampered women and in no way reflects the mental work intrinsic to a true self-care practice.

Additionally, studies show that #selfcare is creating yet another arena for public display and competition, contributing to a negative self-image in those judging themselves lacking in Instagrammable self-care practices (Lieberman, 2018). Competitive #selfcare practices are by definition not self-care. Sharing and teaching your self-care practices with others is an excellent way to expand the positive effects of the practices in this book. But to the extent that #selfcare promotes another metric telling you how you are falling short in comparison to your peers, it's destructive and the antithesis of true self-care practices.

So how do you respond to the #selfcare movement? As an initial step, differentiating for yourself self-care practices you use to reduce school and work stress from pop culture practices is essential. A facial or bingeing on Netflix is not the same as mindfulness-based stress reduction or other self-care practices described in this book. Being able to describe these differences to others is equally important. Unit managers, colleagues, administrators and friends and family may also need help in understanding that the practices you prioritize are not the same as what they see on social media. Sharing the information in this book with them may help them understand the difference and better support your practices.

Mental Health and #selfcare

Another challenge presented by the #selfcare movement is the unintended undermining of serious mental health concerns. Although self-care practices can reduce feelings of anxiety and depression, they alone are not the answer to all mental health concerns. After years of trying to destigmatize mental health concerns, the #selfcare movement may be unintentionally restigmatizing those who need professional support by suggesting you can meditate away a mental illness. This movement also suggests that addressing mental health concerns is quick, cheap, and easy. Although adopting healthy practices that relieve stress can be an important part of responding to anxiety and depression, seeking professional care is also often necessary. Indeed, there is growing concern among mental health counselors that clients, especially young adults, are choosing #selfcare practices as what they perceive as a more expedient way to address serious mental health issues (Goodman, 2019).

The hyper-feminization of #selfcare may also exacerbate the gender gap that already exists between men and women seeking professional mental health treatment, as men are statistically less likely to seek mental healthcare than women (Pattyn et al., 2015). If the #selfcare movement sends even the subtle message that facials, bubble baths, and manicures are an effective way to treat anxiety and depression, then anyone who does not resonate with these practices may feel further isolated from healthy ways to address their mental health needs.

What can you do to push back against these unhelpful stereotypes enmeshed in the #selfcare movement? As a role model for your patients and peers, you play an important part in normalizing professional mental health treatment and dispelling the idea that personal self-care practices alone can effectively treat all mental health concerns (Feist et al., 2020).

> ## In Real Practice
>
> One way to improve working conditions for nurses is through advocacy. Tomajan (2012) provides a detailed description of the skills and steps required to engage in successful advocacy for yourself, your colleagues, and your patients. Important skills include problem-solving, communication, influence, and collaboration. In this time of rapid change in healthcare, nurses are a valuable voice in point-of-care, healthy work environment, and appropriate resource advocacy. Nurse educators have a powerful role to play in advocacy for the profession, as well.

Closing Thoughts

As the other chapters in this book describe, adopting self-care practices is essential to your roles as nursing student and nurse. However, your self-care practices alone cannot change the systemic problems currently causing high levels of burnout among healthcare workers, particularly new nurses. Systemic problems such as understaffing, as well as lack of interprofessional collaboration, professional autonomy, and adequate resources, require advocacy and critical problem-solving beyond individual self-care practices.

An overreliance on nurse resiliency training or mindfulness-focused programs by healthcare institutions can mask the need for system-level responses. Your self-care practices can support you in advocating for changes that support a safe and healthy work environment; they just cannot solve all the problems nurses face. Moreover, the rise of the #selfcare movement has cast a shadow over self-care practices. Educating others about your practices and their value to your well-being as distinct from the #self-care movement can help dispel this shadow. This is particularly important because #selfcare is often portrayed as a hyper-feminine and simplistic way to address not only daily stress but mental health concerns that require professional support. When we say that you are not alone in your self-care practice, we are acknowledging the necessity of seeking help when needed. So as all good things do, self-care practices come with a warning—they can't fix everything, but they can help sustain you so you can advocate for the changes the world needs.

Key Points

- Self-care practices alone cannot change systems problems.

- Systems problems lead to burnout and moral distress, particularly in new nurses.

- Combine self-care practices with advocacy to effect positive system changes.

- Differentiate self-care practices from the #selfcare movement.

References

Brown, S., Whichello, R., & Price, S. (2018). The impact of resiliency on nurse burnout: An integrative literature review. *MEDSURG Nursing, 27*(6), 349–378.

Epstein, E. G., Whitehead, P. B., Prompahakul, C., Thacker, L. R., & Hamric, A. B. (2019). Enhancing understanding of moral distress: The measure of moral distress for health care professionals. *AJOB Empirical Bioethics, 10*(2), 113–124. https://doi.org/10.1080/23294515.2019.1586008

Feist, J. B., Feist, J. C., & Cipriano, P. (2020). Stigma Compounds the Consequences of Clinician Burnout During COVID-19: A Call to Action to Break the Culture of Silence. *NAM Perspectives*.

Goodman, W. (2019, July 12). When self-care becomes a weapon. *Psychology Today*. https://www.psychologytoday.com/us/blog/healing-together/201907/when-self-care-becomes-weapon

Gordon, S., & Nelson, S. (2005). And end to angels: Moving away from the 'virtue' script toward a knowledge-based identity for nurses. *American Journal of Nursing, 105*(5), 62–69.

Halm, M. (2019). The influence of appropriate staffing and healthy work environments on patient and nurse outcomes. *American Journal of Critical Care*, 28(2), 152–156. https://doi.org/10.4037/ajcc2019938

Lampen, C. (2020, January 30). World's busiest career woman finally engages in self-care. *The Cut*. https://www.thecut.com/2020/01/wellness-barbie-introduced-to-teach-kids-about-self-care.html#_ga=2.158804346.1546021492.1583856305-299397566.1583856305

Lieberman, C. (2018, August 10). How self-care became so much work. *Harvard Business Review*. https://hbr.org/2018/08/how-self-care-became-so-much-work

Lorde, A. (2017). *A burst of light: And other essays*. Courier Dover Publications.

Mudallal, R. H., Othman, W. M., & Al Hassan, N. F. (2017). Nurses' burnout: The influence of leader empowering behaviors, work conditions, and demographic traits. *Inquiry: A Journal of Medical Care Organization, Provision, and Financing*, 54. https://doi.org/10.1177/0046958017724944

National Academies of Sciences, Engineering, and Medicine. (2019). *Taking action against clinician burnout: A systems approach to professional well being*. The National Academies Press. https://doi.org/10.17226/25521

National Academy of Medicine. (n.d.a). Expressions of clinician well-being: an art exhibition. Retrieved from: https://nam.edu/expressclinicianwellbeing/#/artwork/197

National Academy of Medicine. (n.d.b). Expressions of clinician well-being: an art exhibition. Retrieved from: https://nam.edu/expressclinicianwellbeing/#/artwork/199

Occupational Safety and Health Administration. (n.d.). *Workplace violence in healthcare: Understanding the challenge*. U.S. Department of Labor. https://www.osha.gov/Publications/OSHA3826.pdf

Pattyn, E., Verhaeghe, M., & Bracke, P. (2015). The gender gap in mental health service use. *Social Psychiatry and Psychiatric Epidemiology, 50*(7), 1089–1095. https://doi.org/10.1007/s00127-015-1038-x

Rees, C. S., Heritage, B., Osseiran-Moisson, R., Chamberlain, D., Cusack, L., Anderson, J., Terry, V., Rogers, C., Hemsworth, D., Cross, W., & Hegney, D. G. (2016). Can we predict burnout among student nurses? An exploration of the ICWR-1 Model of Individual Psychological Resilience. *Frontiers in Psychology, 7*, 1072. https://doi.org/10.3389/fpsyg.2016.01072

Reinhart, R. J. (2020, January 6). Nurses continue to rate highest in honesty, ethics. *Gallup*. https://news.gallup.com/poll/274673/nurses-continue-rate-highest-honesty-ethics.aspx

Rushton, C. H., Batcheller, J., Schroeder, K., & Donohue, P. (2015). Burnout and resilience among nurses practicing in high-intensity settings. *American Journal of Critical Care*, 24(5), 412–421. https://doi.org/10.4037/ajcc2015291

Shanafelt, T. D., & Noseworthy, J. H. (2017). Executive leadership and physician well-being: Nine organizational strategies to promote engagement and reduce burnout. *Mayo Clinic Proceedings*, 92(1), 129–146. https://www.mayoclinicproceedings.org/article/S0025-6196(16)30625-5/pdf

Silva, C. (2017, June 4). *The millennial obsession with self-care*. NPR. https://www.npr.org/2017/06/04/531051473/the-millennial-obsession-with-self-care

Tomajan, K. (January 31, 2012). Advocating for nurses and nursing. *OJIN: The Online Journal of Issues in Nursing, 17*, (1), Manuscript 4.

Whitehead, P. B., Herbertson, R. K., Hamric, A. B., Epstein, E. G., & Fisher, J. M. (2015). Moral distress among healthcare professionals: Report of an institution-wide survey. *Journal of Nursing Scholarship, 47*(2), 117–125. https://doi.org/10.1111/jnu.12115

11

Strengths-Based Self-Care: Good Enough, Strong Enough, Wise Enough

Tim Cunningham
pronouns: He/Him

Tim Cunningham began his professional career as an actor, then a hospital clown. He began doing international humanitarian work with Clowns Without Borders. While a clown, he fell in love with nurses' ability to connect with patients and families, even in times of terrible suffering—so he became an emergency nurse. The rest is history.

"Someone who has experienced trauma also has gifts to offer all of us—in their depth, their knowledge of our universal vulnerability, and their experience of the power of compassion."

—Sharon Salzburg

By this point in the book you may be feeling overwhelmed about all the options you have to practice self-care. There is a lot on your plate. If you don't feel over-whelmed, excellent! If you do—there is nothing wrong with that, by the way—this chapter is especially for you. The take-home message here is simple: You are good enough, strong enough, capable enough to succeed. Succeed at what? At your career, in your relationships, and, in context of this book, in practicing self-care.

Florence Nightingale said the role of the nurse is to "put the patient in the best condition for nature to act upon him" (Nightingale, 1861, p. 94). In other words, she believed that medical care is designed to support a patient so that they may heal according to nature—sometimes we just need a little boost to do so. The same holds true with self-care and resilience. We have it within ourselves already; we are strong enough, good enough, and wise enough.

When it comes to resilience, findings in the National Academies of Sciences, Engi-neering, and Medicine report, *Taking Action Against Clinician Burnout: A Systems Approach to Professional Well-Being* (2019), suggest that compared to the rest of our country's population, nurses have as much resilience as anyone else, at base-line. We recognize that because of the nature of our work, however, it is crucial to build more resilience so that we may face the challenges of our work head-on. We need to build up our resilience to support the natural base of resilience that we are all born with. In order to build from this base, we may examine how strong we already are. To build this resilience, first take a breath, feel your feet on the floor, and ground yourself. Then pay attention.

First, Pay Attention

The author Pema Chödrön suggests, "Meditation practice isn't about trying to throw ourselves away and become something better. It's about befriending who we are already" (2010, p. 2). There is something within you, within me, within all of us that serves as a singular point of strength, the strongest roots of the tree. It is from this source that we may grow strong, emotionally. Many people call it differ-ent things, such as "essence," "spirit," or "inner-being," to name only a few names.

This "essence" is both unique to each individual and universal in that all living people have it. The challenge is finding it, acknowledging it, and allowing it space to flourish—it's even more of a challenge to connect with it when the storms of life, school, and work swirl around you. Many of the self-care practices that we've discussed in this book center on the practice of paying attention. By paying attention, we recognize our inner strength, who we really are.

So, what can we pay attention to? The list is endless. The trick is finding what the point of attention needs to be, in the moment, so that you can focus on your task at hand or take a brief break to practice self-care.

In his book *Better: A Surgeon's Notes on Performance*, Atul Gawande (2007) shares essays about the deep perfectionism, albeit also tragic at times, in the surgical professions. The key, though, to being a strong clinician is clear: It is the ability to pay attention. You can practice this any time, to improve, to be "better," or to relax. Consider, for a moment, focusing on your breath. Or you can focus on the sensations of your feet on the floor. You can squeeze and release your hands, focusing on the changes in sensation. You can focus on a color and how often you see it as you walk outside for five minutes. The practice of paying attention, of building the capacity to pay attention, begins with choosing a point of focus. You've got this.

The Victim Narrative and How to Recognize It

In some instances, including how we respond to stressors at work, we can choose to be victims. Sometimes it is the easiest choice. When the stressors of nursing school feel as if they are about to become paralyzing, or your new role as a clinician feels overwhelming—which can be a normal sensation for many learners and new nurses—you have the option to choose how you interpret those stressors. You can become angry and blame "the system." You can put your head down and "power through." You can also take the role of the victim and tell yourself that because of circumstances beyond your control, you are now not going to succeed.

Of course, there are many other ways to interpret and face these stressors, some obviously emotionally healthy and some not. The "victim's approach" or victim's narrative is a pitfall that can very quickly make your experience as a student or new nurse intolerable. Be careful of that. We also know that this "victim narrative"—in other words allowing yourself to believe that you are stymied by factors far beyond your control, and worse, that you can just give up because of them—can become quite detrimental over time (Edwards et al., 2010).

Dr. Cynda Rushton, author of *Moral Resilience* (2018), warns us not to fall into the "victim narrative" of burnout and posttraumatic stress disorder (PTSD). In this context, a victim narrative of burnout could look like this:

Because I feel symptoms of burnout based on my work stress, I will continue to withdraw from work, my colleagues, and friends—there is nothing that I can do to fix it, and the system has broken me. I give up.

A victim narrative stemming from PTSD might look similarly:

The traumas I have witnessed in the past have made me unable to feel any longer. I can no longer find meaningful connections with friends, family, and colleagues, I will just come into work, do my job, go home, and repeat. I do not feel like I have meaning in what I do.

We understand that trauma, especially, can have profound impacts on how you experience your life. It is essential that you seek support if you experience challenges in your life that arise with symptoms of PTSD.

The seminal study on adverse childhood experiences (ACEs) by Felitti et al. (1998) revolutionized the way we view high-level and low-level traumas that children experience and how these traumas affect well-being and health for our entire lifetimes. This is to say that if you have experienced trauma, we realize that your history does affect the way you view the world and interact with it—we see you and hear you. We also recognize there are choices you can make about how you choose to view the significant experiences and barriers of the past and how you choose to move forward in the present. Triggers that stir challenging and sometimes incomprehensible emotions from past traumatic events can feel debilitating at times (Salmon & Morehead, 2019). We encourage you to be kind with yourself and gentle as you work with such experiences.

We can use our inherent resilience, strengthened through self-care, so that we can grow from our experiences of stress, suffering, and trauma. Falling victim to ourselves and our experience can prohibit us from growing. It could possibly even lead us down a path toward suffering PTSD or worsening our PTSD symptoms if we already experience them.

Posttraumatic Growth

Drs. Lawrence Calhoun and Richard Tedeschi have evolved a process that pushes against the victim narrative of PTSD with a concept called posttraumatic growth (PTG) (Calhoun & Tedeschi, 2014). In essence, PTG encourages people to consider what they have learned from past traumatic experiences, how they have grown emotionally, and how have they become psychologically stronger after stressful or traumatic experiences. Perhaps the trauma or stress has been chronic, ongoing for some time, and if so, has that made the person even stronger? Consider how many of our classmates and colleagues may have grown up in a community or country that judged them, incessantly and unjustly, by the color of their skin, the person they choose to love, their religious beliefs, their ability status, or their citizenship status.

For many of us, trauma can be a daily occurrence. The PTG model does not diminish the traumas someone has gone through, nor does it disregard them as insignificant. Rather, it focuses first on what wisdom, growth, and knowledge have come from the traumatic events. In Figure 11.1, which illustrates Calhoun and Tedeschi's consideration of PTG, you see the term "narrative" used a couple of times. A key element to PTG is how you develop your narrative of growth (Calhoun & Tedeschi, 2014). You may share this narrative with others through conversation or writing, or you may find yourself just contemplating it within. It is this narrative that arises, in its own unique way, as unique as you are, that helps build this strength from your stressful experiences.

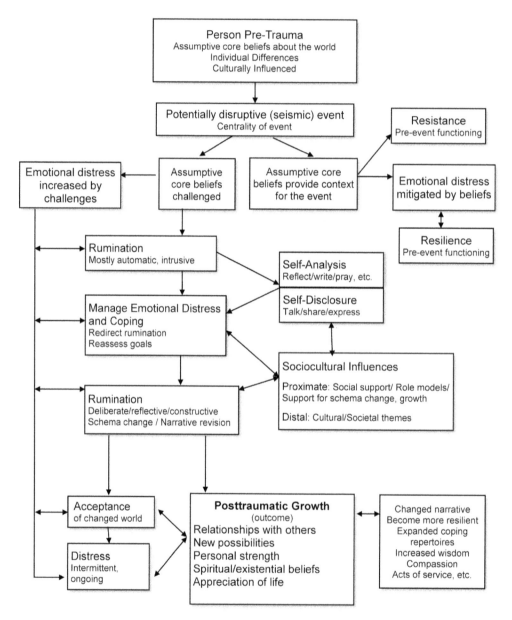

FIGURE 11.1 A comprehensive model of PTG.
From Tedeschi et al., 2018. Reprinted with permission.

This growth narrative naturally opposes the victim narrative. It gives agency to the person having experienced trauma; it reminds us that we might be better, stronger, and even kinder based on what we have witnessed. PTG reminds us that strength can grow from within (Calhoun & Tedeschi, 2014). This "within" is rooted in your "essence, spirit, or inner source." You may compare building up your own PTG to emotional exercises. Reflecting on PTG regularly, you can build up your resilience similarly to how you build strength when you exercise. Pay attention, focus, see who you are, and focus on the five key dimensions of PTG, over and over again, until these aspects of growth come to mind second-nature to you. You'll find yourself building upon your inherent strength, your posttraumatic growth, and your emotional intelligence, which we'll discuss in the next section.

Five Elements of Posttraumatic Growth
(Jayawickreme & Blackie, 2014)

1. *Personal strength*: How do you see yourself as changed because of the traumas you've experienced, and how have you become stronger because of them?

2. *Closer relationships*: When you think about the relationships that have withstood the traumas in your life, how have they changed? Which ones have lasted, and what strength do you find in them?

3. *Greater appreciation for life*: How do you see life differently now as a result of your traumas? What do you value more now? What in life brings you joy?

4. *New possibilities*: Do you think about certain aspects of your life differently now, and in doing so, how have those perspective changes inspired you to experience innovative ideas? What do you do differently now in your life that builds resilience for yourself and others?

5. *Spiritual development*: What are your new views on spirituality, having withstood the traumas in your life? How have these views changed, and what sort of spiritual wisdom have you noticed in your own self?

Posttraumatic growth offers a lens through which we can examine aspects of our traumas. It provides a platform from which we can, if we choose, reflect upon how we've gotten stronger based on the challenges we've faced in life. Much evidence suggests that the suffering we witness as nurses, though it is not our own suffering, can begin to create symptoms of PTSD. This is called *secondary trauma* or *vicarious trauma* (Von Rueden et al., 2010). PTG offers a way to examine our traumas and focus on the growth that comes from the suffering we've experienced or witnessed. In that, we find strength, thus our strength's-based approach in understanding how we've become stronger and understanding what self-care practices we should engage in to support this strength. Ultimately, as we care for ourselves and our strengths, we are building emotional intelligence. Figure 11.1 (Tedeschi et al., 2018) walks you through aspects of posttraumatic growth. Pause for a moment, read through it and consider, in your own experience, how this relates to your personal and professional journey.

Emotional Intelligence

Inspired by the work of researchers John Mayer and Peter Salovey, Daniel Goleman became a leading expert in the US on emotional intelligence (EI) (Goleman, 2006). This concept strives to understand how we can recognize our own emotions and the emotions of others; it also helps us understand how we react to those perceived emotions (Caruso et al., 2019).

What does emotional intelligence look like?

Table 11.1 details five aspects of high emotional intelligence (Goleman, 2006; Goleman 2009).

Table 11.1 Five Aspects of High Emotional Intelligence

Characteristic of EI	Example
Self-Awareness	As a nurse, you know some of your emotional triggers, and you understand when they are occurring. You make efforts to remove yourself from triggering situations, or you ask for help from a colleague when you feel emotionally unstable.
Self-Regulation	This is about pacing yourself, committing to what you can but not overdoing it either. When you feel tiredness coming on, take a break, take a breath, and take a day off to recharge and refresh if you can.
Motivation	This is about remembering what inspired you to become a nurse and relying on that when things get tough.
Empathy	When you see someone suffering, you connect with that suffering. For a moment, you are able to walk in that person's shoes.
Social Skills	Think about this as "reading the room." How do you make subtle changes to the way you communicate with people in your lives? Do you speak with patients different than with family members, partners, or friends? How do you use self-awareness to make those changes so that you can connect with people and patients on their level?

High EI Clinical Scenario

Consider a nurse with arguably high EI working in a crowded emergency department (ED). He is nearing the end of his 12-hour shift, and it has been a very busy day. At around 18:00 a mother comes in with her child, and the child is screaming in pain because he has an ear infection. The child's mother has never had to take any of her children to an ED before, and the nurse recognizes that the mother is as nervous as her child. Sadly, the ED is so full that the mother will have to wait in the waiting room until a bed space is available. The mother does not take that news well. She begins to yell at the nurse. She even berates him and tells him that he does not know how to do his job, that he is incompetent. She tells him that the hospital is a complete disaster and that she'll never bring her son here again. She is so scared and angry that she begins to cry while yelling at the nurse.

Remember, this nurse has high emotional intelligence. He listens to the aggravated mother, and he waits until she finishes (even though he is very busy and knows that he may get behind on the other patients that he needs to triage). He does not take her words personally, even though she has said mean, even hurtful, things about him.

Finally, she says, "What right do you even have to call yourself a nurse?"

He calmly and slowly explains to her the process that her son will go through in being examined by a physician and what the likely outcomes will be—that the physician will prescribe an antibiotic, likely amoxicillin, a nurse will give the first dose to the child here at the ED, and then she will go home with a prescription for the rest. The nurse goes on to explain why they have to wait in the waiting room and then gives a dose of ibuprofen to the child to help with the pain while they wait. The child stops crying after taking the medication, and the mother calms down.

This is a real-life example of EI in action. The nurse, though exhausted from a long shift, was able to recognize that if he took the words of this angry mother personally, he too would find himself angry and possibly even yelling back at her. He also saw that the mother was not angry at him, as a person; he was able to use his inherent (and learned) EI to see that she was afraid and felt very insecure about her son's situation. This nurse was not a mind reader to any extent; however, he was able to put emotional, physical, and verbal cues together to understand that the mother just wanted to take care of her son. In fact, the nurse, of course, did too. Within just a few seconds during this interaction, this nurse was able to improve the situation for the mother, the child, and himself by decreasing everyone's stress. This is high EI in action. EI is something that is inherent to us all and it is also something, like resilience, that takes practice, can be learned, and can improve over time (Mattingly & Krager, 2019). Strengths-based self-care practices can help us recognize our EI and, kindly, recognize where we have room to improve upon our EI.

Low EI Clinical Scenario

Now think about what low emotional intelligence would look like in the same situation. Perhaps a nurse with low EI would be easily triggered by the angry mother who was simply trying to do what she thought was best for her child. A nurse with low EI might snap back at the mother, might yell at her or, worse, might even call security on her to calm her down. All these actions would only elevate the mother's anger, frighten her child, and negatively escalate this situation. What's more, a nurse with lower EI might not have taken the time to give the child a dose of ibuprofen before sending the mother and child back into the waiting room.

The nurse with high EI was able to use his EI, which Goleman points out comes from self-awareness, empathy, and social skills (Goleman, 2009) to help the mother and child. The nurse used these skills, all of which we can foster over time. Plus, if the nurse experienced any trauma or stress from being yelled at by this mother, he could also apply posttraumatic growth to this situation so that when it happens again, he can remember how this past interaction worked and provide even better care for future patients in similar situations.

PTG and EI evolve through iterative processes, which is to say that you can build your own EI and experience PTG by having an experience (positive or negative), evaluating what it means to you (internally and externally—contemplating it or sharing the experience with others through conversation or writing), and then using those evaluations to find strength moving forward toward the next experience (Tuck & Patlamazoglou, 2019). As I mentioned before, it's like exercise.

A common aspect of both PTG and EI is that they begin from within. You have them within yourself, even if they are sometimes hard to find.

Recognize That You've Already "Made It"

In 2010, I attended a talk by the founder of mindfulness-based stress reduction, Dr. Jon Kabat-Zinn (Kabat-Zinn, 2010). In his presentation, he asked us to imagine, for a moment, that we had "arrived." What he meant by that was what if we had already succeeded in meeting all our goals and all our dreams? What if, he espoused, we could just be present in *this moment* and realize that we accomplished all we needed to accomplish simply because we were *here*? That's still a bit hard to wrap my head around, but I remember that when I heard those words, for a moment, I relaxed and felt good about myself. I was astonished.

We know that if we choose not to take the victim narrative when heavy stressors load us down we can more clearly recognize our strengths and our resilience. We also know that self-care practices can help build up those strengths (Austin et al., 2009).

You May Already Be Practicing Self-Care

Something that I have found astonishing about the concept of self-care is that many people already practice it—and they are good at it—without even knowing they are doing it. In 2017, I was curious to learn more about how some of my colleagues practiced and thought about self-care, so I ran a small study among the nurses that I worked with. The findings were fascinating.

In brief, this is what happened: My team built a survey to examine two core concepts.

The first concept was a question: *What is self-care to you?* In asking that question, we wanted to understand what nurses in our health system did to take care of themselves.

The second concept was a bit more complex. Here we hypothesized that nurses with frequent self-care practices (a dose effect) would score lower on scales that represented perceived stress. We were astonished by a couple of things.

You can see in Table 11.2 that the nurses we surveyed talked about a variety of forms of self-care. At the onset of our project, my research team believed that most of our nurses would mention doing forms of self-care that are more common in published literature (like exercise, meditation, and yoga)—well, we were incorrect! Some nurses did say they engaged in those practices, but many more listed other ways that they choose to practice self-care, such as reading, knitting, napping, gardening, and spending time with family. Our study reminded us that self-care is an ongoing practice and not a one-off event. We learned from these data that the definition of self-care should remain broad and that many of our nurses were already practicing self-care even if it did not fit the "traditional" definition. It begs the question: Do we even need a traditional definition of self-care if we run the risk of excluding people from practicing it?

Table 11.2 Pilot Data Addressing the Use and Impacts of Self-Care, Resilience, and Compassion

					Percent					
					(1)	(2)	(3)	(4)	(5)	(6)
	#	%	Mean	SD	Daily	4-6x/wk	2-3x/wk	1x/wk	<1x/wk	1-2x/mo
Meditation	53	13.9%	2.9	1.6	22.6	20.8	20.8	20.8	5.7	9.4
Breathing exercises	86	22.5%	2.4	1.4	38.4	16.3	26.7	10.5	5.8	2.3
Prayer	119	31.2%	1.5	0.9	72.3	12.6	11.8	1.7	1.7	0.0
Yoga	82	21.5%	3.6	1.1	4.9	8.5	31.7	40.2	7.3	7.3
Exercise (including walking/ hiking)	205	53.7%	2.5	0.9	14.1	36.1	42.9	3.9	1.5	1.5
Martial arts	2	0.5%	3.5	0.7	0.0	0.0	50.0	50.0	0.0	0.0
Writing	38	9.9%	3.7	1.4	5.3	15.8	21.1	34.2	10.5	13.2
Visual arts	25	6.5%	4.6	1.4	0.0	8.0	16.0	24.0	16.0	36.0
Music	118	30.9%	1.4	0.9	77.1	11.0	9.3	0.8	0.0	1.7
Other*	79	20.7%	2.6	1.5	34.2	17.7	22.8	15.2	1.3	8.9

Cunningham et al. (2017)

Most importantly, we learned that many of our colleagues were practicing self-care—they just chose to think of it differently than what was commonly thought of as self-care. *Just because it's not published does not mean it doesn't exist or it is not valid*—you should keep that concept in mind, especially when it comes to self-care.

Secondly, from this project, we learned that nurses who did practice self-care did it regularly. These results are meaningful because they back up the existent evidence that self-care practices must be practiced regularly over time in order to build positive impacts (Crane & Ward, 2016).

Self-care might be happening right in front of you already. We learned that in our small study, and further we have learned that self-care can be far more sustainable if you first support ongoing practices that you or your colleagues do, rather than telling yourself or others to add another thing to your plate. Again, begin from a place of thinking: "I'm already doing enough." That is a place of strength.

Pay It Forward

When you see your classmate or colleague practicing self-care, point it out. Let them know that what they are doing is good for them in ways that they may not even yet understand. Know that when you practice self-care, you are building on your own inherent strengths and wisdom, you may be nourishing your posttraumatic growth (PTG), and you're certainly building emotional intelligence (EI). If you have a practice that feels like self-care to you—it helps you feel relaxed, grounded, present, more engaged, and even energized sometimes—keep it up, and share it with others.

Dr. Mike Wessells, a humanitarian, peace builder, and psychologist who has worked extensively for decades with child soldiers, families who have faced forced displacement, war, and deadly disease, is a proponent of PTG. He proposes that no matter what has happened to us, we still have the ability to come together with others in a sense of community and use our inherent strengths to grow (Wessells & van Ommeren, 2008). Self-care is your inherent strength; it can help you thrive. When you recognize that, it is important to share with others. Self-care begins with the self, but then it moves outward and nourishes your community, too.

In Real Practice

At the time of this publication, the concept of posttraumatic growth is still relatively new in the nursing profession. The COVID pandemic has changed that drastically. Chen et al. (2020) published a large cross-sectional survey examining burnout and posttraumatic growth among a sample of 12,596 nurses during the COVID pandemic. It is important to note that not all of these nurses in the sample treated people with COVID directly; however, those that did showed higher levels of posttraumatic growth as compared to those who did not. This finding suggests that when we find meaning in our work, as challenging as it may be, we might be primed to experience the effects of posttraumatic growth in our lives. Researchers also learned that critical care nurses and female nurses were slightly more likely to experience symptoms of burnout.

This paper is important because it is one of the first published papers looking at posttraumatic growth among nurses as it relates to the COVID pandemic. Conversely, this study is just a cross-sectional study and therefore does not reflect change, intervention, or any sort of randomization, thus making it less robust. It is a good start, however, as we continue to learn about strengths that arise from experiencing traumatic situations in healthcare settings.

Closing Thoughts

Self-care can feel daunting at times, and the desire to practice self-care can make you feel "not good enough," if you don't feel like you're doing it right. You may also feel that you have to do more, add more to your already full plate to figure out ways to practice self-care. You can think about this differently and from a place of personal strength. You can consider the challenges you've had in your life, traumas that you've experienced or traumas that you've witnessed, and focus on how you've grown from them. This form of self-care uses posttraumatic growth and emotional intelligence as ways to recognize the inherent strengths you've developed over your lifetime. Reflecting on those strengths that are already there is a form of self-care. So, put simply: Pay attention, recognize that you've already "made it," and pay it forward.

Key Points

- Many of us already practice self-care, but we don't realize it's self-care. By recognizing what self-care you already practice, you can develop a sense of strength.

- We can learn and grow from traumas and stressors in life; we do not have to become victims to them and can nourish posttraumatic growth as well as emotional intelligence.

- As you learn about your own inner strength, share it with others so that they can learn from you and recognize that self-care is inherent and unique to us all.

References

Austin, W., Goble, E., Leier, B., & Byrne, P. (2009). Compassion fatigue: The experience of nurses. *Ethics and Social Welfare, 3*(2), 195–214.

Calhoun, L. G., & Tedeschi, R. G. (Eds.). (2014). *Handbook of posttraumatic growth: Research and practice.* Routledge.

Caruso, D. R., Mayer, J. D., Bryan, V., Phillips, K. G., & Salovey, P. (2019). Measuring emotional and personal intelligence. In M. W. Gallagher & S. J. Lopez (Eds.), *Positive psychological assessment: A handbook of models and measures* (pp. 233–245). American Psychological Association. https://doi.org/10.1037/0000138-015

Chen, R., Sun, C., Chen, J. J., Jen, H. J., Kang, X. L., Kao, C. C., & Chou, K. R. (2020). A large-scale survey on trauma, burnout, and posttraumatic growth among nurses during the COVID-19 pandemic. *International Journal of Mental Health Nursing.* https://doi.org/10.1111/inm.12796

Chödrön, P. (2010). *The wisdom of no escape: And the path of loving-kindness.* Shambhala Publications.

Crane, P. J., & Ward, S. F. (2016). Self-healing and self-care for nurses. *AORN Journal, 104*(5), 386–400. https://doi.org/10.1016/j.aorn.2016.09.007

Cunningham, T. Inkelas, K. K., & Trail, J. (2017). *Pilot data addressing the use and impacts of self-care, resilience and compassion at a level-one trauma center and school of nursing.* Abstract presentation. CENTILE Conference, Washington, DC, 2017.

Edwards, D., Burnard, P., Bennett, K., & Hebden, U. (2010). A longitudinal study of stress and self-esteem in student nurses. *Nurse education today, 30*(1), 78–84.

Felitti, V. J., Anda, R. F., Nordernberg, D., Williamson, D. F., Spitz, A. M., Edwards, V., Koss, M. P., & Marks, J. S. (1998). Relationship of childhood abuse to many of the leading causes of death in adults: The adverse childhood experiences (ACE) study. *American Journal of Preventive Medicine, 14*(3), 245–258. https://doi.org/10.1016/S0749-3797(98)00017-8

Gawande, A. (2007). *Better: A surgeon's notes on performance.* Picador.

Goleman, D. (2006). *Emotional intelligence*. Bantam.

Goleman, D. (2009). *Working with emotional intelligence*. A&C Black.

Jayawickreme, E., & Blackie, L. E. (2014). Post-traumatic growth as positive personality change: Evidence, controversies and future directions. *European Journal of Personality*, 28(4), 312–331. https://doi.org/10.1002/per.1963

Kabat-Zinn, J. (2010, March). *Mindfulness in medicine and psychology: Its transformative and healing potential in living and in dying*. Talk presented at the University of Virginia, Virginia, US.

Mattingly, V., & Kraiger, K. (2019). Can emotional intelligence be trained? A meta-analytical investigation. *Human Resource Management Review*, 29(2), 140–155. https://doi.org/10.1016/j.hrmr.2018.03.002

National Academies of Sciences, Engineering, and Medicine. (2019). *Taking action against clinician burnout: A systems approach to professional well-being*. National Academies Press.

Nightingale, F. (1861). *Notes on nursing for the labouring classes*. Harrison.

Rushton, C. H. (Ed.). (2018). *Moral resilience: Transforming moral suffering in healthcare*. Oxford University Press.

Salmon, G., & Morehead, A. (2019). Posttraumatic Stress Syndrome and Implications for Practice in Critical Care Nurses. *Critical care nursing clinics of North America*, 31(4), 517–526.

Tedeschi, R. G., Shakespeare-Finch, J., Taku, K., & Calhoun, L. G. (2018). *Posttraumatic growth: Theory, research, and applications*. Routledge.

Tuck, D., & Patlamazoglou, L. (2019). The relationship between traumatic stress, emotional intelligence, and posttraumatic growth. *Journal of Loss and Trauma*, 24(8), 721–735.

Von Rueden, K. T., Hinderer, K. A., McQuillan, K. A., Murray, M., Logan, T., Kramer, B., Gilmore, R., & Friedmann, E. (2010). Secondary traumatic stress in trauma nurses: Prevalence and exposure, coping, and personal/environmental characteristics. *Journal of Trauma Nursing*, 17(4), 191–200. https://doi.org/10.1097/JTN.0b013e3181ff2607

Wessells, M., & van Ommeren, M. (2008). Developing inter-agency guidelines on mental health and psychosocial support in emergency settings. *Intervention*, 6(3/4), 199–218. https://doi.org/10.1097/WTF.0b013e328321e142

section III
The Body and Spirit of a Nurse

12

Reclaiming, Recalling, and Remembering: Spirituality and Self-Care

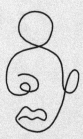

Robin C. Brown-Haithco
pronouns: She/Her

Robin C. Brown-Haithco is a chaplain, educator, and ordained Baptist minister. A meeting with a chaplain in the hospital where she worked as a psychiatric aide solidified her calling to ministry and ultimately led her to seminary and clinical pastoral education. Her passion for caring for suffering persons and educating chaplains in healthcare contexts has been her life's work. A mother and partner, she loves reading, communing with nature, and watching British detective mysteries.

"In the stillness of the quiet, if we listen,
we can hear the whisper of the heart
giving strength to weakness,
courage to fear, hope to despair."

–Howard Thurman

As I write this chapter, our country and our world are in the middle of the COVID-19 pandemic that has dramatically changed the way we live, breathe, and socialize. Never in my life would I have imagined we would find ourselves faced with the devastation this virus has brought. The rituals and traditions we have relied on to help us face death, dying, grief, and loss are turned upside down. We now rely on technology as our primary means of relating to each other. Zoom and FaceTime have become the norm. As a chaplain whose primary way of relating depends on face-to-face encounters, and physical touch the primary way of expressing empathy and compassion, this new normal is challenging everything I know about who I am vocationally and spiritually.

Several months before the COVID-19 virus crossed the borders into the United States, my mom died. She was the person who shaped my understanding of spirituality and who taught me how to live in the midst of adversity and great suffering. She was the one who blessed my call to ministry and pushed me to follow my dreams and live out my God-given potential despite messages I received to the contrary. My grief is still very fresh, and some days I wonder how I will go on without her. Then I remember who she was and the lessons she taught me.

I will never forget her last eight months and her strength as she "lived her dying," a term first introduced to me in a book, *Living Our Dying* (Sharp, 1996). In my mom, I saw a woman who loved life and who lived each day with vibrancy and passion, despite her physical condition. She never complained even though there were times when she was in pain and times when she was physically and emotionally exhausted. She wasn't living in denial. She knew she was dying, but she always wanted us to know that she would live as fully as she could until she took her final breath. The image of her strength is forever etched in my memory and reminds me to stay hopeful, even as the numbers of those impacted by the virus continue to increase and the death rate continues to climb.

When I think back to what created this grounding and foundation in my mom (and also my dad), I must look back to my family's story and my parent's history. They were born two years after the Great Depression, lived through segregation, and raised their family during the civil rights movement, a time of fear and danger for Blacks in America. We grew up with less than enough, but despite these circumstances my family always found a way to see through the difficulties and rise above our circumstances. I believe that much of this was related to the faith of my parents, who instilled in us a trust in the One who created us and who promised to supply our needs. When life has thrown me curveballs, when challenges have pushed me to the edge, and when hope at times has turned into despair, remembering the messages I received growing up calls me back to the faith that sustains and nurtures me. That faith has been grounded in community and in relationship.

This chapter is informed by my rich cultural and spiritual story, viewed first through the lens of my family and the community that nurtured and cared for me, and second through the lens of my vocational-self and the abundant experiences in my profession as a chaplain working in academic healthcare contexts and trauma centers. It is my hope that you will join me in this chapter in exploring your own rich cultural and spiritual story to see more fully how that story has invited you to nursing, and how that story can sustain you in times of crisis and challenge in your clinical work, both as a student and in your nursing career.

Spirituality and Vocation

I believe that the ways we nurture and sustain ourselves in the critical moments of caring for suffering persons is linked to and informed by our *spirituality*. It is in and through our connection to that which is within and beyond ourselves that we find the courage, strength, and commitment to continue doing what we are called to do. You could probably talk to hundreds of people, and each of them will have a different understanding of what spirituality means to them. Throughout my life and vocation, the word has taken on different meanings for me. For the purposes of this chapter, *spirituality* is that which sustains and nurtures us in the critical, chaotic, suffering moments in our lives. It is not necessarily related to (but certainly could be) any particular religious belief or theological understanding. It is defined by those things that give us meaning in life, the core beliefs and values that ground and center us, and the relationships that we trust and depend on to hold us when we can no longer hold ourselves. It is what invites us to find joy in the midst of sorrow and sadness, and it is what allows us to move toward gratitude and hope when what we love most is about to slip away from us. Archbishop Desmond Tutu in conversation with the Dalai Lama tells us:

> We are fragile creatures, and it is from this weakness, not despite it, that we discover the possibility of true joy . . . Life is filled with challenges and adversity . . . Fear is inevitable, as is pain and eventually death . . . Discovering more joy does not . . . save us from the inevitability of hardship and heartbreak. In fact, we may cry more easily, but we will laugh more easily, too. Perhaps we are just more alive. Yet as we discover more joy, we can face suffering in a way that ennobles rather than embitters. We have hardship without becoming hard. We have heartbreak without being broken. (Lama et al., 2016, pp. 11–12)

The *vocations* we choose, and that at times may choose us, are intimately linked to our spirituality. The work we do should flow out of our inner landscape and core values. When what we do matches the joy and passion within us, whatever bumps in the road we may encounter will not deter us from our commitment and purpose in life. Our life's task is to listen for what that call is in our lives. Buechner says it like this:

> Vocare, 'to call,' . . . is the work that [we are] called to in this world, the thing that [we are] summoned to spend [our] life doing. We can speak of . . . choosing . . . vocation, but perhaps it is at least as accurate to speak of a vocation's choosing [us], of a call's being given and . . . hearing it, or not hearing it. And maybe that is the place to start: the place of listening and hearing. (Buechner, 1985, p. 27)

> *Note*: The author uses masculine language in the original text.

Howard Thurman uses the language of dreams or hopes to speak of this vocational call. He writes:

> As long as [we have] a dream in [our] heart, [we] cannot lose the significance of living . . . [We] cannot continue long to live if the

dream in the heart has perished. It is then that [we] stop hoping, stop looking, and the last embers of [our] anticipations fade away . . . The dream is the quiet persistence in the heart that enables [us] to ride out the storms of [our] churning experiences. It is the exciting whisper moving through the aisles of [our] spirit . . . The dream is no outward thing. It does not take its rise from the environment in which one moves or functions. It lives in the inward parts, it is deep within, where the issues of life and death are ultimately determined. Keep alive the dream; for as long as [we have] a dream in [our] heart, [we] cannot lose the significance of living. (Thurman, 1976, pp. 36–37)

Note: The author uses masculine language in the original text.

Both Buechner and Thurman suggest the same theme. One's vocation is internal to one's being. It does not come from outside of us. That does not mean it cannot be affirmed by those who know us well and have listened to our hearts. Vocation is a voice calling from within inviting us to do that which brings us joy while at the same time meeting the deepest needs of those in the world (Buechner, 1993, p. 119). I fully believe that our vocation calls us, and when we listen deeply to our heart's desires, we will respond to that call with excitement and passion. Wicks affirms this notion of vocation:

The interior life . . . is a place of self-knowledge, self-nurturance, challenge, and solid peace. It is a place that will not only be our strength but also one that we can offer to others. When our interior life is strong, our attitude toward others is gentle. When our inner life feels nourished, our hearts can be open to others' pain. (Wicks, 2008, p. 107)

Spirituality and Self-Care

It is only when we lose sight of our core values and beliefs and stop listening to our inner voice that we struggle to nurture and sustain ourselves amid life's challenges. In the clinical context, giving daily attention to your own self-care is therefore key to continuing to live out your vocation with joy, gratitude, and hope. As patient acuity increases, and family members create challenges and tension in the care of critically ill patients, finding ways to shield yourself from the suffering you witness is vital to maintaining your health and wholeness. Thus, much of what I hope to do as I move about my hospital is to educate staff regarding the vital need for self-care: "managing our lives in such a way that we consistently maintain our physical, emotional, intellectual and spiritual well-being" (Oswald, 1991, p. 10).

It seems that in order to talk about self-care we must understand its goal, which is to nurture *true self*. Parker Palmer speaks wonderfully about true self in his understanding of vocation. He writes:

> . . . Discovering vocation does not mean scrambling toward some prize just beyond my reach but accepting the treasure of true self I already possess. Vocation does not come from a voice 'out there' calling me to become something I am not. It comes from a voice 'in here' calling me to be the person I was born to be, to fulfill the original selfhood given me at birth . . . (Palmer, 2000, p. 10)

Many of us spend our lives seeking to find who we are and where we belong by looking outside of ourselves. Palmer is saying it is already in you—listen for the voice calling you to your original selfhood. In the Christian text, the Apostle Paul reminds Timothy, his mentee, to "stir up the gift" that is within him (2 Timothy 1:6 King James Version). This is the *treasure of true self*. The Dalai Lama says it this way:

> One great question underlies our existence . . . What is the purpose of life? . . . I believe that the purpose of life is to find happiness. . . The ultimate source of happiness is within us. Not money, not power, not status. Power and money fail to bring inner peace. Outward attainment will not bring real inner joyfulness. We must look inside. (Lama et al., 2016, p. 14)

A Call to Remember

Through an intentional exploration of my own life narrative, I have come to know myself in ways I would never have imagined. As I have reflected on my personal story, I have been invited to "recall" and "remember" life experiences that are only now leading to transformation. In my work with healthcare staff, I always begin with their story. As they lean into my invitation to share their story with me, often there is an "aha!" moment; their face will light up, and they will say something like, "That's where that comes from—that's why I do what I do."

Twice a year I am invited to lead a training on resilience in the workplace for new grad nurses. As I begin the training, I invite the new nurses to recall the event, moment, or story when they knew this vocation of nursing summoned them, and the moment when they accepted that call in all its uncertainty and joy. As they recall and remember, I invite them to hold on to that memory, that point of connection with their spirit that will sustain them when the moments of suffering are overwhelming, when their own grief in the midst of suffering might lead them to question their vocation.

My own personal experience has provided wisdom for my vocation of staff support. There have been moments in my vocational life when I have wondered, "Can I keep doing this work?" There have been moments when I have known that if I did not find ways to nurture myself physically, emotionally, spiritually, and mentally, then this work of caring for others would deplete me and steal my joy. One such moment was when my mom died. In the days following her funeral, my grief was so great I found it difficult to get up each day and go to work, knowing that in my day I would have to encounter more death and dying, suffering and pain. My daily walks in the park meditating, and my time in therapy doing my grief work, helped to call me back to a place of resilience and well-being, a place of hope.

When I stop in those moments of questioning to remind myself why I chose this vocation and why it chose me, I realize that this work I am engaged in is something I can't *not* do. It is in the fabric of my being. It is who I was created to be. It is that to which I was called to at birth by the One who created me. Could I do something else? Yes, absolutely. But would that something else nurture my spirit? Probably not.

It is my belief that at certain points in our lives, this work of remembering is key to health and wholeness because it calls us back to our true self, to that place within that often we cannot explain to ourselves or others. But what we do know is that place of soul and spirit, gratitude, joy, and hope is what allows us to live with freedom and flexibility in the vocations to which we have been called.

Cultivating Resilience

So how do we maintain mental, physical, and spiritual health? How do we care for ourselves while caring for others? What are the things in our lives that help to nurture us? Where is that one place that calls to us when life becomes too much—that place that refreshes us and calms us and calls us back to our center?

In my thirty years of training chaplains and providing emotional and spiritual support of clinicians in healthcare, I have learned the importance of identifying where in the body stress resides. This is primary for me in helping persons to cultivate resilience. Are you aware of it when you are stressed? What is the feeling attached to the stress your body is holding? I have learned in my work with staff that many of us are able to identify when we are stressed. We may even be able to identify the symptoms that very often reside in our bodies, such as heart palpitations, gastrointestinal issues, high blood pressure, and headaches. Many of us are even able to identify behavioral changes related to our stress, like impatience, withdrawal, appetite changes, and sleep disruptions. I have learned that what is most difficult to pin down (not just for nurses but for most of us in the world) are the emotions that we feel and the behavior we demonstrate in relationship to the stresses our bodies are carrying. The work of maintaining health and wholeness requires that we have an intimate connection to our bodies, that we listen to what our bodies speak to us. The work requires that we name, feel, and embrace the emotions related to the suffering and trauma we experience in the work of caring for suffering persons.

Our Bodies Are Trying to Tell Us Something

Let me share a personal story. In 2010, I found myself in the emergency department with symptoms of what I believed was a heart attack. It turned out to be an anxiety attack. I did not even know I was anxious until the friend who had come to the hospital with me pointed out behaviors she had noticed for several weeks: eye twitching, inability to focus, difficulty staying in one place, and pressured speech.

This is when I learned the importance of paying attention to the ways my body speaks to me. I now know where in my body stress resides. I now know ways to better manage that stress so it does not lead to physical and mental distress. I have learned what nurtures me most when I'm feeling most anxious, such as walking in the park listening to gospel music or jazz. As I walk, I can feel the stress and anxiety begin to roll off and a sense of calm and joy find its place within my spirit again.

There is an intimate connection between our spiritual selves and our emotional, physical, and mental selves. Many in traditional religions (I will speak to my Christian tradition primarily, since it is what I know best) tend to separate spirit from body, sacred from secular, thereby creating a divide within us. Self-care can only happen when we allow all aspects of ourselves to speak to the other. Our Western thinking often sees through the lens of dichotomous thinking—either/or, black/white, male/female. Spirituality invites us to see through the lens of paradoxical thinking—both/and, and all the areas of gray in between.

I have learned in my work with clinicians that the work of healthcare is becoming more and more stressful. Patients seem to be arriving sicker and sicker, and families are arriving with heightened emotions that often get directed toward the staff who are caring for their loved ones. Some staff are able to go beneath the surface emotion (often anger) and see the deeper emotion (fear of losing their loved one). When this translation of the surface emotion occurs, staff are able to live in the tension between the two. This is what I mean by *paradoxical thinking*—holding two contradictory thoughts or opinions or emotions simultaneously—living in the tension of the both/and. The family is angry and afraid at the same time. The emotion most easily recognized is the anger; the one that can go unnoticed is the fear, the emotion that makes us more vulnerable.

I am always amazed when I am called to a clinical area to assist staff who are working with a challenging patient and family situation. There is almost always at least one staff member who seems to be unfazed by the situation, who seems to have found a way to engage with the family despite the challenge and tension. When invited to share the difference in their response, they will usually say something like, "I try to find a way to align with them in their anxiety and fear. When I can do that the family sees my care and not my judgment." This, I believe, is the way they also tend to their own self-care. Staying centered within themselves allows them to clearly see and empathize with the other without taking in fully the emotions of the other into themselves.

When our life spirals out of control and we find ourselves in the gray, nothing seems to be neat and clean, there is no clear black or white, everything has been turned upside down. Our ability to expand the boundaries, move outside the box, and reframe what we see allows us to move toward the unknown with a sense of surety that "all things work together for good" (Romans 8:28 New Revised Standard Version). Our world does not have to collapse. Howard Thurman's writings suggest that knowing who I am and to whom I belong gives me the courage to face the uncertain days of tomorrow. (Howard Thurman's *Deep Is the Hunger* is one of my favorite books.)

My staff support work with nurses spans the spectrum of new to experienced and seasoned staff. I would like to share a story from a neurosurgical critical care nurse who is now over 20 years into her nursing vocation. As we sat together at a table in the hospital hallway distributing information on advance directives to patients and visitors who passed by, I invited her to share with me what brought her to this work of nursing and what sustains her in this work. Here is what she said:

> I first knew I wanted to be a nurse when I went into the hospital to deliver my daughter at a young age. The nurse who cared for me during and after the birth showed such compassion and kindness. I remembered thinking, 'I want to be able to give back this kindness and compassion to others.' I have remained in nursing because of the people I work with. Our support of each other and care for each other keeps me returning to work each day. I am in nursing because I cannot see myself doing anything else. This is who I am.
>
> –Tracy, RN
> Neurosurgical ICU

In Real Practice

Spirituality and religion are different concepts, and although one or the other or both may be helpful to some students' and nurses' personal well-being, that may not be the case for others. That said, it is important to recognize that spirituality and religion may play important roles in the lives, healing, and dying of your patients. O'Brien et al. (2019) study the effectiveness of a spirituality and end-of-life training for healthcare clinicians to help them better meet the spiritual needs of their patients. Learners came to understand the difference between spirituality and religion and why they matter to patients at end-of-life. They gained new skills, including the ability to recognize a patient's spiritual distress; to appreciate the value of silence and active listening; and to understand that a nurse or physician's role is not to "fix" things for patients, but rather to help them think through solutions. The article underscores the value of overcoming our own discomfort with spirituality and religion in order to better care for our patients.

Closing Thoughts

Put simply, life is "a web of connections" (Malhotra, 2016, para. 1). These connections shape and inform our spirituality—the values and beliefs we hold, the relationships that invite us to our best selves, the rituals that sustain and nurture us, the breath (spirit) that enlivens and brings us joy and invites us to gratitude in times of suffering and happiness. Spirituality links us to our vocational call—the true self within us that calls us to the work that "we can't not do."

When we lose sight of who we are and to whom we belong, the work that once gave us life loses its significance, that which gave us a full heart becomes heavy, until we eventually find ourselves with an empty heart (Todaro-Francheschi, 2013). Our task throughout life is to recall the "true self" given to us at birth. This reclaiming, recalling, remembering must happen at various points throughout our lives. And it is this recalling that will invite us to live fully into our gifts and reclaim our health and wholeness when life's circumstances tempt us to forget who we are and to whom we belong.

When I counsel nursing staff, whether they are new or experienced, to help them explore and examine self-care, I always end our sessions with a meditative moment. I invite them to listen to their hearts by creating a space for that listening to occur. I dim the lights and invite them to sit in a comfortable and relaxing position and then ask them to imagine that they are in their favorite nurturing place (sitting by a lake, walking along the beach, sitting on their deck with a glass of wine after a long day, enjoying dinner with friends, or a yoga class)—whatever that space or place is that calls them back to themselves and helps them to re-center. I then turn on quiet music, bamboo flute and Celtic harp, specifically *Love and Peace* by Lisa Lynne and George Tortorelli (1997). For five minutes it is their time to catch their breath—to breathe out the distractions, disruptions, and stress and breathe in the peace that they are imagining as they sit in their space of nurturing. As the music ends, I offer this blessing:

> As you leave this place to go about your day-to-day work of
> compassionate caring, stir up the passion within you—stir up that
> which you know within your heart is the reason why you do this

work; and when the intensity and stress become too much, allow this "passion" or "gift" to sustain and nurture you in your work. Whatever is lovely, whatever is good, think on these things. Peace and Blessings!

Key Points

- Spirituality invites us to find joy. It is what allows us to move toward gratitude and hope.

- When our interior life is strong, our attitude toward others is gentle. When our inner life feels nourished, our hearts can be open to others' pain (Wicks, 2008).

- The work we do should flow out of our inner landscape and core values.

- Our task throughout life is to recall the "true self" given to us at birth. It is this recalling that will invite us to live fully into our gifts and reclaim our health and wholeness.

References

Buechner, F. (1985). *The hungering dark*. HarperSanFrancisco.

Buechner, F. (1993). *Wishful thinking*. HarperOne.

Lama, D., Tutu, D., & Abrams, D. C. (2016). *The book of joy: Lasting happiness in a changing world*. Penguin.

Lynne, L., & Tortorelli, G. (1997). *Love and peace CD*. Lavender Sky Records.

Malhotra, R. (2016, 27 August). The Vedic metaphor of Indra's net. *Pragyata*. https://pragyata.com/the-vedic-metaphor-of-indras-net/

O'Brien, M. R., Kinloch, K., Groves, K. E., & Jack, B. A. (2019). Meeting patients' spiritual needs during end-of-life care: A qualitative study of nurses' and healthcare professionals' perceptions of spiritual care training. *Journal of Clinical Nursing*, 28(1–2): 182–189. doi:10.1111/jocn.14648

Oswald, R. (1991). *Clergy self-care*. The Alban Institute.

Palmer, P. (2000). *Let your life speak*. Jossey-Bass.

Sharp, J. (1996). *Living our dying*. Hyperion.

Thurman, H. (1976). *Meditations of the heart*. Friends United Press.

Todaro-Franceschi, V. (2013). *Compassion fatigue and burnout in nursing*. Springer Publishing Company.

Wicks, R. J. (2008). *The resilient clinician*. Oxford University Press.

From a Space of Fullness: Anchoring in Spirituality

–Victoria Tucker

Hello,

You were on my mind. Today is Sunday, and the September sun shines unapologetically as I write to you. Everything collides as I look up; the sun's brightness makes it difficult to differentiate between the clouds and the sky. It is 83 degrees with low humidity, and just as I get warm from the sun, a breeze greets my skin and reminds me that I am still. The birds are chirping out of view; their sounds are company. This is my escape. I get to bring my full self here, away from the noise, lists, expectations, judgment, performance, and pressure. Here I get to simply be "me." *Do you have a place like this?*

My escape is in my parent's backyard. I must admit that their backyard is accessible, but it has been about five years since I stepped outside of my routine to sit there and be present. I unintentionally dismissed the need for this space in the hustle of my routine. Today, I am reminded that I can always return here no matter how far I journey away. *And, you can too.* Please do not misconstrue my absence in this sacred space as tolerance for my lifestyle; I lost my way here. I physically pass it almost daily by necessity, rarely with intention to be present. My pace the past five years has consisted of mindless movement, frantic travel, and mind-numbing commutes. I am an off-campus graduate student in a doctoral program, a palliative care nurse, and community caregiver for a widowed neighbor with dementia. I know I am not alone in having responsibilities or competing priorities. I am in the good company of empathetic souls who are also at the crossroads of life's intersecting paths while treading the road to education.

If no one else says it this week, let me affirm that I see you. I recognize that seeing you does not lessen the load that you may carry, or eradicate the systemic injustices within our communities. I do hope that in acknowledging your wholeness we can collectively see our innate value in and beyond our professional roles. You are siblings, parents, partners, community members, caregivers, nurses, providers, as well as students. There are many other roles and titles that could be added here. Students are not unidimensional beings devoid of a past with a present connected solely to their books and exams. We are multidimensional learners who bring perspectives, experiences, lessons, losses, and wisdom to our work and study. Yes, we receive knowledge, but we give it as well. The synergistic rhythm of pouring out and pouring in requires an awareness of the mind, body, and, most intimately, the spirit. I will pause here to ask two nonjudgmental questions:

How is your heart? How full is your spirit?

How did you answer these questions?

I have often conflated the notion of filling my cup with filling my spirit, only to find that the needs for both are different. My cup can be refilled through getting adequate rest, eating a well-balanced meal, exercise, and positive social engagement. My spirit requires authentic connection to God and a daily nurturing practice. Honestly, my spirit as a student has fluctuated from full to empty.

I define *emptiness* as a perpetual depletion of my spirit that occurs through sustained discon-nection and exposure to stressors, pressure, and expectations. The exposure may be self-inflicted or come from relationships and systems that I navigate. My spiritual depletion was normalized as my roles were upheld and my reputation was maintained. I am blessed with a community that deeply knows me; they often sense this emptiness before I recognize it. Unaddressed, the emptiness manifested as anxiety, exhaustion, bitterness, fear, anger, and physical illness.

I define *fullness* as connection and showing up wholeheartedly to learn, teach, serve, care, and receive with an acknowledgement of my own needs and an awareness of others. Progress toward a full spirit takes considerable time, conscious effort, and vulnerability. My spiritual practice directly shapes my ability to be present in seasons of plenty and drought.

Faith, for me, is a radical form of self-love and self-care. I am a Christian. At a young age, I discovered that God is omnipresent in my life. My mom demonstrated the importance of inti-mate connection and relationship with God that extended beyond a day of the week or physical building. She modeled a daily spiritual practice for me and my brother. My mom communes with God without the need of a formal invitation, setting, or instruction. She nurtures her spirit through prayer, singing, scriptures, solitude, gathering, resting, dancing, and being in nature. Her vigilance to her spirit means that when her cup is empty, she is not depleted; she can replenish in times of stress because her deficits are physiological, not spiritual.

Spiritual practice looks different for everyone. My spiritual practice influences my core values and commitment to my studies, research, work, and service. In 2016 I attended the Upaya Institute and Zen Center's Being with Dying: Professional Training Program for Clinicians in Compassion-ate Care of the Seriously Ill and Dying. This experience, along with every death, has revealed to me that being with the dying teaches us so much more about how to be with the living.

My spiritual walk with God is honest, imperfect, and intimate. I get to show up as I am with my questions, convictions, and doubts. I am beautiful, loved, created with purpose—and so are you. At 30, I still shrink and tremble when life presents threats to my security. I cannot turn a blind eye to the systemic injustices across policy, policing, education, housing, and healthcare institu-tions. As a nurse, I am devoted to providing equitable, dignified, and compassionate care to each patient. Nursing is my form of activism and resistance.

I wish I could invite you to join me in my parents' backyard. Consider this a call to vigilance wherever and in whatever season you are. My desire for us all is to move forward from a space of fullness.

With love and gratitude,

Victoria Tucker

13

Sleep, Exercise, and Nutrition: Self-Care the Kaizen Way

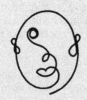

Tim Cunningham
pronouns: He/Him

Tim Cunningham began his professional career as an actor, then a hospital clown. He began doing international humanitarian work with Clowns Without Borders. While a clown, he fell in love with nurses' ability to connect with patients and families, even in times of terrible suffering—so he became an emergency nurse. The rest is history.

"I may not be there yet, but I am closer than I was yesterday."

—Misty Copeland

I remember in 2010, just one year after beginning my professional practice as a nurse, I had the opportunity to listen to His Holiness the 14th Dalai Lama give a speech. There I stood, in a crowd of hundreds of people, listening to the world-renowned figure. What I remember most about his talk are two things. For one, he laughed frequently and authentically. He spoke with a sense of levity, which made us all smile while he spoke about love, compassion, suffering, and how we can make this world a better place.

Toward the end of his speech, an audience member asked him, "What is the secret to a good life?"

The Dalai Lama laughed so hard that his body shook.

"I don't know," he told us.

Then he laughed again and said, "I think if you had to choose one thing that you could do to have a good life, it would be to make sure you get enough sleep!" The crowd roared with applause and laughter. Laughter and sleep. Sounds simple. But as we know, it's not always that easy.

An overarching theme of this book, and one that is critically important for this chapter, is that change in self-care practices takes time, and that's completely normal. For example, if you decide you want to run a marathon (26.2 miles) and you've never run more than a mile or two, you're not going to be able to start training one day and then run the whole marathon the next. Think similarly about self-care practices like sleep, nutrition, and exercise.

The Philosophy of Kaizen

I recommend a philosophy to guide you through this chapter called *Kaizen*. Kaizen is a core value of *Lean methodologies* that health systems increasingly use to build high reliability (Oster & Braaten, 2016). *Kaizen* is a Japanese term that means "good change." Car manufacturing companies, like Toyota, have used this concept to identify small problems and feasible changes that can be made to fix them (Hosono, 2020). By taking a "bite-sized" approach to change, rather than trying to fix and change everything at once, change can happen, sustainably, over time. What's best about Kaizen is that change is manageable. You don't have to climb the mountain today or finish the whole marathon right away—you just have to take one step forward. When you think of Kaizen, think about incremental change and remember that self-care is a practice. It needs repetition, and it can become easier over time.

Florence Nightingale might agree. Her words reflect the notion that in order to grow strong and wise, you first must begin with a small, manageable or feasible, step: "So never lose an opportunity of urging a practical beginning, however small, for it is wonderful how often in such matters the mustard-seed germinates and roots itself" (Brainy Quote, n.d.).

Small, manageable steps. This chapter examines the three critical roots of self-care—sleep, exercise, and nutrition—and explores simple ways to approach how you care for your physical well-being.

Sleep. Plain and Simple.

Sleep. Do you feel like you get enough of it? I can say that I often wish I could get more of it, and I'm not alone. In financially wealthy nations worldwide, two-thirds of adults don't get the recommended eight hours of sleep each night (Walker, 2017). Inadequate sleep (less than six or seven hours per night) can wreak havoc on your immune system; shorten your life expectancy; make you more susceptible to Alzheimer's disease, cancer, heart disease, diabetes, memory impairment, depression, anxiety, and suicidality; and stimulate your body's hunger hormones and increase your weight (Walker, 2017). We don't perform as well at work when we are tired, and we are less likely to exercise or eat well when we're struggling with exhaustion. This is just the tip of the why-we-need-sleep iceberg. As Matthew Walker writes in his book, *Why We Sleep*, there are no biological functions "that do not benefit from a good night's sleep" (Walker, 2017, p. 8).

Sleep Hygiene

The Centers for Disease Control and Prevention (CDC) defines sleep hygiene as a set of activities that you can do to improve the quality and regularity of your sleep (CDC, n.d.). Physiologically, we know that regular sleep cycles are key to one's health and self-care; however, in the nursing profession, especially with shifts that rotate from days to nights, that kind of regularity of sleeping hours is not always possible. Here, the CDC offers some other things that you can do, whether you have regular sleep cycles or not, to support your sleep hygiene (CDC, n.d.):

- Make sure your bedroom is quiet, dark, relaxing, and at a comfortable temperature.

- Remove electronic devices, such as TVs, computers, and smartphones, from the bedroom.

- Avoid large meals, caffeine, and alcohol before bedtime.

- Get some exercise. Being physically active during the day can help you fall asleep more easily at night.

Good sleep hygiene is important to us all, and it is especially so for nurses. The nature of our work requires that we be alert and able to concentrate. We need to safely operate equipment, including our cars on the drive home. Work stress, hectic schedules, and night shifts are just a few of the sleep disruptors nurses typically face.

Shift Work Disorder

An important element of good sleep hygiene is sticking to a consistent sleep schedule (Walker, 2017), but that isn't always possible for nurses. Shift work disorder is a condition that manifests as chronic drowsiness, frequent inability to concentrate, and generalized low energy during the waking hours. It is most common among people who work changing shifts, which is to say, people who work some dayshifts, some night or evening shifts, on a constantly rotating schedule. Many new nurses in US hospitals are scheduled on rotating or nights-only shifts as they begin their careers. One study suggests that up to 30% of shift workers experience shift work disorder (Booker et al., 2020). It goes on to say that the key factor that makes symptoms of shift work disorder worse, when controlling for exercise, alcohol, and medication intake, is simply inconsistent sleep patterns. We know that it often does not feel "simple" to achieve consistent sleep patterns; your body even fights against you with rising cortisol levels during the day, signaling your body to wake up just as you need to fall asleep.

Nonpharmacological Interventions for Sleep

It is my opinion and the result of much scientific research (Walker, 2017) that the healthiest way to get a good sleep is to use natural methods. Granted, there are some conditions in which sleep medication is essential, so keep that in mind and do not feel discouraged if you are prescribed sleep medications. But what can you do to avoid having to take sleep medications, even if you are working multiple night shifts or (even more challenging) on a rotating schedule of days to nights?

Reduce Light

Certainly a physiological challenge to nearly half of our clinical nursing, hospital-based workforce is that the presence of light encourages us to stay awake. Melatonin, a natural hormone, is released more extensively in our bodies when there is limited natural sunlight (Brown, 1994). Released from the pineal gland, melatonin interplays with our circadian rhythms, influencing us to sleep when the sun has gone down (Wams et al., 2017). The challenge, then, as you work night shifts and have to sleep during the day when the sun is out, can be finding ways to reduce the ambient light around you.

Blackout curtains or other window covers that completely block the light from your room can trick your body into thinking that it's nighttime, even if it is high noon outside. Eye masks can also block out extra light. There is good evidence that they work for our hospitalized patients who need to sleep and rest (Sweity et al., 2019); they are likely to work for you, too. Many nurses use earplugs to block out distracting noise. You can find very effective ones at your drugstore; be sure to read the directions to maximize their effectiveness.

Support of friends and family is another way to improve your sleep hygiene. Let the people you live with know how important sleep is to you, and ask them for quiet times in your apartment or house during your sleep hours.

And finally, there are preventive things you can do throughout the day. In addition to the list above from the CDC for good sleep hygiene, here are a few more (Walker, 2017):

- Limit your caffeine intake during the day.
- Avoid exercise late in the day.
- Don't smoke.
- Take a hot bath or shower before bed.
- Keep your bedroom cool.
- Turn the clock face away from your bed so you don't "watch the clock" when you're having trouble sleeping.
- Try to get 30 minutes of natural sunlight each day.

Aromatherapy

Some evidence suggests that the herb lavender can be helpful in supporting good sleep patterns. More commonly grown in arid parts of the US and the globe, lavender can be grown in pots most anywhere, when attended to properly. Its essence, whether fresh from its blooms or in liquid tinctures, is thought to help improve sleep. Not only is lavender considered to support healthy sleep hygiene, it is thought to help reduce anxiety (Lillehei et al., 2015; McCaffrey et al., 2009). The risks of using lavender safely to help with sleep are very low, and negative side effects are minimal to nonexistent.

Napping

We have another option when it comes to good sleep hygiene: the power of napping. When is the last time you took a nap? People in some countries take a siesta in the middle of the day, every day. We know that napping, even for 10–15 minutes, can reduce stress and energize you to keep moving forward during your day (or night shift). Even though there is convincing evidence that taking naps can help people with their attention spans, energy levels, and overall well-being (Fallis et al., 2011; Zion & Shochat, 2019), many employers are unwilling to allow their staff to take naps on the job. Of course, you don't want to find yourself napping at the nurses' station; however, there are some healthcare employers who designate private, staff-only areas where you can prop up your feet and take a nap. Some people can wake up from naps easily and be back to themselves and on their game pretty quickly. If your employer provides this option, see how the power of napping works for you.

Medications for Sleeplessness

Practice sleep hygiene so that you can develop patterns and habits that will allow you to sleep well, despite the challenging hours and schedules of nursing. Unfortunately, no matter how vigorously you follow all the quality sleep suggestions, you may experience periods of sleeplessness. Insomnia sucks.

Be cautious if you choose to take sleeping medication. Yes, they can help sometimes, but we've also learned about the deleterious effects of some sleeping medications (Walker, 2017). Talk to your primary care physician or nurse practitioner, and the two of you can make the decision together. Intense sleeping medications, like zolpidem (brand name: Ambien), can cause aggressive and unpredictable behavioral changes (Dinges et al., 2019). Sleepwalking and nighttime binge eating have also been associated with the use of this drug. A randomized trial on zolpidem found that it can lead to "emergent awakenings" during the night and decreased performance during the day (Dinges et al., 2019).

Some over-the-counter cough and cold medications and the antihistamine diphen-hydramine (brand name: Benadryl) have been used for aids in sleeping as well (Per-kins, 2001). Again, anytime you consider taking a medication to help with sleep, first speak with a trusted nurse practitioner or physician to seek advice on whether medicinal sleep aids are right for you.

There is some evidence that ingesting a small dose of *melatonin* can help make sleep more restful (Sadeghniiat-Haghighi et al., 2008). As discussed earlier in the chapter, melatonin is a hormone produced in the pineal gland that increases when ambient light decreases (the onset of nighttime) and decreases with sunlight. You might find some positive benefits to taking a dose of melatonin, especially if you are a night-shift worker and you have to sleep during the day. Further, some evidence suggests that melatonin can serve as an anti-inflammatory agent (Nabavi et al., 2019).

If you struggle with sleep, try to approach some of the suggestions below as a Kaizen practice. Take small steps. Pay attention to your body. Experiment until you find something that works for you. For example, rather than scrolling through your phone right before bed, intentionally take five minutes to read a book or magazine. Or you could take one minute before you fall asleep to close your eyes and do a breathing exercise or body scan. If this small change feels helpful, you might try stepping away from your phone for ten minutes before sleep and do a five-minute body scan. Gradually adjust the balance of time-away-from-the phone and relaxation techniques until you find the ideal mix.

Restorative sleep is so critical to your well-being, it is definitely worth the effort.

Exercise

If you have a chance to do some exercise during the day, falling asleep at night will likely be easier (Uchida et al., 2012). But exercise provides many more benefits than as a sleep enhancer. Exercise is ubiquitous as a way to care for ourselves, whether it's playing ping-pong or running a marathon. As nurses, we know the health benefits of movement and physical activity for heart disease prevention, diabetes self-management, and more (Ross et al., 2019). Physical activity produces physical, emotional, and spiritual benefits, and in my own experience, I have found that exercise is the foundation of my self-care practice.

Exercise Doesn't Need to Happen in a Gym

What does exercise mean to you? When someone says, "Go exercise," what is the first thing that comes to mind? Is it running, walking, weight training, swimming, stretching, gardening, playing tennis, or hiking in the woods? There are few wrong answers when it comes to exercise—it's all about what *you* consider to be exercise. The health benefits may be "all in your head."

Harvard researcher Alia Crum led a fascinating study around the question of exercise and the placebo effect. She and her research team studied 84 female hotel housekeepers. They told the intervention group that their work cleaning rooms and making beds met the Surgeon General's recommendations for a healthy lifestyle. Compared to the control group of housekeepers who were *not* told this information, the intervention group not only believed they exercised more, they also had measurably better health outcomes such as reductions in weight and blood pressure. The results suggest that exercise "affects health in part or in whole via the placebo effect" (Crum & Langer, 2007).

What did this study suggest to us? The housekeepers who were told that their work was "doing exercise" improved on certain scores, though nothing had changed but their mindsets. We see in this work that intention or belief can be a powerful tool for health. What if you considered taking the stairs next time you go to work, rather than the elevator, as a way to exercise? Do you think that maybe you'd experience psychological and even physical benefits?

We know that exercise can be many things. One common factor about exercise is that if we *believe* what we are doing is exercise and thus good for us, it might have better impacts on our well-being; thus, it can be a form of self-care. Sometimes there is not enough time to go to the gym, sometimes you just can't fit that yoga class into your schedule, but you can always find a few short minutes during your day. During that time, you could walk outside, take the stairs, or do stretching exercises in a storage closet. Consider those actions as exercise, too.

Personal Perspective

My Time to Unwind

–Nicole Jefferson, BSN, RN (she/her)

Being a nurse is tough, but being a new nurse working in a pandemic is even tougher. At the beginning of the pandemic, I started working on a new floor in an entirely different field of nursing. I had transferred from general medicine to labor and delivery. It was stressful learning so many new skills and procedures along with getting to know my new coworkers, all the while keeping track of policy changes due to COVID-19. In order to practice self-care during this stressful time, there isn't just one thing that I do. I exercise frequently, find a good book to read, and try to cook healthy meals. Since the pandemic started, I've had more time to explore in the kitchen, so I recently started making my own recipe book. I find new recipes to try, and if I liked the meal, I print it and add it to my personal recipe book.

Another self-care practice that I love to indulge in is dancing. Sometimes I'm up at two in the morning dancing in my room or learning a new TikTok dance. I'm able to have fun, get some exercise, and express my artistic side all while moving my body.

However, the most important self-care practice that I've learned is to *listen* to my body. For me this means taking time out to rest. Sometimes I push myself too hard or I try to do everything, and there have been many times where my body is trying to tell me to rest, but I don't listen. Now I'm teaching myself that it's okay to lie in bed for half a day or simply do nothing and relax or take a nap. If my body needs to rest, then I let it. These simple practices have aided me to not only preserve but improve my overall health.

Exercise for Social Connection

Exercise is also a great way to connect with others and build your social network. If you have moved to a new town or city for your job, hanging out with other people in a yoga class or a race training program will help you meet new people while boosting your fitness level. There are also dance clubs, music groups, volunteer projects, and other social groups that can provide human connection while getting you off the couch.

You don't need to be best friends or even talk to them to benefit from their presence. Neuroscientist James Coan has done fascinating research on the power of relationships (Sbarra & Coan, 2018). His work suggests that the presence of another person, whether close friend or just an acquaintance—like the barista at your favorite coffee shop—can stir within you a sense of calm, of belonging, and of safety (Coan et al., 2017). We can foster this connectedness while simultaneously building our bodies in these social groups. I often reflect on a marathon I ran once in which I did not talk to anyone, but I still felt a part of a team, a massive group of 20,000 people with the shared goal of running 26.2 miles. I felt connected to something bigger than myself and felt less alone.

If you're not going to hop out of bed this morning and run a marathon, this might be the perfect time to think about the Kaizen way. I'm reminded of a colleague who works with diabetes patients. She wanted to help one of her patients get a bit of exercise each day to help manage her blood sugar levels. During a clinic visit, she learned that her patient walked her granddaughter to the school bus stop every morning. My friend encouraged her patient to walk to the end of the next block and back after her granddaughter got on the bus. Every day. She already was dressed and out of the house, so making that additional effort was a simple step toward better health.

Let's Talk About Sex

—Michelle S Maust, MD, FAPA

Any truly holistic approach to wellness embraces sexuality. Sex serves vital roles in human behavior beyond procreative purposes. Sexual activity is a valuable form of self-care, and like other important areas of life—relationships, work, exercise, sleep, nutrition—it deserves attention. Tending to our sexual health can in turn optimize our physical and emotional well-being.

First things first: A partner is not a requirement for sexual satisfaction. Masturbation can be a powerful means of stress reduction, and orgasm triggers a release of sexual tension that produces a complex neuroendocrine response (Rowland, 2006). Masturbation has been associated with positive sexual experiences and healthy self-image (Robbins et al., 2011). Taking time to have sex with yourself, while engaging your

continues

continued

senses, appreciating your body, and seeking erotic pleasure is a healthy practice that builds from multiple therapeutic modes including cognitive behavioral therapy, mindfulness, and biological activation (Gordon, 2020).

Sexual activity can buffer the stress of everyday life. In a study examining sexual habits, sex appeared to relieve stress by disrupting the escalation of stress from one day to the next (Ein-Dor & Hirschberger, 2012). Sex also produces health benefits including maintaining circulator, neural, and muscular functionality of genitalia, preventive actions for prostate cancer in men, and counteracting vaginal atrophy in women (Levin, 2007). Further, sexual intimacy can foster the desire needed for durable relationships. Relationships are essential for coping throughout life, and they incur advantages. Satisfying relationships including sexual activity are noted to reduce exposure to stress and even promote recovery from stress (Ein-Dor & Hirschberger, 2012).

Lifestyle choices can enhance sexual well-being (Finley, 2018). Exercise improves mood, protects against depression (Schuch et al., 2018), and supports sexual function. Even a single bout of exercise can boost self-esteem (Ellis et al., 2013), and the positive body image that emerges with regular exercise can increase sexual well-being (Stanton et al., 2018). Cardio workouts prior to sex have been shown to increase sexual desire during sex (Lorenz & Meston, 2014). Sex itself is calorie-burning, dopamine-releasing exercise that reinforces further engagement in sexual activity.

Yoga, the practice of linking breath and movement, produces benefit in multiple neuropsychiatric disorders (Balasubramaniam et al., 2013) and appears to enhance sexual function too. Women who completed a 12-week yoga camp reported improved sexual function in all domains measured (Dhikav et al., 2010). Yoga includes *mindfulness*— the state of being aware in the present moment—which is precisely what is practiced during sensate focus exercises used in sex therapy. Mindfulness has been shown to significantly improve sexual response in women with sexual desire and arousal disorders (Brotto et al., 2008). High levels of chronic stress appear to inhibit sexual arousal in women (Hamilton & Meston, 2013). From these findings it follows that tending to stress, anxiety, and coping skills is a worthwhile habit for sexual function and self-care.

Avoiding certain substances is a critical lifestyle factor to support sexual function. Recreational drug use leads to depression of sexual function, even if acute intoxication heightens sensation or feelings of togetherness, as seen in MDMA or other substances that have come to be known as "love drugs." Regarding alcohol use, while intoxication can promote disinhibition and lead to sexual activity, the effect of higher doses of alcohol is attenuation of the arousal response (Mollaioli et al., 2020).

Obesity and cardiovascular disease worsen sexual function. In men these risks are directly linked to erectile dysfunction, and in women, high body mass index is associated with reduced sexual desire (Mollaioli et al., 2020). Diet can improve sexual function. In women with metabolic syndrome, practicing a Mediterranean diet over two years improved measures of sexual function (Esposito et al., 2017). While there is certainly not one particular diet or regimen that is appropriate for everyone, recognizing the role that lifestyle factors play in sexual function can help motivate individuals to make healthy choices that improve their satisfaction.

Sleep is vital for all body functions, and sex is no exception. Shorter sleep duration is associated with decreased sexual function (Kling et al., 2017), and obstructive sleep apnea is associated with sexual dysfunction in a dose-related fashion (Stavaras et al., 2012). Focusing efforts on healthy sleep habits can be the key to improving sexual function.

Engaging in a course of psychotherapy can provide far-reaching benefits. Reflecting on sexuality in a safe space helps individuals explore their own thoughts and identify any troublesome patterns. Underlying issues like preconceived notions about sexual behavior or negative body image can be worked through in therapy to foster sexual well-being in life. A history of sexual trauma can be especially damaging to sexual health, but psychotherapy can provide a healing process for growth and well-being. Therapy helps people get where they are going. Therapy and many forms of self-care can promote wellness. Keep tending to the most pleasurable part of wellness.

Nutrition

Just as nurses are knowledgeable about the health benefits of sleep and exercise, we have an intellectual understanding of the importance of good nutrition. In Chapter 1, we outlined the many barriers to healthy behaviors that nurses face. These include long work hours and exhaustion, making it difficult to prepare healthy meals. Nurses often work in unhealthy food cultures where baked goods and vending machines are plentiful but healthy options are not. Eating healthy is often a struggle; barriers to exercise and lack of sleep increase hormone imbalances and the risk of weight gain (Motivala et al., 2009).

We hope that eating a nutritious diet is important to you, but how will you figure out what works best for you? As there are a plethora of books, podcasts, websites, and blogs about exercise, we are also overwhelmed by information about nutrition and diet. Every few years new trends and fad diets come along, many claiming to be based on scientific evidence; some are, and some are not. We hear from experts and enthusiasts on the benefits of high-carb diets, low-carb diets, high-fat and low-fat diets, locale diets (e.g., Mediterranean, Sonoma), keto diets, and paleo diets. Others weigh in on the timing of meals, the harms and benefits of snacking, and recently, intermittent fasting. There are diets for people at risk for heart disease, diabetes, and allergies and food sensitivities, such as gluten. And let's not forget whole food diets and the popularity of vegan and vegetarian diets.

These diets may work for some people, but not for everyone (Hill et al., 2005). So how will you create your own eating and nutrition guidelines?

Listen to Your Body

Begin by paying attention to your body. How do you feel after eating certain foods? What does hunger feel like for you on a scale of 1 to 10? At what point while eating do you feel *too* full, and how does that make you feel? What aspects of nutritious eating stress you out the most? Consider the approach of mindful eating, when you think about your nutritional intake (Warren et al., 2017). If you are hungry, take care of yourself, and eat a little bit. Please note if you are fasting for a religious practice, like for the Muslim holy month of Ramadan, or you have given something up in your diet for the Christian practice of Lent, for example, finding meaning in these practices can sometimes increase your ability to focus and home in on your intentions as a caregiver and a nurse.

Snacks can be very beneficial when you are on the move, have a full patient load, and know that your lunch break might not happen. A medical student who had just finished her clinical rotations said the best lesson she learned was to keep hard-boiled eggs in her white coat pocket. She said she could sneak into a restroom and eat one quickly to keep herself going.

Stay Hydrated

Hydration is a key element of good nutrition, so be sure to drink ample water. A glass of water can help you feel less tired as well as less hungry; sometimes fatigue and hunger are signals that our bodies are dehydrated (Grandjean & Grandjean, 2007).

Again, think about approaching your nutritional habits the Kaizen way. Experiment by changing one small behavior at a time, whether that be packing a meal for work before you go to bed, getting up a little earlier so you have time to eat breakfast, or limiting desserts to a few times a week or less. Try your hand at weekly meal prep; there are so many ideas and recipes available online now. Consider healthy take-out options, such as a delicious salad, or consider a home-delivery meal service. Many are modestly priced, cut down on trips to the grocery store, eliminate food waste, and encourage nutritious eating. Finding the best way to keep yourself well-fueled will be a lifetime experiment; you'll adjust and adapt as you learn more about your body and as your lifestyle and schedule change. The following sidebar shares two comfort food stories from two international nursing colleagues.

Personal Perspective

Comfort Food and Self Care

–Daniel Jeong, DNAP, RN, CRNA (he/him)

Making and eating home-cooked meals is at the top of my list for self-care activities. Taking time to cook a delicious meal takes my mind away from stressors, plus eating a quality meal warms my heart and body. Being a second-generation Korean American, I often flip between making traditional Korean dishes that I grew up eating with my family, like kimchi stew, and American comfort foods that I learned to cook through US media, like chicken pot pie. I feel being exposed to two different cultures has broadened my options, particularly to the choices of dishes that I consider my comfort foods!

Another one of my prime self-care practices includes traveling around the country, whether with friends or by myself. These trips provide a respite from the monotony of daily life and a fresh perspective to tackle problems that I face. On my solo trips, I'm often mindful of the surrounding environment, exploring the unique culture of each place that I visit—each city has its own soul. Unsurprisingly, one of my favorite pastimes is trying local restaurants and foods and seeing how to incorporate some of these new eats into my growing menu of comfort foods.

–Eric Ng, BSN Nursing Student (he/him)

Although the ideal of becoming a physician has become a part of the model minority myth surrounding Asian Americans, I chose to enter nursing because it seemed more personable, and I enjoyed the idea of spending more time interacting with patients. For my self-care, I tend to play video games or treat myself to a nice meal. Specifically, eating Cantonese food was commonplace at home, reflecting my parents' upbringing in southern China and providing me with a sense of familiarity. One of my favorite meals to eat is hot pot!

There is no one right way to do nutrition, so listen to your body and what it seeks. Treat yourself with nutritious and delicious foods, and of course, comfort foods that remind you of family, friends, loved ones, and home.

Evaluate Your Alcohol Usage

I would be remiss if I didn't say something about the pros and cons of alcoholic beverages as a form of self-care. Having a drink with friends can be a great way to relax and unwind. However, as we've already mentioned in this chapter, alcohol, especially near bedtime, can disrupt your sleep (Devenney et al., 2019). Alcohol can lead to even more dangerous consequences, especially if you are at high risk of addiction.

A glass of wine at the end of a shift, for example, can be a form of self-care for *some* people. Pay attention to your drinking behaviors and how you feel before and after you drink. If that nightly glass of wine becomes multiple glasses or even a nightly bottle of wine, try a Kaizen approach such as only drinking one glass a day, then working down to weekends only, and then perhaps to just on special occasions. Notice if reducing your alcohol intake improves how you feel. If you still crave alcohol or can't cut back, then please consider talking with a trusted physician or nurse practitioner. Signs of alcohol dependence include (Powell et al., 2007):

- An ongoing need to drink more to obtain an optimal level of intoxication
- Drinking to manage a hangover or feelings of alcohol withdrawal
- A desire to drink less or change drinking habits or the inability to do so
- Giving up important social or occupational activities so that you can drink

And it follows that alcohol abuse could look like (Powell et al., 2007):

- Ongoing use of alcohol despite the failure to accomplish academic, occupational, social responsibilities;

- Using alcohol regularly during situations when it is physically dangerous (such as driving or operating heavy machinery);
- Ongoing alcohol use in spite of social disruptions;
- Legal actions taken against you while you were under the influence of alcohol

There are many resources available both online and in your community. The AUDIT (Alcohol Use Disorders Identification Test) can be self-administered online (https://www.drugabuse.gov/sites/default/files/audit.pdf). If you work in a hospital, you should have access to an Employee Assistance Program, or you can call your insurance provider for a referral to a therapist or substance use disorder program. One of the most well-known organizations in the US that has shown very good results for many of its participants is Alcoholics Anonymous (AA) (Humphreys et al., 2014). There are AA chapters in most cities and towns across the US, so if you would like to learn more about them, you can seek your local chapter at www. aa.org. The health, personal, and professional consequences of excessive alcohol intake are too great for you to ignore. I encourage you to care for yourself with healthy alcohol consumption.

Stress and the Sleep-Exercise-Nutrition Triangle

Although we know about the importance of self-care when it comes to supporting resilience and being our best selves, when stress arises, we can easily lose touch with our self-care practices. The three topics of this chapter are usually the first self-care practices that we abandon when we face stress. Unfortunately, when the wheels come off one side of the self-care triangle of sleep, exercise, and nutrition, they are likely to come off the others as well. For example, if you have a large paper due or a stressful situation at work, you may lose sleep over it due to worry. Now you're stressed *and* tired, so healthy eating takes too much effort. Despite knowing that certain foods can increase inflammation and make stress in our bodies even worse (Spritzler, 2019), those are the very foods we turn to when the going gets tough. Sweet, salty, and processed foods are the common culprits we eat in order to "manage" our stress. Now all sides of the triangle are crushed; the last thing you'll want to do after getting a terrible night's sleep and eating too much pizza is go to the gym or head out for a run.

We cannot always take care of ourselves the way we need to, and that is normal and okay. This is the perfect time to practice self-compassion. Talk to yourself the way you would talk to a dear friend who was doing their best under difficult circumstances. Here's the most important thing: No one is perfect.

Closing Thoughts

There is no one who understands the demands of nursing like another nurse. I encourage you to find colleagues who seem to have a handle on some of these sleep, nutrition, and exercise self-care practices. Ask them what they have learned over the years about sleep hygiene, how they fit exercise into their schedule, or what their meal planning strategies look like. I bet they will be flattered to be acknowledged for their expertise, and they are sure to have some good ideas to share with you.

Most importantly, be forgiving and kind to yourself. If you don't reach your sleep, exercise, and nutrition goals right away or if you feel like you're not always doing a good job of self-care, take a deep breath. You're just like me and so many others on that. I've been writing about self-care and studying it for years, and I *still* struggle with it. That is one big reason why I love the idea of Kaizen; a little bit goes a long way.

In Real Practice

A retrospective, observational study of nurses and their sleep habits—namely, hours of sleep before shifts—shows important data that help us advocate for the need of sleep. This study by Stimphfel, Fatehi, & Kovner (2020) is robust due to its large sample size, thus supporting its generalizability. Nurses (N=1,568) from across the US provided information for this study. Researchers compared nurse sleep hours to various aspects of patient care quality. Of note, researchers found that short sleep duration before a shift had a direct relationship with patient quality of care and safety outcomes. Thus, in this study, less sleep before a shift suggested decreased safety and lower quality of care for patients. Alternatively, more sleep improved quality of care. This paper reminds us of the utmost importance of good sleep.

Key Points

- In this chapter we talked about the Japanese term Kaizen—or the small, measurable, and feasible steps that we can make to bring about positive change. The Kaizen (or "good change") method is one way you can approach the sleep, exercise, and nutrition aspects of self-care. Try making small changes to improve your daily health habits and see how they work. Make adjustments and improvements as needed.

- Sleep is critical to your health and well-being. There are many recommendations to improve your sleep hygiene, but they commonly include reducing caffeine, alcohol, and screen time before bed; sleeping in a cool, dark, quiet room; and exercising and being physically active during your waking hours.

- Exercise prevents chronic disease and maintains and even improves your emotional health. There are infinite activities that constitute exercise, so don't get discouraged because you don't like to run or go to the gym. Exercising in groups, such as a dance class, bowling team, or hiking club, has the added benefit of social connectivity, which also fosters well-being.

- Be creative in your approach to nutrition. Fuel your body with foods you love but that also make you feel good. Our bodies have a lot to tell us if we choose to listen. Experiment with Kaizen strategies that address your unique food preferences, schedule, and lifestyle needs.

References

Balasubramaniam, M., Telles, S., & Doraiswamy, P. M. (2013). Yoga on our minds: A systematic review of yoga for neuropsychiatric disorders. *Frontiers in Psychiatry*, 3, 117. https://doi.org/10.3389/fpsyt.2012.00117

Booker, L. A., Barnes, M., Alvaro, P., Collins, A., Chai-Coetzer, C. L., McMahon, M., Lockley, S. W., Rajaratnam, S. M. W., Howard, M. E., & Sletten, T. L. (2020). The role of sleep hygiene in the risk of Shift Work Disorder in nurses. *Sleep*, 43(2), zsz228. https://doi.org/10.1093/sleep/zsz228

Brainy Quote. (n.d.). *Florence Nightingale quotes.* https://www.brainyquote.com/quotes/florence_nightingale_121022

Brotto, L. A., Krychman, M., & Jacobson, P. (2008). Eastern approaches for enhancing women's sexuality: Mindfulness, acupuncture, and yoga (CME). *Journal of Sexual Medicine*, 5(12), 2741–2748. https://doi.org/10.1111/j.1743-6109.2008.01071.x

Brown, G. M. (1994). Light, melatonin and the sleep-wake cycle. *Journal of Psychiatry and Neuroscience*, *19*(5), 345.

Centers for Disease Control and Prevention. (n.d.). *Sleep and sleep disorders*. Retrieved from https://www.cdc.gov/sleep/about_sleep/sleep_hygiene.html

Coan, J. A., Beckes, L., Gonzalez, M. Z., Maresh, E. L., Brown, C. L., & Hasselmo, K. (2017). Relationship status and perceived support in the social regulation of neural responses to threat. *Social cognitive and affective neuroscience*, *12*(10), 1574–1583. https://doi.org/10.1093/scan/nsx091

Crum, A. J., & Langer, E. J. (2007). Mind-set matters: Exercise and the placebo effect. *Psychological Science*, *18*(2), 165–171.

Devenney, L. E., Coyle, K. B., Roth, T., & Verster, J. C. (2019). Sleep after heavy alcohol consumption and physical activity levels during alcohol hangover. *Journal of clinical medicine*, *8*(5), 752.

Dhikav, V., Karmarkar, G., Gupta, R., Verma, M., Gupta, R., Gupta, S., & Anand, K. S. (2010). Yoga in female sexual functions. *Journal of Sexual Medicine*, *7*(2), 964–970. https://doi.org/10.1111/j.1743-6109.2009.01580.x

Dinges, D. F., Basner, M., Ecker, A. J., Baskin, P., & Johnston, S. L. (2019). Effects of zolpidem and zaleplon on cognitive performance after emergent morning awakenings at Tmax: A randomized placebo-controlled trial. *Sleep*, *42*(3), zsy258. https://doi.org/10.1093/sleep/zsy258

Ein-Dor, T., & Hirschberger, G. (2012). Sexual healing: Daily diary evidence that sex relieves stress for men and women in satisfying relationships. *Journal of Social and Personal Relationships*, *29*(1), 126–139. https://doi.org/10.1177/0265407511431185

Ellis, N., Randall, J., & Punnett, G. (2013). The effects of a single bout of exercise on mood and self-esteem in clinically diagnosed mental health patients. *Open Journal of Medical Psychology*, *2*(3), 81–85. http://dx.doi.org/10.4236/ojmp.2013.23013

Esposito, K., Ciotola, M., Giugliano, F., Schisano, B., Autorino, R., Iuliano, S., Vietri, M. T., Cioffi, M., De Sio, M., & Giugliano, D. (2007). Mediterranean diet improves sexual function in women with the metabolic syndrome. *International Journal of Impotence Research*, *19*(5), 486–491. https://doi.org/10.1038/sj.ijir.3901555

Fallis, W. M., McMillan, D. E., & Edwards, M. P. (2011). Napping during night shift: Practices, preferences, and perceptions of critical care and emergency department nurses. *Critical Care Nurse*, *31*(2), e1–e11. https://doi.org/10.4037/ccn2011710

Finley, N. (2018). Lifestyle choices can augment female sexual well-being. *American Journal of Lifestyle Medicine*, *12*(1), 38–41. https://doi.org/10.1177/1559827617740823

Gordon, E. (2020, April 25). Solitary sex: How self pleasure will get you through sheltering alone. *Volonté*. https://www.lelo.com/blog/solitary-sex/

Grandjean, A. C., & Grandjean, N. R. (2007). Dehydration and cognitive performance. *Journal of the American College of Nutrition*, *26*(sup5), 549S–554S.

Hamilton, L. D., & Meston, C. M. (2013). Chronic stress and sexual function in women. *Journal of Sexual Medicine*, *10*(10), 2443–2454. https://doi.org/10.1111/jsm.12249

Hill, J. O., Thompson, H., & Wyatt, H. (2005). Weight maintenance: what's missing? *Journal of the American Dietetic Association*, *105*(5), 63–66.

Hosono, A. (2020). Kaizen toward learning, transformation, and high-quality growth: Insights from outstanding experiences. In *Workers, Managers, Productivity* (pp. 45–67). Palgrave Macmillan, Singapore.

Humphreys, K., Blodgett, J. C., & Wagner, T. H. (2014). Estimating the efficacy of Alcoholics Anonymous without self-selection bias: An instrumental variables re-analysis of randomized clinical trials. *Alcoholism: Clinical and Experimental Research, 38*(11), 2688–2694.

Kling, J. M., Manson, J. E., Naughton, M. J., Temkit, M., Sullivan, S. D., Gower, E. W., Hale, L., Weitlauf, J. C., Nowakowski, S., & Crandall, C. J. (2017). Association of sleep disturbance and sexual function in postmenopausal women. *Menopause, 24*(6), 604–612. https://doi.org/10.1097/GME.0000000000000824

Levin, R. J. (2007). Sexual activity, health and well-being—The beneficial roles of coitus and masturbation. *Sexual and Relationship Therapy, 22*(1), 135–148. https://doi.org/10.1080/14681990601149197

Lillehei, A. S., Halcón, L. L., Savik, K., & Reis, R. (2015). Effect of inhaled lavender and sleep hygiene on self-reported sleep issues: A randomized controlled trial. *Journal of Alternative and Complementary Medicine, 21*(7), 430–438. https://doi.org/10.1089/acm.2014.0327

Lorenz, T. A., & Meston, C. M. (2014). Exercise improves sexual function in women taking antidepressants: Results from a randomized crossover trial. *Depression and Anxiety, 31*(3), 188–195. https://doi.org/10.1002/da.22208

McCaffrey, R., Thomas, D. J., & Kinzelman, A. O. (2009). The effects of lavender and rosemary essential oils on test-taking anxiety among graduate nursing students. *Holistic Nursing Practice, 23*(2), 88–93. https://doi.org/10.1097/HNP.0b013e3181a110aa

Mollaioli, D., Ciocca, G., Limoncin, E., Di Sante, S., Gravina, G. L., Carosa, E., Lenzi, A., & Jannini, E. A. F. (2020). Lifestyles and sexuality in men and women: The gender perspective in sexual medicine. *Reproductive Biology and Endocrinology, 18*(1), 1–11. https://doi.org/10.1186/s12958-019-0557-9

Motivala, S. J., Tomiyama, A. J., Ziegler, M., Khandrika, S., & Irwin, M. R. (2009). Nocturnal levels of ghrelin and leptin and sleep in chronic insomnia. *Psychoneuroendocrinology, 34*(4), 540–545.

Nabavi, S. M., Nabavi, S. F., Sureda, A., Xiao, J., Dehpour, A. R., Shirooie, S., Silva, A. S., Baldi, A., Khan, H., & Daglia, M. (2019). Anti-inflammatory effects of Melatonin: A mechanistic review. *Critical Reviews in Food Science and Nutrition, 59*(sup1), S4–S16. https://doi.org/10.1080/10408398.2018.1487927

Oster, C., & Braaten, J. (2016). *High reliability organizations: A healthcare handbook for patient safety & quality.* Sigma Theta Tau.

Perkins, L. A. (2001). Is the night shift worth the risk? *RN, 64*(8), 65–65.

Powell, P. A., Faden, V. B., & Wing, S. (2007). The Surgeon General's Call to Action to Prevent and Reduce Underage Drinking, 2007. US Department of Health and Human Services.

Robbins, C. L., Schick, V., Reece, M., Herbenick, D., Sanders, S. A., Dodge, B., & Fortenberry, J. D. (2011). Prevalence, frequency, and associations of masturbation with partnered sexual behaviors among US adolescents. *Archives of Pediatrics & Adolescent Medicine, 165*(12), 1087–1093. https://doi.org/10.1001/archpediatrics.2011.142

Ross, A., Touchton-Leonard, K., Perez, A., Wehrlen, L., Kazmi, N., & Gibbons, S. (2019). Factors that influence health-promoting self-care in registered nurses: Barriers and facilitators. *Advances in Nursing Science, 42*(4), 358–373.

Rowland, D. L. (2006). Neurobiology of sexual response in men and women. *CNS Spectrums, 11*(S9), 6–12. https://doi.org/10.1017/S1092852900026705

Sadeghniiat-Haghighi, K., Aminian, O., Pouryaghoub, G., & Yazdi, Z. (2008). Efficacy and hypnotic effects of melatonin in shift-work nurses: Double-blind, placebo-controlled crossover trial. *Journal of Circadian Rhythms*, 6(1), 10. https://doi.org/10.1186/1740-3391-6-10

Sbarra, D. A., & Coan, J. A. (2018). Relationships and health: The critical role of affective science. *Emotion Review*, 10(1), 40–54. https://doi.org/10.1177/1754073917696584

Schuch, F. B., Vancampfort, D., Firth, J., Rosenbaum, S., Ward, P. B., Silva, E. S., Hallgren, M., Ponce De Leon, A., Dunn, A. L., Deslandes, A. C., Fleck, M. P., Carvalho, A. F., & Stubbs, B. (2018). Physical activity and incident depression: A meta-analysis of prospective cohort studies. *American Journal of Psychiatry*, 175(7), 631–648. https://doi.org/10.1176/appi.ajp.2018.17111194

Spritzler, F. (2019). 6 foods that cause inflammation. Healthline Media. Retrieved from https://www.healthline.com/nutrition/6-foods-that-cause-inflammation#Food-Fix:-Beat-The-Bloat

Stanton, A. M., Handy, A. B., & Meston, C. M. (2018). The effects of exercise on sexual function in women. *Sexual Medicine Reviews*, 6(4), 548–557. https://doi.org/10.1016/j.sxmr.2018.02.004

Stavaras, C., Pastaka, C., Papala, M., Gravas, S., Tzortzis, V., Melekos, M., Seitanidis, G., & Gourgoulianis, K. I. (2012). Sexual function in pre-and post-menopausal women with obstructive sleep apnea syndrome. *International Journal of Impotence Research*, 24(6), 228–233. https://doi.org/10.1038/ijir.2012.20

Stimpfel, A. W., Fatehi, F., & Kovner, C. (2020). Nurses' sleep, work hours, and patient care quality, and safety. *Sleep health*, 6(3), 314–320. https://doi.org/10.1016/j.sleh.2019.11.001

Sweity, S., Finlay, A., Lees, C., Monk, A., Sherpa, T., & Wade, D. (2019). SleepSure: A pilot randomized-controlled trial to assess the effects of eye masks and earplugs on the quality of sleep for patients in hospital. *Clinical Rehabilitation*, 33(2), 253–261. https://doi.org/10.1177/0269215518806041

Uchida, S., Shioda, K., Morita, Y., Kubota, C., Ganeko, M., & Takeda, N. (2012). Exercise effects on sleep physiology. *Frontiers in neurology*, 3, 48.

Walker, M. (2017). *Why we sleep: Unlocking the power of sleep and dreams*. Scribner.

Wams, E. J., Woelders, T., Marring, I., van Rosmalen, L., Beersma, D. G., Gordijn, M. C., & Hut, R. A. (2017). Linking light exposure and subsequent sleep: A field polysomnography study in humans. *Sleep*, 40(12), zsx165.

Warren, J. M., Smith, N., & Ashwell, M. (2017). A structured literature review on the role of mindfulness, mindful eating and intuitive eating in changing eating behaviours: effectiveness and associated potential mechanisms. *Nutrition research reviews*, 30(2), 272–283.

Zion, N., & Shochat, T. (2019). Let them sleep: The effects of a scheduled nap during the night shift on sleepiness and cognition in hospital nurses. *Journal of Advanced Nursing*, 75(11), 2603–2615. https://doi.org/10.1111/jan.14031

14

Six Steps to Compassion: Practicing T'ai Chi in a Healthcare Setting

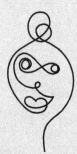

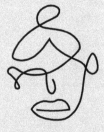

Hiromi Hangai Johnson
pronouns: She/Her

Hiromi H. Johnson started practicing T'ai Chi as part of a rehabilitation program following knee surgery in Japan. After experiencing the benefits and pursuing the martial art for more than 40 years, she feels that sharing T'ai Chi is her calling. She has also practiced Vipassana meditation and Japanese tea ceremony since 1978. In her spare time, she enjoys making silk scarves from vintage Japanese kimonos.

Kath Weston
pronouns: Agnostic

Kath Weston, a professor and anthropologist, survived graduate school by playing conga drums, training as an auto mechanic, and making wooden toys for children. She began studying T'ai Chi and became an accidental gardener while grieving the loss of a beloved aunt. For one of her books, *Traveling Light: On the Road with America's Poor,* she rode buses across the United States for several years.

"It doesn't matter what is happening.
What matters is how we are relating
to our experience."

–Tara Brach

Note to reader:

The authors are grateful to the Compassionate Care Initiative at the UVA School of Nursing for expanding the options available to nurses-in-training and people in all areas of the healthcare system. Special thanks to Susan Bauer-Wu and Dean Dorrie Fontaine for perceiving the benefits of T'ai Chi and organizing institutional support for the class at the UVA School of Nursing. Thanks also to Martin Johnson, who offered helpful comments on earlier drafts of this essay, and to Thomas Ball, Katherine Hoffman, and Martha Taylor for their generosity in sharing their personal and professional experiences with T'ai Chi in the hope that others who work in medical settings will benefit. As an ambassador for CCI, Taylor helped jump-start the initial series of T'ai Chi sessions at UVA Medical Center's Emily Couric Cancer Center.

Exhausted nurses and doctors, their metabolism disrupted by long hours, rotating shifts, high-pressure working conditions, and emergency calls in the dead of night. Hospital administrators torn between the need to meet deadlines for grants that they know will impact the lives of patients and the need to restore themselves so that they can live to write another proposal. Stressed-out nursing and medical students, cramming for exams, coaxing their bodies into alertness with vending machine snacks, crashing after they reach the inevitable limits, then gearing up to start the cycle all over again. What if there was a way to do more than treat these symptoms of a healthcare system that too often compromises the well-being of its care providers? What if there was something deeper than palliative care available to calm and strengthen their bodies while simultaneously teaching them how to cultivate compassion?

In 2015, with the support of the University of Virginia School of Nursing, Hiromi Hangai Johnson, one of the authors, offered a Six-Step T'ai Chi course to serve medical care providers who confront these challenges daily. The weekly course, located in the university's health complex, had a drop-in format. Its mission was to give care providers an opportunity to experience the benefits of T'ai Chi in a medical setting.

The opportunity to share T'ai Chi in a healthcare context was especially meaningful to Johnson, whose mother received a diagnosis of Stage IV breast cancer at the age of 66, had a mastectomy, and suffered side effects from chemotherapy. After her mother passed away in 1988, Johnson started practicing T'ai Chi seriously. With more than 30 years of practice under the guidance of several T'ai Chi Masters, she is a now herself a Master in the Cheng Ming martial arts lineage, as well as the Founder and Director of the nonprofit Charlottesville T'ai Chi Center, where class participants can learn T'ai Chi and related internal martial arts and then go on to explore more advanced T'ai Chi techniques. She dreamed of being able to do something good for patients, doctors, and nurses like the ones who had worked so hard to ease the pain of her mother.

If you are reading this chapter because you have practiced T'ai Chi for years without thinking much about how it relates to compassion or healthcare practice, read on. You will get a glimpse of what happens during a Six-Step class session, gain a better understanding of how T'ai Chi can become a form of care for the caregiver, and learn more about how group T'ai Chi classes cultivate compassion. You will also encounter a discussion of T'ai Chi's potential to transform the high-pressure workplaces in which many medical professionals work. If you are a medical professional who has no idea what T'ai Chi is, that's fine, too. Even the most advanced T'ai Chi practitioners value "beginner's mind."

Welcome to Class

As the clock approaches 5:00 p.m. on a Wednesday, people begin to trickle into the Compassionate Care Room at the school of nursing. Meditation cushions, yoga mats, and blankets are stacked neatly in racks against the wall. Next to them is a sign of gratitude: "Thank you for using this space and taking time to reflect, rest, and care for yourself."

Master Hiromi and the students bow to one another, in a gesture of respect deeply embedded in martial arts traditions. Even before participants make a circle and introductions begin, bowing establishes an orientation to others in the room. After introductions come warm-ups, supported by gentle verbal cues from the instructor. "Palm to the hip and from there up to the solar plexus. Push forward. When you finish the push don't lock your elbow. You are still bending." Then, during the double push: "Feel the rolling, like a wave." Each warm-up is designed to do more than stretch the muscles while loosening and lubricating the joints. These slow movements coax bodies into stances that become integral to more formal T'ai Chi practice. Although teachers can lead warm-ups silently to help establish a peaceful atmosphere, especially after the movements become familiar, an instructor can also take the opportunity to remind participants to attend closely to themselves, much as they would attend a patient. "Weight shift, forward-back, forward-back. Spine turns. When you do the warm-ups, listen to your body. When you turn your spine, what are you feeling?"

There are many different T'ai Chi forms, each composed of a set series of movements. After a period of T'ai Chi Walking, a type of meditation, the Six-Step form practiced in this class begins.

Everyone steps out to the left, feet shoulder width apart, finding unity in difference because "shoulder width" depends upon the body. Knees bend. Shoulders relax. Hands rotate in slightly until the "tiger's mouth" between thumb and forefinger aligns on each side of the body. Arms begin to float steadily, softly upward until they reach the opening position. Together.

The next five steps unfold smoothly, symmetrically. The horse's mane is parted, so to speak, in two directions, as open palms glide past one another, first to one corner, then the next, always coming gently back to the center between movements, maintaining balance. There is time for three repetitions of the entire form, enough to reinforce learning and allow everyone to sink deeper into the experience. Master

Hiromi guides the first round, then turns over the repetitions to participants who have come to class often enough to know how to do the steps themselves. These students work in pairs at the head of the group, synchronizing their motions and giving each other the confidence to lead.

The class accommodates students of all levels by positioning beginners in the middle of the group and more advanced students at the four corners. All six steps easily adapt for differently abled bodies. Students can complete the entire sequence while seated, remain in the middle of the group if they have trouble seeing or hearing, or receive instruction that uses simple analogies ("Throw the frisbee!") to make things easier to grasp.

The Six Steps that comprise the form taught in the class are, in order:

- Beginning
- Opening T'ai Chi
- Part the Horse's Mane
- Play the Lute
- Kick with Heel
- Closing

These Six Steps incorporate the slow, flowing movements and even tempo characteristic of T'ai Chi, yet there is much more going on than learning new motions, or even the self-defense applications embedded within a form. There's a reason T'ai Chi constitutes an *internal* martial art. Its most profound effects—mental, physical, spiritual—happen in ways the eye cannot see. Martha Taylor, a nurse who began studying with Master Hiromi in 2013, originally decided to check out T'ai Chi as a way of addressing the chronic job-related stress she was suffering after decades of working as a hospital nurse. Martha entered her first class "feeling severe depression, hopelessness, overwhelming fatigue." Sixty minutes later, she said, "I felt like I had been plugged into a charger overnight and I was ready to have a fabulous day." Her experience is not unique.

Many people initially try T'ai Chi in order to "de-stress," "get some exercise," or "calm down," then stay because they discover something more powerful. What is it about this centuries-old practice that allows even beginners to improve their health, connect more compassionately with the world, and feel restored, whether or not they go on to learn a more intricate long form like the 100 Steps cherished by the Cheng Ming lineage?

Wellness Benefits of T'ai Chi

It often comes as a surprise to beginners that they can work up a sweat and feel thoroughly refreshed after an hour of performing what looks (from the outside, at least) like very gentle, extremely slow movements. If all they know about T'ai Chi comes from films, or a glimpse of people practicing in a park, they arrive with questions. Does this really count as a workout? Is there any science to back up the claims about health benefits? And what's the point of moving like molasses?

T'ai Chi differs from fitness programs such as weightlifting that sculpt and tone bodies in ways that make it easy to mistake fitness for health (Wayne & Fuerst, 2013). From her perspective as a nurse, Martha saw T'ai Chi as a path to "creating future health instead of being at the mercy of it," a form of preventive and *proactive* medicine, if you like. As a form of bodywork and self-care that doubles as a martial art, T'ai Chi finds inspiration in what has become codified as Traditional Chinese Medicine (TCM), which has its own distinctive take on how bodies work. "Ch'i" ("Qi") is often translated into English as "energy" or "bioelectricity," but as with many translations, these placeholders fall somewhat short.

In his highly influential book, *The Expressiveness of the Body and the Divergence of Greek and Chinese Medicine*, Shigehisa Kuriyama (1999) explains how different conceptualizations of physiology in Greek ("Western") and Chinese medical practice historically led to radically different perceptions of universal bodily phenomena such as the pulse. Anatomical charts abounded in China, as in Europe, but those charts did not view bodies through the lens of muscularity. Instead of realist depictions of liver and lungs derived from a European history of public dissection, the Chinese medical charts mapped a network of meridians that routed ch'i through the body (see also Beinfeld & Korngold, 2013; Kaptchuk, 2000).

T'ai Chi and Healing

Drawing on this legacy, T'ai Chi focuses on promoting ch'i flow, opening the joints, and dispelling stagnation along the meridians rather than building muscle, although muscles do strengthen considerably along the way. Practicing at a slow and steady pace provides a low-impact workout that strengthens the muscular, skeletal, and internal organ systems (Wayne & Fuerst, 2013). At more advanced levels, practicing slowly also improves reflexes and provides a strong foundation for responding quickly to life's challenges.

As interest rises in what the US National Institutes of Health call "Complementary and Integrative Medicine" (CIM), many hospitals and clinics have begun to offer CIM practices, including T'ai Chi, to patients and staff. "This development is in part a result of growing research on the effectiveness of a broad range of CIM healing practices," write David Hufford and his coauthors (2015) in an article that explores barriers to the acceptance of biofield healing in "mainstream" healthcare. At the same time, researchers have begun to bridge the divergent views of the body described by Kuriyama with investigations of "the body electric": molecular bioelectricity generation via ion channels (Levin, 2014), bioelectric signaling in gene regulatory networks (Pietak & Levin, 2017), and so forth.

A brief search of a major medical database such as PubMed will turn up scores of studies that have subjected the health claims associated with T'ai Chi to scientific scrutiny. *The Harvard Medical School Guide to Tai Chi* (Wayne & Fuerst, 2013) is another good place to begin. Some of these studies have small sample sizes or arrive at inconclusive results. Yet there is now enough evidence to support an emerging medical consensus that regular T'ai Chi practice can contribute significantly to health in a range of preventive, palliative, and curative ways.

One of the most widely studied health impacts of T'ai Chi concerns balance. A randomized clinical trial with 670 adults aged 70 or older found that a therapeutic T'ai Chi intervention reduced falls by 58% compared with stretching and by 31% compared with a multimodal exercise program (Li et al., 2018). Consistently positive results have encouraged primary care providers to recommend T'ai Chi to seniors as a method of fall prevention. Studies have also demonstrated T'ai Chi's salutary effects on a range of chronic conditions, from Type 2 diabetes to osteoarthritis (Wang et al., 2016; Yeh et al., 2009). One review of the literature found that regular T'ai Chi practice can lower blood pressure, allowing T'ai Chi "to serve as a practical, nonpharmacologic adjunct to conventional hypertension management" (Yeh et al., 2008, p. 845). Another study concluded that T'ai Chi improved renal and cardiac functions of patients with chronic kidney and cardiovascular diseases, possibly through regulation of lipid metabolism (Shi et al., 2014).

The range of research on T'ai Chi's health benefits has now widened to include documentation of enhanced motor function in Parkinson's patients (Yang et al., 2014), alleviation of insomnia in breast cancer survivors (Irwin et al., 2017), and improved exercise capacity and quality of life for patients with chronic obstructive pulmonary disease (Chen et al., 2016). T'ai Chi has yielded better results than aerobic exercise for people suffering from fibromyalgia (Yang et al., 2014) and proved more effective for treating cancer-related fatigue than physical exercise or psychological support (Song et al., 2018). Physical therapists have started integrating T'ai Chi into rehabilitation programs for arthroscopy patients and stroke survivors (Lyu et al., 2018). Some studies have noted that T'ai Chi offers an especially suitable form of exercise for patients with conditions such as cancer who might otherwise become too sedentary (Chen et al., 2016).

T'ai Chi as Care for the Caregiver

As evidence mounts for the targeted effectiveness of T'ai Chi as a medical intervention, more and more medical practitioners have begun to think of a basic 12-week T'ai Chi course as something they can dispense alongside pharmaceuticals. The title of an article in the *Journal of Transcultural Nursing*, "How to Prescribe Tai Chi Therapy," reflects this shift (Allen & Meires, 2011), as does a story run by the BBC under the headline, "Tai Chi 'Could Be Prescribed' for Illnesses" (BBC News, 2015).

Of course, the benefits discussed in the previous section could apply to anyone. Improved health and quality of life testify to the power of T'ai Chi as a form of self-care, but what transforms T'ai Chi into an especially dynamic form of care for the caregiver? First and foremost, T'ai Chi reacquaints medical practitioners with their own bodies after years of learning to subordinate their bodies' signals to the demands of healing others. Secondly, T'ai Chi's simple, low-cost requirements allow courses to be offered on-site in medical facilities, which in turn permits employees to drop in, "recharge," and return to work if necessary. Last but not least, T'ai Chi has the potential to help caregivers who find themselves struggling with clinical burnout, as they come to understand in an embodied way how compassionate awareness of self and other is inextricably intertwined. A few words from healthcare practitioners who have studied T'ai Chi with Master Hiromi will serve to illustrate these points:

> "The work environment of a major medical center breeds dissociation with the body," explained Martha Taylor, the nurse quoted earlier in this chapter, as she zeroed in on one of the great ironies experienced by those who sacrifice their own health in the course of taking care of the health of others. Martha continued:

> "There are intermittent periods of poor staffing and unpredictable shifts in patient census. Peak performers are identified as people who can work at max capacity for long hours without breaks . . . The toll that this stress takes on the health of hospital employees is monumental . . . Even though I went to the gym regularly and I ate a very healthy diet, I had significant hypertension."

T'ai Chi gave Martha new tools to address the cumulative effects of years of work-related stress that treadmills, salads, and whole grains could not provide. Slowing down, noticing small shifts in her body's orientation, learning from sensations she had become habituated to brushing away, and that was just the start.

Katherine B. Hoffman, a participant in the Six-Step class, worked as a Grants and Contracts Administrator. One of the things she appreciated about the Six-Step class was its convenient location within the health system. That made it easier for her to integrate T'ai Chi into a demanding schedule in which filing grants on time translates into better outcomes for patients. In one instance, a little bit of T'ai Chi went a long way to help Katherine meet an important deadline:

> "The day had been crazy, the deadlines were real. I was pressing on, tired, tight, anxious, as not enough was done and I needed to keep going until it was completed. It occurred to me I could run over and go just that one hour to the T'ai Chi class and come back. I followed the movements. . . The stress and tightness and head spinning with ideas evaporated. I was calm, quiet, and felt relaxed and solid as I returned to work. What a gift! I went back and on with what I needed to do. Everything was easier. I felt good. Work got done and submitted by the deadline."

Rather than continue sacrificing her own health for the benefit of patients, she had discovered a way to support one by supporting the other.

For Thomas Ball, then a second-year physician resident, T'ai Chi had become an antidote to clinical burnout:

> "T'ai Chi is a practice that contributes to my capacity to be present, to be aware of what is going on inside me and those around me, to focus and to stay resilient in the face of day after day in the hospital of caring for patients in severe mental and emotional distress. It helps me to resist the anger, burnout, and jadedness that can come from medical training and practice."

It is this invitation to explore the integration of "inside me" with "those around me" that extends T'ai Chi's benefits well beyond better balance or cardiovascular health. Some might call it a bridge to compassion.

Cultivating Compassion, Sensing the Gap

Imagine a room where a group of people gather to practice T'ai Chi together. When they first enter the room, one by one, on a drop-in basis, they are not yet a group. Beginners, especially, often move to their own rhythm, forgetting to notice what others are doing, forging ahead when they think they remember something and later falling behind. The class goes on. Without really trying, people start to synchronize, moving at the same pace regardless of level of experience. As they sink into their bodies, a sense of community, an effortless orientation to others in the room, something peaceful and shared, emerges. How does this happen?

At times, teachers cultivate a foundation for compassion by giving verbal instructions. After a period of Walking T'ai Chi in the Six-Step class, for example, the instructor might say something like, "There is always some sort of sensation in your body, but you're just not noticing it. If you are being observant about yourself, that will affect other people." In small but explicit ways, they call attention to the link between awareness of self and awareness of others, preparing students to understand why compassion cannot grow in the absence of a compassionate stance toward oneself. They also remind leaders in "the corners" to closely coordinate their movements. More advanced students are positioned at the corners of the group so that less experienced students will always have someone to follow as they turn. If the corners move at different speeds, it becomes confusing for people in the middle, who wonder which one to follow.

The pedagogical methodology of teaching by demonstrating and learning by following also helps integrate people into a larger whole. They soon find themselves moving in parallel, yet somehow as one. This cannot happen without setting aside all the things in a busy workday that lead to self-absorption in a particular set of tasks or problems. They enter a realm of quiet and respite where time is measured not in hours, minutes, or appointments, but in breaths. Breaths taken together.

Compassion? Not yet. Or at best, a lesson in how fleeting compassionate engagement can be, and how quickly awareness can turn away from the open-hearted stance of compassion toward judgment. Once students begin to notice and value the difference attunement makes, they often find themselves becoming critical. "Hey, that person is going too fast/too slow!" they think to themselves. They may start to compare, congratulating themselves on knowing more than the next person or disparaging themselves for making mistakes. Such thoughts create subtle rifts in the form that distract other people and interrupt their own practice.

Skillful instructors will turn these moments, too, into occasions for growth and reflection: "Now that you have noticed judgment creeping in, how will you handle it?" They redirect students away from the competitive, agonistic stance to which students have become habituated, whether through medical training or other sorts of life experiences. They remind students that everyone is there to help one another learn. That includes instructors who pass down the art and its associated benefits in a spirit of compassion for their students and for generations to come. It is often said that a master does not just teach the form: A master shows students how to live.

Soft Overcomes Hard

Internal martial arts such as T'ai Chi work with the counterintuitive principle that soft overcomes hard. Unless the body is relaxed, it cannot effectively redirect the force of an attacker. Unless students can approach themselves compassionately, they will struggle to treat others with genuine compassion. As T'ai Chi practitioners discover more about their bodies during training, they yield to the inevitability of making mistakes *and* watching other people make mistakes. They contemplate what went wrong, gain clarity, and consider more effective ways to practice. They encourage one another. They learn to forgive themselves in order to move on.

Between any open-hearted moment and the rush to judgment there is a subtle gap, where one stance gives way to another. The transitional "spaces" between seemingly discrete movements in a T'ai Chi form mirror the sorts of gaps that constantly open up in the course of a day: gaps between thoughts, between emotional states, between impulse and reaction, between people. Rather than trying to smooth over gaps by eliminating them, T'ai Chi helps people notice the gaps and draws attention to their productive possibilities.

Another way to perceive the gap is by noticing that there is a difference between when you finish and when you actually finish. One thing ends before another begins, but in between there is that subtle pause, an opportunity, a rest, that might otherwise be ignored if a person is in a rush. Only by slowing down long enough to dwell in the gap between assumption and conclusion, for example, can medical practitioners recognize self-sacrifice as a misguided form of compassion that harms self and others alike. The way to move beyond burnout becomes clearer and the path begins to smooth out. Why should this be? Because the ability to sense that gap allows caregivers to direct a more truly compassionate question toward themselves: "Now that you have noticed self-sacrifice creeping in, how will you handle it?"

Learning to sense, or even provide, a gap is equally important for relationships with patients. Foster ways to maintain a sense of connection with patients during transitional moments such as shift changes and room transfers. Let patients finish their sentences and listen carefully. Think back to the feeling in the room during T'ai Chi class and remember how a patient's silence, too, can be filled with meaning. The nurse has to give the patient a space; then the patient will give the nurse the space to be a nurse.

What T'ai Chi Teaches About Patient Care

Hospitals and clinics are places for care and healing, but for employees they can also become conflict zones. Staffing shortages, unpredictable scheduling, multiple shifts, skyrocketing costs, increased paperwork, reduced consultation time, and the emotional burden of delivering news of a poor prognosis take their toll on staff and patients alike. AIIMS (All India Institute of Medical Sciences), a major hospital in New Delhi, began offering martial arts training to its staff as a form of self-protection from abuse when patients' relatives become frustrated, irate, and occasionally violent after coping with the effects of these sorts of conditions (Dutt, 2017). Because T'ai Chi teaches the body to relax in the face of conflict, it helps caregivers stay present, assess situations while remaining emotionally connected to themselves and to their patients, and make better decisions under stress. In this sense, even those who practice the art as a form of self-care rather than self-defense can benefit from its martial aspects.

It is this more subtle and expansive impact of T'ai Chi training that Thomas, the second-year medical resident, emphasized when he explained that T'ai Chi had taught him "principles about how to treat others, how to work, play, and live." This final section introduces three key T'ai Chi principles—slowing down, humility, and patience—with a focus on how they can enhance compassionate care in medical settings.

Practice Slowing Down

In an episode of the podcast *Sincerely, X*, a medical professional speaks anonymously about how clinical burnout contributed to the death of one of her patients (Triff & Campbell, 2017). The patient was fed up with being in the hospital and determined to go home. It was clear to her, as his doctor, that he had not yet recovered. Hospital staff duly dispensed the warnings customarily given to patients when they check themselves out against medical advice, including an explicit statement that informed him that if he took this action, he might die. He went home anyway. Within 48 hours, he was readmitted to the hospital with a gastrointestinal bleed that progressed faster than he could be transfused, and in the course of things, he did indeed soon die. What was it about this situation that made the doctor feel she had, in her words, "killed" her patient, and how might the T'ai Chi principle of slowing down have altered an outcome that still haunted her years later?

Here's how the doctor herself came to see things, after she learned something about the emotional exhaustion and depersonalization that the World Health Organization calls clinician burnout:

> A better version of myself could have caught the small thing that
> became the big thing that led to the hemorrhage. I could have had

the opportunity because that better version of myself would have engaged with him, heard him out, and tried to convince him to stay . . . I didn't exactly make a mistake in the usual sense of the word. I didn't ignore a vital sign or forget to order a medication. I just didn't try very hard. I didn't really try at all with this patient . . . I knew better. I just couldn't manage to care about him. It's a pretty fundamental thing to expect from a doctor: that the doctor who is taking care of you in the hospital or in the office will care *about* you, not just for you.

Somewhere along the way, "Dr. Burnout" had lost the ability to fulfill that trust.

People make mistakes, broadly conceived; that is one of T'ai Chi's first lessons. Humans even *need* to make mistakes to learn. To serve others effectively, they also need to develop a compassionate response to themselves when they fail. But as every nurse, doctor, and lab technician knows, mistakes in medical settings can be costly, life-or-death matters, with significant potential to harm. The podcast guest who sought refuge in anonymity was trying to draw attention to the fact that medical practitioners who convince themselves they are too busy to double-check things are not the only ones who represent a danger to those they serve. It can be just as problematic to lack the wherewithal to make the extra effort it takes to speak from the heart, as it were, to a recalcitrant patient.

Medical institutions have taken many steps to get their error rates down and educate staff about clinician burnout, but few have considered the potential of T'ai Chi to assist in this effort. To do T'ai Chi, you must be aware of your body, in order to guide your body with intention. Maintaining an alienated distance is not an option. This more contemplative side of the martial art has led some to dub T'ai Chi "moving meditation." Insights bubble up that a person moving at breakneck speed would otherwise have brushed aside: "My stomach is gurgling. I guess I forgot to have lunch." "Hmm, I saw that patient for 15 minutes, but did I really *see* that patient?" Slowing down trains people in a kind of focused, present attention that transfers to other areas of life.

In T'ai Chi, as in medical practice, details matter. A slight difference in the height of a block, the path of motion, or the angle of approach can render a move supremely effective or, alternatively, a weak version of self-defense. The same precision that makes all the difference for a surgical cut or accurate dosage is highly valued in the martial arts. Going slow allows people to notice the consequences of small details and make adjustments. Slowing down also allows details that are important—for reasons a student still does not understand—to cross the threshold of awareness. When an instructor reminds students to "turn your center," experienced students turn the upper body around the axis of the spine, while beginners tend to turn their heads. It takes a while for beginners to notice they are not doing the same thing.

In the Six-Step class, people discovered to their surprise that time could go by rather quickly once they stopped rushing around. Settling into their bodies while noticing what was happening "inside" often meant that class was over before they knew it. Another common observation during T'ai Chi practice that translates readily into medical settings is that slowing down may not take as long as you think. It only takes seconds to pause long enough to encourage a patient to voice a concern or to look up from notes on a patient, connecting person-to-person instead of caregiver-to-chart. The alternative is to lapse into the disembodied state of alienation that "Dr. Burnout" learned to recognize only after she lost someone entrusted to her care. "I had stopped seeing patients as people," she explained in the opening to her podcast. "They were just diseases and lab values, test results. And I thought, 'What on earth is wrong with me?'"

The Six-Step class opens a door through which medical practitioners can begin to ask and answer that question. In the beginning, some students think they are moving slowly and grasping all the details when they are not. "This is the slowest I can go!" a student will exclaim as her instructor watches her zip quickly through the form. "How slowly do I have to move?" They may falsely believe that they have mastered a form once they can repeat the movements on their own, without needing to go deeper. Medical practitioners who cling to the illusion that technical competence equals a mastery of medical science, or that personal well-being can have no significant impact on patients, are afflicted with a similar kind of hubris. Hubris is what the second T'ai Chi principle, humility, seeks to address.

Practice Humility

At its root, humility is another instance of soft overcoming hard. In medical settings in the United States, humility tends to be undervalued and may be mistaken for lack of competence, or weakness. Yet without a certain humility, it becomes difficult to show gratitude and respect—for the instructor, the patient, the training, or oneself. People can feel the difference between working together in a manner that is superficially correct while everyone feeds their egos by treating others harshly, and working together in a manner infused with humility and respect. With humility, an interlocking set of medical specialties can coalesce into a whole that is greater than its parts, creating a more peaceful environment like the one established when people practice T'ai Chi together.

One way that T'ai Chi *dōjōs* (training spaces) foster humility and respect is by implementing a code of etiquette. At the opening of a class, everyone bows to a picture of the lineage founder, followed by bows between students and the instructor teaching the class, and again when students lead parts of the warm-ups. There is a deeper purpose to all the bowing that elevates it beyond mere formality. These routine gestures of respect draw a line between student and teacher that allows each to approach the other with compassion. Students are reminded not to presume to teach other students without authorization, like overeager medical students who have not yet qualified in their fields. Instructors are reminded that students appreciate their efforts. Respect gives both sides a little bit of space—another gap—so that knowledge can flow. It becomes easier to dwell in humility regardless of skill level.

Of course, it is important to honor achievements. Every Six-Step class ends with praise and a collective round of applause. But there is an important difference between taking pride in work well done and the kind of pride that seductively whispers, "You have finished your training. You are an expert now. You know more than the patient about certain matters, so you know more than the patient in all things." The latter kind of pride puts people in jeopardy. It encourages caregivers to stop listening. It can trick them into treating test results with more respect than the patient.

Master Hiromi sometimes shares a story with her students about what her own teacher said to her after she learned the final step in a long T'ai Chi form. "When I finished the form, my teacher told me, 'Congratulations on reaching the gate!'" Finishing is beginning. The "same" procedures generate new things to inspect when practiced on another day. Without practice, remembering slides easily into forgetting, no matter how accomplished you are. That realization should be enough to keep anyone humble.

Practice Patience

In medical settings, it is tempting to conclude that the patient is the one who has to be patient. After all, it is the patient who waits for the nurse, the anesthesiologist, and the doctor, not the other way around. In compassionate practice, though, patience turns out to be an essential quality for caregivers. Who would ever get through nursing or medical school if they succumbed to the "compare and despair" syndrome of evaluating their own prospects in light of what others who came before them have already achieved? Who would ever stick with the training required to learn a 100-step T'ai Chi form? They must welcome and accept the fact that the journey takes time and becomes all the more interesting for it.

Patience is also a key to developing the kind of rapport with patients that rests on more than an easygoing manner and a smile. By gaining a better understanding

In Real Practice

Anxiety is a serious mental health issue, and if you have not experienced it yourself, you most certainly know someone who has. Of the many benefits discussed in this chapter, T'ai Chi has also demonstrated effectiveness in reducing anxiety symptoms in nursing students. In the Dinani et al. study (2019), 64 nursing students were randomized into a group that received 40 minutes of T'ai Chi training, three times a week for 8 weeks. Compared to a control group, these students experienced a significant decrease in stress, anxiety, and depression; they also saw an increase in self-confidence. In the Mulcahy et al. study (2020), 63 BSN students were randomized into two groups prior to performing a simulation. The first group prepared for their simulation as usual; the second group practiced 30 minutes of T'ai Chi, following the movements shown in a YouTube video. The experimental group students experienced lower cognitive and somatic anxiety as well as increased self-efficacy and performance in the simulation.

of their internal states through T'ai Chi practice, people learn to pacify their own mental agitation and to respond patiently and appropriately to others without fear, anxiety, confusion, anger, or distraction. All those repetitions—of injections, incisions, and Part the Horse's Mane—yield more than the technical ability to perform a medical procedure or a T'ai Chi form when they cultivate patience.

Like humility and the capacity to slow down, patience grows best when tended. Master Hiromi takes the long view, determined to plant a seed of T'ai Chi every day, 365 days a year.

Closing Thoughts

You cannot force people to practice T'ai Chi, Master Hiromi says, but you can invite them. A few years ago, while shopping in an Asian grocery store in a nearby city, she heard someone calling her name. When she turned around, she saw a tall young man with a happy expression on his face. He looked shy, but Johnson could sense his enthusiasm. The man explained that he had attended a T'ai Chi workshop she gave at his high school. He still remembered the calming and meditative effect of the flowing movements. Although he had not practiced since, he said he planned to study T'ai Chi when the right moment comes. Johnson was impressed by his honesty and his positive attitude toward future practice. A seed of T'ai Chi she had planted was still there, waiting to germinate.

If one out of 365 people takes the first steps on the path of T'ai Chi practice, that is a big change in the world. If those first steps happen in a nursing school or a medical center, the ripple effects ensure that it will be a bigger change than most.

Key Points

- T'ai Chi is a form of Complementary and Integrative Medicine, an internal martial art, that can provide tremendous health and well-being benefits to healthcare workers who are busy and under stress.

- The slow and steady pace of T'ai Chi practice provides a low-impact workout that strengthens the muscular, skeletal, and internal organ systems. Other physical benefits include improved balance and flexibility, reduced stress, and increased body awareness.

- Research indicates that T'ai Chi can be beneficial to patients suffering from chronic diseases, including hypertension, type 2 diabetes, and osteoarthritis, and can enhance motor function in patients with Parkinson's disease.

- T'ai Chi practice cultivates compassion. One way this learning occurs is through attunement to others in the group, moving together while fostering an awareness of any tendency toward judgment.

- T'ai Chi principles are particularly powerful reminders to healthcare professionals: slowing down, humility, and patience.

References

Allen, J., & Meires, J. (2011). How to prescribe Tai Chi therapy. *Journal of Transcultural Nursing, 22*(2), 201–204. https://doi.org/10.1177/1043659610395770

BBC News. (2015, September 18). *Tai Chi "could be prescribed" for illnesses.* https://www.bbc.co.uk/news/health-34279190

Beinfeld, H., & Korngold, E. (2013). *Between heaven and earth: A guide to Chinese medicine.* Ballantine Books.

Chen, Yi-Wen, Hunt, M. A., Campbell, K. L., Peill, K., & Reid, W. D. (2016). The effect of Tai Chi on four chronic conditions—cancer, osteoarthritis, heart failure and chronic obstructive pulmonary disease: A systematic review and meta-analyses. *British Journal of Sports Medicine, 50,* 397–407. https://doi.org/10.1136/bjsports-2014-094388

Dinani, S. K., Mehrabi, T., & Sadeghi, R. (2019). The effect of Tai Chi exercise on stress, anxiety, depression, and self confidence of nursing students. *Jundishapur Journal of Chronic Disease Care, 8*(3). doi:10.5812/jjcdc.92854

Dutt, A. (2017, May 3). Delhi: AIIMS docs learn taekwondo to defend themselves from kin of patients. *Hindustan Times.* https://www.hindustantimes.com/delhi/delhi-sick-of-violence-by-kin-of-patients-1500-aiims-doctors-to-learn-taekwondo/story-MGGo29ttrNBnu6JttG8XIM.html

Hufford, D. J., Sprengel, M., Ives, J. A., & Jonas, W. (2015). Barriers to the entry of biofield healing into "mainstream" healthcare. *Global Advances in Health and Medicine, 4*(Suppl.), 79–88. https://doi.org/10.7453/gahmj.2015.025.suppl

Irwin, M. R., Olmstead, R., Carrillo, C., Sadeghi, N., Nicassio, P., Ganz, P. A., & Bower, J. E. (2017). Tai Chi Chih compared with cognitive behavioral therapy for the treatment of insomnia in survivors of breast cancer: A randomized, partially blinded, noninferiority trial. *Journal of Clinical Oncology, 35*(23), 2656–2665. https://doi.org/10.1200/JCO.2016.71.0285

Kaptchuk, T. (2000). *The web that has no weaver: Understanding Chinese medicine* (2nd ed.). McGraw-Hill.

Kuriyama, S. (1999). *The expressiveness of the body and the divergence of Greek and Chinese medicine.* Zone Books.

Levin, M. (2014). Molecular bioelectricity: How endogenous voltage potentials control cell behavior and instruct pattern regulation in vivo. *Molecular Biology of the Cell, 25*(24), 3835–3850. https://doi.org/10.1091/mbc.e13-12-0708

Li, F., Harmer, P., & Fitzgerald, K. (2018). Effectiveness of a therapeutic Tai Ji Quan intervention vs. a multimodal exercise intervention to prevent falls among older adults at high risk of falling: A randomized clinical trial. *JAMA Internal Medicine, 178*(10), 1301–1310. https://doi.org/10.1001/jamainternmed.2018.3915

Lyu, D., Lyu, X., Zhang, Y., Ren, Y., Yang, F., Zhou, L. Zou, Y., & Li, Z. (2018). Tai Chi for stroke rehabilitation: A systematic review and meta-analysis of randomized controlled trials. *Frontiers of Physiology, 9,* 983. https://doi.org/10.3389/fphys.2018.00983

Mulcahy, A., Holland, B., Gosselin, K., & Pittman, A. (2020). The use of Tai-Chi to reduce anxiety among nursing students undergoing simulation. *Nursing Education Perspectives, 41*(3), 183–184. doi:10.1097/01.NEP.0000000000000495

Pietak, A., & Levin, M. (2017). Bioelectric gene and reaction networks: Computational modelling of genetic, biochemical and bioelectrical dynamics in pattern regulation. *Journal of the Royal Society Interface, 14*(134). https://doi.org/10.1098/rsif.2017.0425

Shi, Z.-M., Wen, H.-P., Liu, F.-R., & Yao, C.-X. (2014). The effects of Tai Chi on the renal and cardiac functions of patients with chronic kidney and cardiovascular diseases. *Journal of Physical Therapy Science, 11,* 1733–1736. https://doi.org/10.1589/jpts.26.1733

Song, S., Yu, J., Ruan, Y., Liu, X., & Yue, X. (2018). Ameliorative effects of Tai Chi on cancer-related fatigue: A meta-analysis of randomized controlled trials. *Supportive Care in Cancer, 7,* 2091–2102. https://doi.org/10.1007/s00520-018-4136-y

Triff, D., & Campbell, C. (Producers). (2017, July 19). Sincerely, X. [Audio podcast]. *Dr. Burnout.* Apple podcasts. https://podcasts.apple.com/us/podcast/dr-burnout/id1238801741?i=1000390072745

Wang, C., Schmid, C. H., Iversen, M. D., Harvey, W. F., Fielding, R. A., Driban, J. B., Price, L. L., Wong, J. B., Reid, K. F., Rones, R., & McAlindon, T. (2016). Comparative effectiveness of Tai Chi versus physical therapy for knee osteoarthritis: A randomized trial. *Annals of Internal Medicine, 165*(2), 77–86. https://doi.org/10.7326/M15-2143

Wayne, P. M., & Fuerst, M. L. (2013). *The Harvard Medical School guide to Tai Chi.* Shambhala Publications.

Yang, Y., Li, X.-Y., Gong, L., Zhu, Y.-L., & Hao, Y.-L. (2014). Tai Chi for improvement of motor function, balance and gait in Parkinson's disease: A systematic review and meta-analysis. *PLOS ONE, 9*(7), e102942. https://doi.org/10.1371/journal.pone.0102942

Yeh, G. Y., Wang, C., Wayne, P. M., & Phillips, R. S. (2008). The effect of Tai Chi exercise on blood pressure: A systematic review. *Preventive Cardiology, 11*(2), 82–89. https://pubmed.ncbi.nlm.nih.gov/18401235/

Yeh, S.-H.., Chuang, H., Lin, L.-W., Hsiao, C.-Y., Wang, P.-W., Liu, R.-T., & Yang, K. D. (2009). Regular Tai Chi Chuan exercise improves T cell helper function of patients with type 2 diabetes mellitus with an increase in T-bet transcription factor and IL-12 production. *British Journal of Sports Medicine, 43*(11), 845–850. http://dx.doi.org/10.1136/bjsm.2007.043562

15

Reflections on Self-Care and Your Clinical Practice

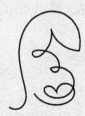

Joy Miller
pronouns: She/Her

Joy Miller, a pediatric nurse practitioner, specializes in pediatric palliative care. She is a tireless advocate for children and families facing medical complexity and life-threatening illness, bearing witness to their resilience with equal parts grace and humility. When Joy isn't working, she refills her tank by spending time with her two children and husband. She loves seeing the world through their eyes.

"Self-care is giving the world the best of you, instead of what's left of you."

–Katie Reed

Nursing is the art of caring and the practice of offering yourself in service to others who are in need. This profession has called you, and you will soon transition from your education and training to a clinical practice. I suspect, if you are like I was, you are wondering how you will realistically be able to manage a self-care practice on top of remembering all the skills you will need in your first nursing role. I thought the same thing. But in my years of nursing I have found opportunities to practice self-care in ways that help sustain me while simultaneously benefitting the patients and families I serve in a pediatric palliative care setting. My hope is that this chapter will provide ideas for you to consider for your own clinical practice. I share what has worked for me, but you will develop techniques that are appropriate to your needs and experiences. The foundation of every practice is self-awareness.

Reflections on Self-Awareness

To begin, find ways that you can check in with yourself throughout the day. When I first started working as a nurse, I realized I needed a transition ritual to start and end my shifts. My way to do this is through journaling. By writing, I honor and validate my feelings, and without judgment, I can move through the emotions I am experiencing at the start of my day. This allows me to be more focused on my patients and families. As I leave work, particularly after a long and stressful shift, I sometimes do the same thing. This provides a positive transition to being at home with my family.

Often, our natural response is to ignore or bury certain feelings instead of naming and validating them, especially if those feelings are difficult. Grief, shame, loneliness, and exhaustion are just a few feelings that are difficult to fully experience. Over time, the burden becomes overwhelming as these feelings pile up, and they can lead to empathy fatigue and burnout (Kozlowska et al., 2015). As nurses, we allow others to borrow strength from us as we bear witness to suffering. If we are generous in sharing our strength, we need a strong sense of self to share.

Sometimes I cringe, looking back at my early days as a nurse. I was not always self-aware, and I projected my feelings in a way that didn't serve me or my patients. In my desire to be helpful, I was certain I knew how someone felt and therefore, what they needed. I quickly came up with *my* truth about what they were experiencing, and even though I was well intentioned, I couldn't possibly know. I was serving my truth over theirs.

As time passed, I learned, grew, and honed my self-reflection practice. I continue to keep a journal to help me process my feelings. There are many interactions with patients and others that I want to remember. There are also moments that I would rather not remember, but that I learned from with humility and grace. Putting the difficult moments to paper makes them a little less painful and helps me begin my recovery process.

My journaling isn't always exhaustive or filled with profound reflection, but sometimes it is. Sometimes I'm completely overwhelmed and exhausted and I don't want to do one more thing, but I do it. Most of the time, I go to my essence—I write down what feels essential to me in that moment. I always start with my check-in question, "How am I feeling?" Then I might go further and ask myself, "What resonated with me today? Was it a song I heard playing in a patient's room? A shared smile with a patient, family member, or colleague? Was it a difficult struggle or bearing witness to suffering? What do these joys and sorrows feel like?"

Honoring your feelings by naming them and writing them down doesn't have to be or feel burdensome. Think of it as a commitment to yourself and your well-being. If you are feeling at a loss for words and don't know what to write, that's okay. Acknowledge that feeling of uncertainty by writing it down and getting it out. My journaling practice has given me the space to reflect on and move through my professional and personal lives with self-compassion, and I believe this has helped me provide compassionate care to my patients.

Reflections on Self-Care in Clinical Practice

What does it mean to take care of myself?

I'm sure you've grappled with this question as a student, and certainly as you've read this book. I can assure you that a self-care practice when you are a working nurse will be so important. There is a misperception that self-care takes a lot of time and money or has to happen in a beautiful space. In this section, I would like to share ways to care for yourself in the middle of a busy clinical practice.

As we move through our day, we are gifted with many "mini-moments" we can devote to self-care. We have a choice in how we respond to any situation, maybe one that we would generally view as an inconvenience or annoyance, like waiting for an elevator or getting stuck in traffic. In those moments, we can choose to shift our focus toward self and consider the gift of awareness, compassion, and gratitude. Maybe that is through deep breathing or recalling a happy memory. It doesn't take much effort or time to center yourself, offer kindness, and move through the rest of your day.

Right now, as I write this chapter and show up to work each day in the middle of a global pandemic, anxious, uncertain, and scared, I choose to ground myself in gratitude while I set an intention for my day at work. I make eye contact with each person I pass on my way in, smiling behind my mask, hoping they can "see" my smile through my eyes. I thank them for being there, for showing up. In one moment, a brief exchange of gratitude and kindness, I can transform my anxious energy into something that I hope serves another person but also serves me.

Many research studies have examined the effects of kindness, offering compassion, and gratitude. In one study, Rowland and Curry (2019) studied the impact of performing acts of kindness on the person performing the kind acts. Study participants who performed (or observed) different acts of kindness increased their own happiness. They also found that the more acts of kindness a person performed or observed, the happier they were. Thanking the hospital parking attendant, helping the housekeeper open a door, and smiling with or without a mask are all reliable self-care practices.

Personal Perspective

What Self-Care Means to Me: Reflections by a New Grad Nurse

—Jennifer deFaria, BSN, RN (she/her)

I thrive on productivity. The biggest challenge for me to properly care for myself is recognizing that the time I spend doing things for me is productive. I have learned that productivity, in this stage of my life, is no longer crossing off homework assignments in my agenda. I am productive when I go to work, but also when I clean my room, call an old friend, or practice a skin care routine. Self-care to me has a lot to do with my mindset. I could scroll through my phone for 10 minutes and feel as if that time was wasted, or I could intentionally allocate 10 minutes for me to go on my phone and then feel ready to focus.

When I change my mindset and create a positive intention, I am able to de-stress and rejuvenate. Self-care is intentionally doing something for myself, recognizing that time is important, and in return I feel revitalized. Self-care is acknowledging my feelings after work, evaluating what I need, and allowing myself to accept my need for rest, exercise, time with friends, or time alone. Self-care is not feeling guilty for allocating time for myself because it will help in the long run for me to give to others.

As a nurse, I work three 12-hour shifts a week, which allows me to have several days off in a row. This time off can be overwhelming, and I have learned to use my time off wisely and intentionally in order to feel energized and ready to work my long shifts. My self-care begins with making a list of goals and mini achievements to complete during the week. This list gives my days off more structure and allows me to feel productive with my time. My list may consist of grocery store runs, chores around the house, new yoga classes, spending time with a friend, journaling, reading a book, and going for a walk. This list keeps me reminded of activities outside of work that help me de-stress and stay organized. As I cross these tasks off my list, I earn my sense of productivity and feel ready to give back to others around me.

Reflections on My Professional Journey

As a nurse and now as a nurse practitioner, the intimate aspects of nursing speak to my soul. These aspects include relationship building, trust, grace under pressure, and the countless opportunities for empathy. My practice is in pediatric palliative care, and my path here was unexpected. As I was completing my master's program, I began applying for pediatric nurse practitioner positions. In one of a series of interviews, I'll never forget being thrown a curveball when the interviewer asked, "Would you be interested in a position in our new pediatric palliative care program?" I didn't hesitate to say yes even though I had no idea what the position would entail. But I knew in my heart that children and families deserved the level of care that this new program would provide.

I accepted the position, and my life changed in ways I didn't know it needed to. It was like a switch flipped. Suddenly I belonged to a group of thoughtful, curious, dedicated, and wise individuals. We show up to support one another because we want to, not because we have to. Everyone's intention is to serve. I also became a clinical ambassador with the new Compassionate Care Initiative, the program that helped initiate the pediatric palliative care program. (You can read more about Compassionate Care Ambassador programs in Chapter 20.)

Since I was thrown that "curveball" in the job interview, I have been afforded incredible opportunities and have built meaningful relationships with colleagues who are dedicated to resiliency, gratitude, and compassion. I think back to that meeting all the time and am so incredibly grateful that the universe brought me there, to that moment, to that opportunity, and to the journeys I've walked with hundreds of children and their families. In many more ways than I can explain here, being a member of this group has in itself been a form of self-care for me.

In-the-Moment Self-Care Practices

If you can take even a brief moment to center to self, that practice can transform your mood and presence and improve your physical state, allowing you to be fully engaged and primed for any encounter.

Grounding

During the most stressful of situations, we are naturally activated. Our sympathetic nervous system or "gas pedal" is thrown into overdrive through signaling by our amygdala and hypothalamus. We may exhibit physical symptoms such as our face getting flushed, heart racing, sweating, shaking, or all of the above. This can feel paralyzing, and it can negatively affect our judgement and inhibit important cognitive processing. Beyond the immediate effects of this activation, there are long-term chronic stress effects of repeated activation of the stress response that can take a toll on our body, including physical damage to blood vessels and arteries, increased blood pressure, an increased risk of heart attacks or strokes, as well as elevated cortisol levels that contribute to the buildup of fat tissue and weight gain.

Our parasympathetic nervous system or the "brake" will eventually kick in and help us de-escalate, tempering our "flight or fight" response. While this is a natural phenomenon, we can choose how activated we become through a grounding practice, right then and there in the moment of our activation. Evidence has identified relaxation, physical exercise, and social support as useful tools to call upon to counteract both the short- and the long-term effects of stress (Dusek et al., 2008).

It is helpful to identify this "activation" state early, pause, and then engage in a mindful practice to down-regulate this arousal state (Kozlowska et al., 2015). A way that I regularly practice down-regulation is with a process called "grounding." (You also read about this in Chapter 4.) This down-regulation technique means tuning into the feeling of my feet on the ground, whether I'm sitting or standing. I focus totally on this sensation, and I instantly feel supported by my feet on the floor. I will move my feet back and forth in my shoe to reset my stance, all in an effort to stimulate the feeling of support.

I ground myself in every chaotic moment that comes my way, and I move from a state of activation to calm. I may have to do this dozens of times in that moment, but the practice of grounding is something I can call upon anytime, anywhere. This applies to all types of stressful situations, and the more you can learn to autopilot to grounding yourself in the moment, the more natural it will become and the more down-regulation effectiveness it will provide.

Deflect and Redirect

Many times, I find myself in very tense and stressful situations in my clinical work. These are situations when no one can predict what will come next, and everyone around me will be so activated they might as well be on the ceiling. As I receive that energy from others, I send it into my grounding practice and try to shift the focus and set the tone for the rest of the room. If I send calm, grounded energy and generosity into the room, my hope is that I will receive that back from others.

In that moment, I am deflecting and redirecting others' energy. As I deflect, I am not ignoring their feelings and responses. I am acknowledging them, and then I pivot and redirect the energy, returning energy that I think will serve in that moment. This cycle of receiving and giving back helps me feel less helpless in the moment and helps me shift to what I *can* do. It is important to remember that in any tense clinical moment, none of us can control what others send our way. However, we can always control how we respond.

Frames of Reference

In your clinical practice, you will have policies, procedures, and protocols to guide your evidence-based practice. You will rely on them in almost every clinical situation. However, you will also need frameworks for approaching those situations in which your patients and families are looking to you for guidance in medical decision-making or goals of care. Frames of reference (Leahy & Feudtner, 2019) are experiential frameworks that you will develop over time, as you gain wisdom and experience. These can help you relate to others, elicit thoughtful consideration, and move with them together toward a common goal.

As I said, you will develop your own, but these are the frames of reference that I have found helpful in my years of clinical practice.

1. **In every encounter, do what will serve.** What can you focus on and do well during this shift, for this patient? Recall your intention in coming into nursing. Lead and set a tone for each encounter with this spirit of compassion, curiosity, and service.

2. **Meet your patients and families where they are.** Take time to gauge where they are in their journey of health or sickness. Set the intention to glean their level of understanding in the current situation. Ask questions such as, "I'm worried about (or I'm hopeful) about this…, are you?" or "This [insert assessment] seems different (or worse or better), would you agree?" Open up dialogues and give your patients and families the opportunity to explore and field questions. Remember it is absolutely okay to say, "I don't know" if you don't have the answers. You don't have to have all the answers. You will come to know your patients best—sometimes better than you know some of your dearest friends and family members. Relationships are borne out of great vulnerability, and the relationships you build in your practice warrant great respect.

3. **Remember the humanity of nursing.** Your patient is more than just a list of comorbidities, diagnoses, and lab values. They're also someone's partner, mother, daughter, sister, father, son, brother, grandchild. They love and are loved. As a wife, daughter, sister, and now mother, I find myself asking, "What would I want for my loved one?" rather than asking, "What would I do if I were in this situation?"

Tonglen Practice

To me, mindfulness is rooted in generosity of spirit. It is taking the current moment and honoring it with grace and kindness. Sometimes it means sending loving-kindness toward one's self, and sometimes it means sending loving-kindness to someone else; this is much of what the practice of Tonglen entails.

Tonglen is Tibetan for the concept of "giving and taking," or sending and receiving (Rinpoche, 2010, p. 222). In the practice, one exchanges the self with another, thus the idea of sending and taking should be practiced alternately. These two practices should follow normal breathing patterns. In Halifax's book, *Being with Dying* (2008), she discusses the practice of Tonglen meditation and leads the reader through the practice through different lenses. The practice starts with self-reflection in our commitment to help others, setting the stage for consideration for and exploration of our own situation, feelings, and heart. This grounding in curiosity allows us to commit to ourselves in our desire to help others and cultivate mercy (Halifax, 2008).

The person practicing Tonglen then focuses on the suffering of another person or living creature (or group of people or living creatures) and imagines inhaling that suffering. Perhaps it is characterized by a black cloud of smoke or some other negative texture. With each exhale, then, the person practicing Tonglen imagines exhaling lightness, love, hope, or health toward the person, creature, or group suffering. Over time, this give and take can help reduce suffering, literally "clearing the air" toward a space of health and love (Halifax, 2008).

When I practice Tonglen with my patients, I find the ability to connect to something tangible, something I could focus on when faced with any kind of suffering. Each person's definition of suffering is different, and we are all showing up to an encounter with our own struggles, successes, views, feelings, biases, and values. It is when we can find a generosity for another and offer them loving-kindness that we can transform how we show up. For example, when I am about to cross the threshold of a patient's room, I take three deep breaths. In those breaths I am receiving and giving loving-kindness before I even interact with the child and family in the room. I'm setting my intention from a foundation of kindness, in anticipation of what I will receive.

Boundaries

As we move through our personal and professional lives, we find circles or communities we gravitate toward, people we enjoy spending time with, and people who inspire us. Conversely, we may also find ourselves in communities that leave us feeling uninspired, angry, or sad. Drawing healthy boundaries can help you learn to recognize what you have the bandwidth for and what you do not. Outside of your work, you need to identify who and what refills your tank and keeps your heart full.

Pratt et al. (2020) reviewed the influence of *engaging authentically* on nurse-patient relationships. Boundaries came up throughout their thematic analyses that revealed four themes: "getting to know the patient as a person," "the complexity of relationship building—it takes time," "the nurse: characteristics and behaviours that support the nurse–patient relationship," and "the patient voice." The ability to authentically engage and relate in an attentive, compassionate and nonjudgmental way built trust and fostered an environment of safe, person-centered outcomes of care. Nurses reported greater satisfaction when they connected with the person they cared for. Conversely, their review of some studies revealed that when nurses became over-involved, it impacted their clinical judgment and ability to provide care. The balance of establishing and maintaining personal and professional is delicate but impactful.

Personal Boundaries

Think of the individuals in your circle. Who do you look forward to spending time with? Who makes you laugh and encourages you to be your authentic self? Who leaves you feeling drained? Of course, your answers won't be the same all the time—some days our friends are exhausting, and sometimes spouses and children drain our energy. A friend may be too much for you to handle today, but in a week or so, you will enjoy their company again. The important thing is to check in with yourself when you are with friends and others outside of work. Pay attention to how you feel before and after you are with them. By doing so, you can weigh the burden and benefit of your relationships and give yourself permission to draw boundaries that serve you.

Social Media Boundaries

This is probably a good time to bring up boundaries and social media. Just as you are well served to spend time with friends and family who refuel your tank, be just as careful with your time and interactions on social media. If you feel happier and more connected to your friends after logging onto social media, wonderful. If your screen time leaves you feeling anxious, angry, or discouraged, try spending less time in those cyber communities or be more selective in your exposure. There are many people and organizations you can follow that offer inspiration online, such as artists and writers. Draw boundaries that include those who uplift you, and limit those who don't nourish your well-being.

Patient Boundaries

Finally, pay attention to boundaries on social media that involve the privacy of your patients and families. As healthcare providers, we are walking journeys with our patients and families that we may be tempted to share in some way with our nonwork people. Be careful, because the lines between work and home can sometimes blur. Although our professional and personal lives may overlap, we must maintain appropriate boundaries.

Closing Thoughts

Self-care for the clinician is rooted in self-awareness, the ability to dig deep and reflect on who we are and how we show up in life. It involves checking in with ourselves and sometimes naming difficult emotions. Our feelings of fear, anxiety, uncertainty, exhaustion, and hopelessness are natural, and we must honor them.

In Real Practice

How effective are interventions designed to improve self-care behaviors among student nurses? It is harder to evaluate the impact of these programs than one might think. The Ashcraft and Gatto study (2018) measured BSN student self-care behaviors, health habits, and perceptions longitudinally, in order to measure the impact of a three-year self-care curriculum. Students were asked to complete a self-care assessment when they began their BSN program and again one week before graduation. The results of the evaluation generally showed a positive impact on health perceptions and several mental health measures. However, it's important to consider that student nurses' stress levels naturally increase over the course of their training; nursing school presents many barriers to self-care behaviors; and alcohol use (one of the study measures) will naturally increase as students become of legal age to drink. The study raises interesting questions about the longer-term impacts of self-care curricula, as student nurses become professionals who will hopefully put their self-care skills to practice and become role models for their patients.

Considering yourself first is not selfish. Rather, it's an essential part of serving others and flourishing in your nursing career. There are many in-the-moment techniques you can use to maintain a healthy balance in your own life, and I have shared my experience with some of these methods here. My hope for you as a new nurse is that you write your own exciting story and develop your own tool kit for maintaining your well-being. Don't feel overwhelmed by all the pressure to "do self-care." Simply pay attention. Listen to what your body, head, and heart are trying to tell you, and then respond with self-compassion. I'm sure that someday you, too, will be able to share your wisdom with new and aspiring nurses.

Key Points

- The transition from student to professional nurse is exciting and nerve-wracking. With so much to remember about clinical skills and patient care, creating a personal self-care practice seems daunting. There are many things you can do "in the moment" while you care for your patients that will keep you well and serve those you care for.

- The foundation of an ongoing self-care practice is self-awareness. Pay attention to your body and accept that it is okay to feel bad at times. Nursing is stressful, and being a new nurse makes you even more vulnerable to stress. One way to create order out of emotional chaos is journaling. A journaling practice will allow you to "dump" the emotions onto paper so you are more focused for work or more available to family.

- It will be helpful to find "mini-moments" in your day, or opportunities to take a deep breath or reflect on gratitude or other positive emotion. Similarly, simple acts of kindness benefit not only those you are kind to, but also you and your own well-being.

- There are many in-the-moment practices you can adopt as healthy responses to difficult or chaotic situations. These include grounding, deflecting and redirecting, practicing Tonglen, and setting boundaries. Again, the key to each of these is choosing in the moment how to respond to a challenging stressor.

References

Ashcraft, P. F., & Gatto, S. L. (2018). Curricular interventions to promote self-care in prelicensure nursing students. *Nurse Educator, 43*(3), 140–144.

Dusek, J. A., Hibberd, P. L., Buczynski, B., Chang, B.-H., Dusek, K. C., Johnston, J. M., Wohlhueter, A. L., Benson, H., & Zusman, R. M. (2008). Stress management versus lifestyle modification on systolic hypertension and medication elimination: A randomized trial. *Journal of Alternative and Complementary Medicine, 14*(2), 129–138. https://doi.org/10.1089/acm.2007.062

Halifax, J. (2008). *Being with dying: Cultivating compassion and fearlessness in the presence of death.* Shambhala Publications, Inc.

Kozlowska, K., Walker, P., McLean, L., & Carrive, P. (2015). Fear and the defense cascade: Clinical implications and management. *Harvard Review of Psychiatry, 23*(4), 263–287. https://doi.org/10.1097/HRP.0000000000000065

Leahy, A., & Feudtner, C. (2019). Outcome dimensions in pediatric palliative care. *Pediatrics,* 143 (1) e20183347. doi:https://doi.org/10.1542/peds.2018-3347

Pratt, H., Moroney, T., & Middleton, R. (2020). The influence of engaging authentically on nurse-patient relationships: a scoping review. *Nursing Inquiry,* 2020;00:e12388. https://doi.org/10.1111/nin.12388

Rinpoche, P. (2010). *Words of my perfect teacher: A complete translation of a classic introduction to Tibetan Buddhism* (Revised edition). Yale University Press.

Rowland, L., & Curry, O. (2019). A range of kindness activities boost happiness. *Journal of Social Psychology, 159*(3), 340–343. https://doi.org/10.1080/00224545.2018.1469461

section IV
The Transition to Nursing Practice

16

Supportive Professional Relationships: Mentoring and Nurse Residency Programs

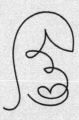

Carrie McDermott
pronouns: She/Her

Carrie McDermott, a registered nurse and clinical nurse specialist, is passionate about evidence-based practice. She specializes in mentoring student nurses and newly graduated nurses in their transition to practice, developing clinical competency, and deflecting incivility in the workplace.

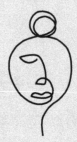

Millie Sattler
pronouns: She/Her

Millie Sattler is a registered nurse whose areas of expertise are nurse retention, career development, and nurse recognition. She is passionate about mentoring nurses at all levels through kindness, consideration, and sharing of knowledge.

> "When I look back at my life, what jumps out is how many variables had to fall in place in order to give me a chance... There were teachers, distant relatives, and friends... Remove any of these people from the equation, and I'm probably screwed."

> —J. D. Vance

As a student nurse or newly graduated nurse, you should anticipate that entry into the nursing profession brings challenges. New nurses need time to develop the technical skills and clinical judgement necessary to care for patients safely. They need patience and support from preceptors, leaders, and peers. Heavy workloads and short staffing can complicate the transition phase during the first year of entry into professional nursing, and some workplace cultures can be quite hostile with toxic negativity. To adapt to the fast-paced, hectic world of nursing, novice nurses should identify opportunities for social support. Mentoring is an excellent mechanism for providing this much-needed support for student nurses and newly licensed registered nurses (NLRNs). Nurses who are new to the profession should consider entering into a mentoring program for their personal/professional development and to ease the transition into their practice.

A report on the future of nursing (Institute of Medicine [IOM], 2011) asserted that there is a need to support nurses entering the profession. They recommend transition to practice programs, such as nurse residency programs, to ease the transition from the student role to the role of professional nurse. Major challenges faced by NLRNs include (Kramer et al., 2012):

- Delegation
- Prioritization
- Managing care delivery
- Decision-making
- Collaboration
- Conflict resolution
- Self-confidence

A structured transition-to-practice nurse residency program (NRP) provides a means of social support and a rich resource for mentoring. These programs are designed to help new nurses adjust to the realities of the nursing profession, support development in the professional role, and provide guidance for self-care during the transition to practice and beyond (Fink et al., 2008; Goode et al., 2016).

Without adequate support, new nurses can become discouraged and quickly leave their first role. Some even leave the profession altogether. Nursing turnover rates are known to be high among NLRNs. Turnover rates have been reported to be as high as 17.5% to 20% within the first 12 months (Kovner et al., 2014; Weathers & Raleigh, 2013). When there are high rates of nursing turnover, high rates of staffing shortages follow, which further discourage nurses remaining in the workforce. With the increasing demands on our healthcare system and high rates of nursing turnover, there is an ever-increasing need to rely on NLRNs to meet workforce needs. Novice nurses entering the profession should seek out prospective employers with the structure to support their transition to practice through a nurse residency program and mentoring.

What Is Mentoring?

Mentoring relationships exist in all aspects of our lives. We instinctively gravitate toward individuals who inspire us. We look to our teachers, family members, and leaders in our community as role models and advisors. When a more experienced person takes the time to offer guidance to a less experienced one, they are giving the gift of mentoring. Mentoring is a demonstration of caring (Vance, 2011). A mentor is someone who takes a genuine interest in your well-being, personally and professionally. The mentoring relationship is one of mutual respect, which, over time, is empowering, affirming, and supports the development of professional excellence (Vance & Olson, 1998).

In nursing, a mentoring relationship is one that occurs between an experienced, seasoned nurse and a novice nurse, one that is structured to support personal and professional development, career advancement, and professional excellence (Vance, 2011). The experienced nurse may be a leader, preceptor, educator, or esteemed colleague. Because of their experience, a mentor can help you adjust to the realities of nursing and support you on your journey to professional excellence. Most importantly, the mentor is someone who has taken an interest in helping you succeed. A mentor can see the potential in you that you have yet to identify for yourself. With their wisdom, a mentor can support your development both personally and professionally. They can act as a coach, a confidant, an advisor, and a role model.

A mentor is a trusted advisor who can guide you on your journey to professional excellence. As you prepare for your entry into the nursing profession, you should consider entering into a mentored relationship.

The Benefits of Mentoring

Mentoring relationships in nursing can have beneficial effects for the mentee, the mentor, and the organization. Navigating through nursing school and the transition to practice as a professional nurse is a taxing and stressful journey. While novice nurses are still learning, they lack confidence in the clinical setting, and this can lead to stress and anxiety. Mentoring can decrease stress levels in new graduate nurses and decrease anxiety in student nurses by providing socialization and emotional support (Kim et al., 2013; Van Patten & Bartone, 2019). Student nurses have reported that mentoring has given them insight into the world of nursing, increased their confidence, increased their understanding of how to deal with difficult situations, and better prepared them for the realities of nursing (Lavoie-Tremblay et al., 2018).

Mentoring programs are also beneficial for the mentors. Nurse mentors have reported that mentoring was an enriching experience, that they gained insight into themselves as well as a better understanding of how to support new nurses. Mentoring can increase sensitivity to the challenges faced by new nurses (Lavoie-Tremblay et al., 2018). Mentors feel gratified by the mentoring relationship and valued for the wisdom they have to offer. They feel like they *matter* to other nurses and to the organization. (You'll read more about the importance of mattering in Chapter 21.) Their mentoring is reciprocated in the things they learn from their mentee. Some mentors have reported that mentoring reenergized their passion for nursing (Clausen et al., 2011).

Mentoring programs can have a positive influence on the work environment by contributing to a healthy, supportive culture. Mentoring has beneficial effects on engagement and organizational commitment (Topa et al., 2014). Studies on mentoring in nursing suggest that mentoring can increase feelings of belonging. Other benefits of mentoring include career optimism, professional growth, and competence (Weese et al., 2015). Mentoring programs have reported increased motivation and career development in mentees (Lavoie-Tremblay et al., 2018; Weng et al., 2010). Mentoring has also been associated with improved retention and a decrease in turnover (Cottingham et al., 2011; Fox, 2010).

Mentoring in the Nursing Profession

There are numerous mentoring roles in the nursing profession. Nurses rely on each other to support their practice and help them develop new skills. In the work setting you may find that you already have a mentor assigned to you. When you start a new job, you should be assigned a mentor to oversee your orientation. The mentor may be a preceptor or other staff assigned to train and supervise you on the job. Student nurses working as interns or externs will have mentors assigned to them to support them in their role. Newly graduated nurses in NRPs will have preceptors assigned to them in the clinical area and educators to support their professional development in the learning sessions. These mentors are assigned for a time-limited role, and the formal relationship typically ends when the program goals have been met.

Group Mentoring

Mentors can be assigned to a one-on-one mentorship or to a group mentorship. Group mentoring assignments may be a group of less experienced nurses assigned to a more experienced nurse for the purpose of sharing wisdom or developing a particular skill (Clausen et al., 2011). Group mentoring is different from group precepting. In *group mentoring*, an experienced nurse meets regularly with a small group of less experienced nurses to discuss shared experiences (Lavoie-Tremblay, 2018). Group mentoring is useful when there are a number of nurses in the same situation. For example, group mentoring has been used to support student nurses preparing for their transition to practice and to mentor nurses once they have graduated and entered into an NRP (Lavoie-Tremblay et al., 2018; Van Patten & Bartone, 2019). Group mentoring increases access to mentors by requiring fewer mentors than a one-on-one mentoring program and allows the group opportunities for socialization and peer support (Hall et al., 2019).

Matched and Peer Mentoring

Some organizations offer matched mentoring programs. Matching may be facilitated by someone who knows the characteristics of the available mentors and the interested mentees (Vance, 2011). Mentoring programs offered through schools of nursing, professional organizations, and employers may use matching to introduce the mentor/mentee dyad (Vance, 2011). Examples of dyads can include a student nurse matched with an RN in the clinical setting, a graduate student nurse with an undergraduate student nurse, or an upper-class student—like a senior—with an entry level student. Peer mentoring programs are another type of matched mentoring program. In peer mentoring programs, the mentor and the mentee have a similar status in the organization (Hunt & Ellison, 2010).

Mentors who are assigned are usually unassigned after the mentee reaches key milestones. Mentors who are matched may also be available for a limited time depending on the program design. In addition to these mentors, you may want to seek out a mentor for a lasting relationship. Before you begin seeking out a mentor, reflect on what you want from the mentoring relationship (Vance, 2011). Why do you want a mentor, and what do you hope to gain from the relationship? Begin networking, join professional organizations, and attend conferences in the specialty area or topics that interest you. You may well find a mentor in the people and places that reflect your areas of interest. Knowing your personal and professional goals will help you find the right mentor for you (Vance, 2011). Nurses often feel honored when they are asked to be a mentor, so don't hesitate to ask when you meet the person you think would be a good mentor for you!

Qualities of a Mentor

A mentor should be able to provide an entry to professional networks and contact information that would not be available to the mentee otherwise. The mentor brings experience and wisdom (Academy of Medical-Surgical Nursing, 2012).

Mentor qualifications include:

- Commitment to the organizations' mission and goals
- Strong interpersonal skills
- Willingness to assist with mentees' professional development
- Willingness to learn from the mentee
- Ability to think strategically, share credit and successes
- Ability to help the mentee learn from their mistakes
- Ability to embrace diversity

The expectations of the nurse mentor are to serve as a guide to the mentee as they develop new skills. The mentor role is to develop, confirm, and encourage the mentee to progress and strive for excellence professionally. Mentoring is an evolving, encouraging, and empowering relationship that contributes to personal confidence-building and professional excellence (Vance, 2011).

Mentor roles include (Vance, 2011):

- **Coach:** to help strategize your mentee's goals, recognize and analyze their strengths and opportunities for improvement, encourage your mentee to strive for excellence, and assist them with evaluating their progress.

- **Counselor:** to listen carefully to what the mentee is saying about their job, career goals, personal lifestyles, and events. This act will help them with their own decisions that will lead them to the future.

- **Confidant:** to listen without opinion and maintain confidentiality regarding the discussions.

- **Encourager:** to inspire and show the mentee a path that will engage their energy and passion, to assist them if they face challenges in meeting their goals.

- **Friend:** to provide kindness and reassurance, as someone who genuinely cares for and believes in their mentee and wants the best for them.

- **Visionary:** to see where the mentee is initially but to see what they can become.

- **Resource:** to connect the mentee with information, ideas, people, and other resources that can help the mentee advance.

In our experience there are several roles that the mentor should *not* embrace:

- **Advocate:** It is up to the mentee to advocate for themselves. The mentor is to help the mentee learn how to take care of themselves, not do it for them.

- **Mediator:** The mentor is not a mediator between a supervisor and a mentee. Again, it is up to the mentee to speak up for themselves. The mentor may advise, coach, or help strategize, but never can be positioned between a mentee and a supervisor.

- **Judge:** The mentor and mentee may see goals differently from one other. The mentor's role is to help the mentee decide for themselves to see what aligns with the mentee's talents, values and beliefs, and individual goals and not impose the mentor's ideas on the mentee.

- **Boss:** One of the nice things about being a mentor is that you do not have to supervise the mentee, and the mentee does not have to be intimidated by the mentor. The more the mentor removes the hierarchical distinction, the more successful the relationship is likely to be. The mentor should not tell the mentee what to do but should guide them in the right direction and assist the mentee with their decision and what will work best in their own life. The mentee will weigh the mentor's advice against their personal goals. Any decision should be the mentee's decision.

- **Magician:** It is not up to the mentor to "fix" things for the mentee. Encourage the mentee to see that they may have a lot of power over what happens with their career goals and in their work lives, and they do not need a magician to make it happen.

Finding the Right Mentor

Strong mentoring programs have a systematic approach to matching a mentor with a mentee. Ideally, an assigned facilitator has access to the information about the mentor and mentee needed to ensure a learning fit. Factors taken into consideration when matching mentor with mentee are personality, professional interest, proximity, educational background, age, gender, culture, roles in the organization, and compatibility (Vance, 2011). If you plan to participate in a mentoring program, you should reflect on your motivation and goals for seeking a mentor. In preparation for entering a mentoring program, ask yourself the following questions:

1. Why would I like to have a mentor?
2. What am I seeking to learn, and why is this important for my professional growth?
3. Do I have a specific goal that I would like to accomplish through this program?
4. What will be important to me in my mentor/mentee relationship?
5. What characteristics, skills, and experiences am I seeking in a mentor?

Setting Goals With Your Mentor

You and your mentor should establish specific, measurable goals as a pair. These goals serve as a beacon to guide you, essentially a roadmap of where to go and how to get there. These goals are not your ultimate career goals, but rather goals that the two of you have agreed upon for a specific time frame (Vance, 2011). Examples of goals might be to:

- Explore a particular career option
- Establish a career direction
- Ensure that you complete all the needed qualifications for the desired job

- Decide on an academic program to pursue and begin enrollment

- Improve working relationships with the supervisor and coworkers

- Develop technical or professional skills in a growing area

- Initiate and nurture a network of individuals who can help you in a newly identified career

Career goals might include accomplishments such as certification, academic advancement, or receiving a promotion. Goals for professional development may include building and refining skills like presentation skills, conflict management skills, and writing skills.

The mutually agreed upon goals drive the mentoring process, but as the journey continues, the goals may change. The goals should be reviewed and reevaluated throughout the relationship to ensure that they are still meeting your needs (Vance, 2011). Thus, goal setting and evaluation of goals in a mentoring process becomes iterative by nature. You and your mentor will know when you have successfully met these goals. Once goals are met, or a predetermined time frame has passed, the mentoring sessions may conclude. In many cases, the mentor and mentee continue to have a relationship of mutual respect that is supportive and inspirational and may last for a long time, even after the formal mentoring period is over (Vance, 2011).

Transition to Practice Nurse Residency Programs

Mentors can be found within the programs and structures employers have in place to support the transition from student nurse to professional nursing. An NRP is an effective mechanism for supporting the transition from advanced beginner to competent professional nurse (Goode et al., 2016). A structured transition-to-practice NRP is a series of learning opportunities that blend classroom learning with clinical immersion to support the transition to practice (Bleich, 2012). These programs typically last from six to twelve months, and they focus on developing professional nursing practice through reflection, small group activities, and formal presentations (Bleich, 2012). As you prepare to transition from the role of student nurse to that of professional nurse, take time to investigate the programs your prospective employers have in place to support your transition to practice.

Transition to practice NRPs have a positive effect on newly licensed registered nurses' (NLRN) self-confidence, competence, organization, and prioritization (Goode et al., 2013). A structured NRP will encourage mentoring, collegial support, self-care activities, professional development, and group evidence-based practice projects. Nurses completing an NRP report greater job satisfaction, enjoyment of work (Ulrich et al., 2010), better socialization, and integration onto the unit (Kramer et al., 2012). NRPs have also been reported to increase NLRN first-year retention rates to nearly 95% and decrease voluntary turnover rates (Goode et al., 2013). With the support of nursing leaders and the executive team, a structured NRP can increase job satisfaction, reduce work stress, and decrease turnover in new graduates hired to work in acute care settings (Specter et al., 2015).

An Evidence-Based Curriculum

The research on NRPs provides a roadmap for identifying programs designed for maximum support of NLRNs. The curriculum should focus on four areas: developing clinical leadership skills, clinical decision-making skills, competences for quality and patient safety, and developing the professional role (Specter et al., 2015). The topics of patient safety, clinical reasoning, communication and teamwork, patient-centered care, evidence-based practice, quality improvement, and informatics should be included in the NRP curriculum (Specter et al., 2015). Content on delegation, managing conflict, and care coordination should also be included to support development of leadership in the clinical area. Ethical decision-making, end-of-life care, stress management, and cultural competence should also be part of the curriculum to support professional role development. NRPs with the following characteristics have been able to demonstrate better outcomes (Specter et al., 2015):

- Programs should be at least nine to twelve months long

- Program curriculum should include content on evidence-based practice

- Programs should include customization for specialty areas

- Programs should have a highly supportive preceptor program

The length of the NRP may vary from one employer to another. As a new nurse, you should look for a program that is at least nine to twelve months in length. Better outcomes such as job satisfaction, confidence, competence, and retention rates have been associated with longer programs (Goode et al., 2016). One reason that a longer program is more beneficial is because stress levels of NLRNs go up at around six months. At the same time, job satisfaction may go down. By supporting NLRNs for nine to twelve months, their stress levels are able to go back down, and once again job satisfaction is up (Rush et al., 2013; Specter et al., 2015). It is especially important to have the continued support of the NRP during the vulnerable period between months six and twelve.

One pillar of success for an NRP is dedicated time reserved for the resident nurse to learn and reflect on concepts learned in the classroom and at the bedside. Returning to the residency session to reflect on the bedside experiences helps to enrich their understanding and promote development of critical thinking and clinical judgement. This reflective activity, practiced in an environment that is safe and supportive, is a form of self-care and mindfulness. The supportive collegial relationships established with the other resident nurses encourage self-care through social support (Fink et al., 2008). It is particularly helpful to group resident nurses with others from the same or similar departments to share learning activities that are customized for the knowledge and skills required for that specialty area and to extend the bonds of a supportive relationship into the clinical setting.

One way to confirm that an NRP program and curriculum are evidence-based is to look for accredited programs in your search for prospective employers. The Commission on Collegiate Nursing Education (CCNE) and the American Nurses

Credentialing Center (ANCC) are accrediting agencies that will evaluate transition to practice nurse residency programs for their standards. The goal of the accrediting agencies is to ensure that a transition to practice NRP has the structure, processes, and resources necessary to fulfill their mission of supporting new nurses in their transition to practice. You may find a list of accredited programs by going to the accrediting agencies' websites:

- https://www.aacnnursing.org/CCNE
- https://www.nursingworld.org/organizational-programs/accreditation/ptap/

Mentors Within the Nurse Residency Program

A structured NRP should have a designated NRP Coordinator (Krugman et al., 2006). Mentoring by the NRP Coordinator occurs in the classroom, through one-on-one interactions, and behind the scenes as they coordinate the necessary resources to support resident nurses' onboarding. The NRP Coordinator coordinates the classroom learning sessions, schedules guest speakers and panels, and organizes interactive learning activities, including games designed for learning and many other creative teaching methods to make the residency sessions an excellent learning experience. The NRP Coordinator collaborates with nursing leaders and preceptors to plan the resident nurse's onboarding in a deliberate and thoughtful manner. This planning also ensures that the resident nurse has dedicated time to attend classroom residency sessions. The NRP Coordinator will "check-in" with residents in the classroom and ask you to share how things are going in your new role as a professional nurse (Krugman et al., 2006).

In your NRP you may meet an NRP Group Facilitator. The Group Facilitator is assigned to facilitate small group discussions for a group of resident nurses. The Group Facilitator is usually a seasoned nurse who is also in a leadership role as a manager, educator, or advanced practice nurse. These facilitators lead small group discussion using focus questions (Krugman et al., 2006). The discussions are a safe place for resident nurses to share their experiences. A resident may choose to share problems or concerns they have during the small group discussion. These seasoned nurses are able to mentor the resident nurses by facilitating reflective practice and thoughtful discussions. A Group Facilitator is familiar with the organizational culture and can offer guidance on how to handle difficult situations while maintaining the privacy and confidentially of the nurse residents (Krugman et al., 2006).

The role of the preceptor is central to your success in your transition to practice (Hall et al., 2019). A preceptor is an experienced nurse who is assigned to you during your orientation to the clinical area. The role of the preceptor is to prepare you to function independently in your clinical area (Van Patton & Bartone, 2019). Your preceptor will supervise you, evaluate your knowledge, skills, and ability to competently perform all the skills necessary for your role as a professional nurse. The preceptor carefully selects tasks and patient care responsibilities to assign you, progressing those assignments from simple to more complex. As you carry out these assignments, the preceptor evaluates your competence to perform technical skills and your ability to use clinical judgement independently (Hall et al., 2019).

Coaching is a key part of the preceptor role (Van Patton & Bartone, 2019). During the transition to practice, resident nurses are learning and developing their technical and interpersonal skills and their clinical judgement (Krugman et al., 2006). Your preceptor may coach you in ways that help you perform procedures more efficiently. They may have tips to help you stay organized, and they will find opportunities for you to practice repetition of skills so that you develop greater dexterity. A preceptor can enlighten you to the secret body of knowledge—the knowledge that all the seasoned nurses on the unit have but is not in the procedure manual, like physician preferences, interdepartmental communication preferences, and tricks to maintaining your supply chain (Hall et al., 2019).

Mentoring is also a part of the preceptor role (Topa et al., 2014; Hall et al., 2019). A preceptor will help you socialize in your new clinical area by introducing you to your colleagues. When interacting with physicians, your preceptor may introduce you and invite the physician to contribute to your development by taking the time to explain tests, procedures, and treatments. Preceptors will network on behalf of their orientee; they often seek out unique clinical situations in hopes of exposing the resident nurse to more varied experiences while they are still on orientation. Although mentoring is considered part of the preceptor role, it is not a long-term mentoring relationship. Once the orientation is over, the preceptor will step back from the mentoring role unless the resident nurse makes a request for a formalized mentoring relationship (Hall et al., 2019).

Evidence-Based Practice Projects

An important part of the NRP and the transition to practice is the process of learning how to apply evidence from research, and other sources, to your practice at the bedside. As you investigate prospective employers with NRPs, you will want to inquire about the opportunity to complete an evidence-based practice (EBP) project during your residency (Krugman et al., 2006; Specter et al., 2015). In order for nurses of the future to lead change and promote the highest quality, safe patient care NLRNs must learn to apply EBP at the bedside (IOM, 2011). Resident nurses will identify a problem and develop an EBP project that will improve care in their clinical area. This can be done independently or in small groups. Resident nurses seek out evidence from the literature to identify and implement a best practice recommendation. Once complete, the projects are shared publicly through staff meetings, journal clubs, conferences, and poster presentations. This process helps the NLRN learn the EBP process, quality improvement processes, and how to implement a change (Melnyk & Fineout-Overholt, 2019). They also develop experience with dissemination of knowledge when they create a poster and present their completed project.

Collegial Support

Your peers, the other resident nurses, will also play a role in mentoring you during your transition to practice. The period of time during transition to practice can bring on many emotions, including stress and feelings of isolation. Participation in residency sessions allows residents to find the social support that may be missing in their work environment (Fink et al., 2008). During these seminars, resident nurses share their challenges and successes. They listen and support one another through the stories they tell and the feelings they share. For a novice nurse who may feel isolated, the sharing of experiences with one another is reassuring. Realizing that you are facing the same or similar challenges, and feeling the same feelings, validates that you are not alone on your journey.

Over time, a spirit of camaraderie develops. Resident nurses share their trials with their peers and the lessons they've learned at the bedside. During the residency seminars, the topic of self-care is threaded throughout the curriculum. These close-knit groups of residents help each other find ways to cope with their job stressors (Krugman et al., 2006). They share self-care techniques and encourage one another to try different self-care activities. The residency program provides a safe place to share and support one another with advice and encouragement. The spirit of camaraderie extends beyond the residency classroom and into the clinical area as social support and ultimately establishing the resident nurses into the unit's social structure.

Storytelling

NRPs use small-group activities to create an atmosphere of caring, support, and psychological safety. Thoughtfully prepared discussion questions are used to stimulate discussions on recent experiences in the clinical environment (Krugman et al., 2006). These discussions enable the resident nurses to tell stories of their clinical experience and unpack the sequence of events along with the emotions they may have experienced at the same time. The goal is to reinforce the learning that is based on experience and to encourage additional learning that will take place by reflecting on the experience (Bolden et al., 2011).

Nurses learn through stories—the stories they tell and the ones that they hear (Benner, 1984). In an NRP, the resident nurses will share stories of their personal experiences in their small groups and in the larger group. The Residency Coordinators will draw the stories out by asking if anyone wants to share. Once the sharing starts, others usually start to join in. They may have a similar experience to share, a contradictory experience, or a similar experience that had a different outcome. There may be pearls of wisdom in these stories that benefit everyone. By sharing their stories, they are mentoring one another. They are caring for themselves and for their cohort. They are passing on the gift of what they have learned in their own experience.

Supportive Preceptor Program

The NRP that you enter should have highly skilled, supportive preceptors. The preceptor should have no more than one orientee at a time, and you should expect to have one primary preceptor to work with on most shifts. You and your preceptor should be on the same schedule as much as possible and share the same assignment (Specter et al., 2015). Initially, your preceptor may have a reduced clinical assignment to ensure that there is adequate time to introduce you to the clinical setting and explain department routines. You and your preceptor will share an assignment, and your preceptor will supervise you in your delivery of care. Over time you will take on more responsibility until you are able to assume all the responsibilities for a full patient assignment.

Supportive preceptors are essential for a successful transition to practice. In one study, orientees in hospitals with high preceptor support scored higher competence levels than the orientees in hospitals with low preceptor support (Clipper & Cherry, 2015). Supportive preceptor programs are also associated with better retention in the first year of nursing (Blegen et al., 2015). To find the best support for transition to practice in the first year of nursing, new nurses should evaluate the structure of the preceptor program at their prospective employer and select employment settings with a highly supportive preceptor program.

Use the checklist below to guide your inquiry into your prospective employer's NRP.

Checklist for Evaluating NRP Attributes

✓ Program is at least 12 months long.

✓ Orientation is with a dedicated preceptor.

✓ The preceptor has only one orientee at a time.

✓ There is protected time to attend monthly residency seminars.

✓ The program includes access to mentors.

✓ Participation in the program includes completing a mentored evidence-based practice project.

✓ The program is accredited by a nationally recognized accrediting agency.

Closing Thoughts

Mentors are important connections that can help to promote your self-care and your professional development as you transition to practice as a professional nurse. Mentoring relationships are an excellent mechanism for providing the social support that student nurses and newly licensed registered nurses (NLRNs) need as they transition into practice. A mentor is someone who takes a genuine interest in your well-being both personally and professionally. Mentoring relationships in nursing can have beneficial effects for the mentee, the mentor, and the organization. There are a wide variety of mentoring programs for nurses, but the success of the mentoring relationship is dependent upon the mutually structured goals developed by the mentoring dyad (Vance, 2011).

In Real Practice

The impact of stress on learning during clinical placements can have multiple negative impacts on learning, confidence, and mental well-being. In the Grobecker study (2016), the authors hypothesized that a sense of belonging could help mitigate the negative effects of stress during clinical placements among BSN students. Belongingness is the feeling that you are needed, valued, and accepted by a group. If you feel as though you fit in, you are less likely to feel lonely or rejected. You may also be more motivated and able to learn effectively. It makes intuitive sense that nursing students are more likely to flourish in their clinical placements if they feel a sense of connection to nursing staff, patients, and others. This study indicates that a sense of belonging during clinicals has an inverse relationship with stress. It is important for learning, and ultimately for patient care, that nurse educators promote positive, welcoming environments for clinical students.

A structured transition to practice nurse residency program (NRP) provides a means of social support and a rich resource for mentoring. When these programs are evidence-based, they can help new nurses deal with the realities of the nursing profession. To find the best support for your transition to practice in the first year of nursing, you should investigate programs offered by prospective employers to include an NRP, mentoring resources, and a supportive preceptor program.

Key Points

- Mentors are important connections that can provide support for you during your transition to practice through professional excellence, social support, networking, and encouragement.

- Mentoring can be found in nursing school, in nurse residency programs, in clinical leaders, and in formal mentoring programs.

- Before engaging in a mentorship, reflect on your goals. Why do you want a mentor, and what are you seeking in a mentor?

- Take advantage of mentoring programs offered through your school, your employer, or professional organizations.

- Mentoring relationships in nursing can have beneficial effects for the mentee, the mentor, and the organization.

References

Academy of Medical-Surgical Nursing. (2012). *AMSN Mentoring Program site coordinator guide.* AMSN. https://www.amsn.org/professional-development/mentoring

Benner, P. (1984). *From novice to expert.* Prentice Hall.

Blegen, M. A., Spector, N., Ulrich, B. T., Lynn, M. R., Barnsteiner, J., & Silvestre, J. (2015). Preceptor support in hospital transition to practice programs. *Journal of Nursing Administration, 45*(12), 642–649. https://doi.org/10.1097/NNA.0000000000000278

Bleich, M. R. (2012). In praise of nursing residency programs. *American Nurse Today, 7*(5), 47–49. https://www.myamericannurse.com/in-praise-of-nursing-residency-programs/

Bolden, L., Cuevas, N., Raia, L., Meredith, E., & Prince, T. (2011). The use of reflective practice in new graduate registered nurses residency program. *Nursing Administration Quarterly, 35*(2), 134–139. https://doi.org/10.1097/NAQ.0b013e31820feb5e

Clausen, M., Wejr, P., Frost, L., McRae, C., & Straight, H. (2011). Legacy mentors: Translating the wisdom of our senior nurses. *Nurse Education in Practice, 11*(2), 153–158. https://doi.org/10.1016/j.nepr.2010.10.001

Clipper, B., & Cherry, B. (2015). From transition shock to competent practice: Developing preceptors to support new nurse transition. *Journal of Continuing Education in Nursing, 46*(10), 448–454. doi:10.3928/00220124-20150918-02

Cottingham, S., DiBartolo, M. C., Battistoni, S., & Brown, T. (2011). Partners in nursing: A mentoring initiative to enhance nurse retention. *Nursing Education Perspectives, 32*(4), 250–255. https://doi.org/10.5480/1536-5026-32.4.250

Fink, R., Krugman, M., Casey, K., Goode, C. (2008). The graduate nurse experience: qualitative residency program outcomes. *Journal of Nursing Administration.* Jul–Aug;38(7–8):341–348. doi:10.1097/01.NNA.0000323943.82016.48. PMID: 18690125.

Fox, K. C. (2010). Mentor program boosts new nurses' satisfaction and lowers turnover rate. *Journal of Continuing Education in Nursing, 41*(7), 311–316. https://doi.org/10.3928/00220124-20100401-04

Goode, C. J., Lynn, M. R., McElroy, D., Bednash, G. D., & Murray, B. (2013). Lessons learned from 10 years of research on a post-baccalaureate nurse residency program. *Journal of Nursing Administration, 43*(2), 73–79. https://doi.org/10.1097/NNA.0b013e31827f205c

Goode, C. J., Ponte, P. R., & Havens, D. S. (2016). Residency for transition into practice: An essential requirement for new graduates from basic RN programs. *Journal of Nursing Administration,, 46*(2), 82–86. https://doi.org/10.1097/NNA.0000000000000300

Grobecker, P. A. (2016). A sense of belonging and perceived stress among baccalaureate nursing students in clinical placements. *Nurse Education Today, 36*, 178–183. https://doi.org/10.1016/j.nedt.2015.09.015

Hall, S., Taylor, S., & Altobar, C. (2019). Transition to practice: Onboarding components for establishing and sustaining healthy work environments. *AACN Advanced Critical Care, 30*(4), 416–420. https://doi.org/10.4037/aacnacc2019329

Hunt, C. W., & Ellison, K. J. (2010). Enhancing faculty resources through peer mentoring. *Nurse Educator, 35*(5), 192–196. https://doi.org/10.1097/NNE.0b013e3181ed8143

Institute of Medicine. (2011). *The future of nursing: Leading change, advancing health.* National Academies Press. https://doi.org/10.17226/12956

Kim, S. C., Oliveri, D., Riingen, M., Taylor, B., & Rankin, L. (2013). Randomized controlled trial of graduate-to-undergraduate student mentoring program. *Journal of Professional Nursing, 29*(6), e43–e49. https://doi.org/10.1016/j.profnurs.2013.04.003

Kovner, C. T., Brewer, C. S., Fatehi, F., & Jun, J. (2014). What does nurse turnover rate mean and what is the rate? *Policy, Politics, & Nursing Practice, 15*(3/4), 64–71. https://doi.org/10.1177/1527154414547953

Kramer, M., Maguire, P., Halfer, D., Budin, W. C., Hall, D. S., Goodloe, L., Klaristenfeld, J., Teasley, S., Forsey, L., & Lemke, J. (2012). The organizational transformative power of nurse residency programs. *Nursing Administration Quarterly, 36*(2), 155–168. https://doi.org/10.1097/NAQ.0b013e318249fdaa

Krugman, M., Bretschneider, J., Horn, P. B., Krsek, C. A., Moutafis, R. A., & Smith, M. O. The national post-baccalaureate graduate nurse residency program: A model for excellence in transition to practice. *Journal for Nurses in Staff Development.* 2006 Jul–Aug;22(4): 196–205. doi: 10.1097/00124645-200607000-00008. PMID: 16885686

Lavoie-Tremblay, M., Sanzone, L., Primeau, G., & Lavigne, G. L. (2018). Group mentorship programme for graduating nursing students to facilitate their transition: A pilot study. *Journal of Nursing Management, 27*, 66–74. https://pubmed.ncbi.nlm.nih.gov/30198617/

Melnyk, B. M., & Fineout-Overholt, E. (Eds), (2019). *Evidence-based practice in nursing and healthcare: A guide to best practice* (4th Ed). Wolters Kluwer.

Rush, K. L., Adamack, M., Lilly, M., & Janke, R. (2013). Best practices of formal new graduate nurse transition programs: An integrative review. *International Journal of Nursing Studies, 50*(3), 345–356. https://doi.org/10.1016/j.ijnurstu.2012.06.009

Specter, N., Blegen, M. A., Silvestre, J., Barnsteiner, J., Lynn, M. R., Ulrich, B., Fogg, L., & Alexander, M. (2015). Transition to practice study in hospital settings. *Journal of Nursing Regulation, 5*(4), 24–38. https://doi.org/10.1016/S2155-8256(15)30031-4

Topa, G., Guliemi, D., & Depolo, M. (2014). Mentoring and group identification as antecedents of satisfaction and health among nurses: What role do bullying experiences play? *Nurse Education Today, 34*, 507–512. http://dx.doi.org/101016/j.nedt.2013.07.006

Ulrich, B., Krozek, C., Early, S., Ashlock, C. H., Africa, L. M., & Carman, M. L. (2010). Improving retention, confidence and competence of new graduate nurses: Results from a 10-year longitudinal database. *Nursing Economic$, 28*(6), 363–367. https://www.semanticscholar.org/paper/Improving-retention%2C-confidence%2C-and-competence-of-Ulrich-Krozek/2d34496a23f615cc9244bdce83d10c921616c534

Vance, C. (2011). *Fast facts for career success in nursing: Making the most of mentoring in a nutshell.* Springer Publishing Company, LLC.

Vance, C., & Olson, R. (1998). *The mentor connection in nursing.* Springer.

Van Patten, R. R., & Bartone, A. S. (2019). The impact of mentorship, preceptors, and debriefing on the quality of program experiences. *Nurse Education in Practice, 35*, 63–68. https:/doi.org/10.1016/j.nepr.2019.01.007

Weathers, S. M., & Raleigh, E. D. H. (2013). 1-year retention rates and performance ratings: Comparing associate degree, baccalaureate, and accelerated baccalaureate degree nurses. *Journal of Nursing Administration, 43*(9), 468–474. https://doi.org/10.1097/NNA.0b013e3182a23d9f

Weese, M. M., Jakubik, L. D., Eliades, A. B., & Huth, J. J. (2015). Mentoring practices benefiting pediatric nurses. *Journal of Pediatric Nursing, 30*(2), 385–394. https://doi.org/10.1016/j.pedn.2014.07.011

Weng, R. H., Huang, C. Y., Tsai, W. C., Chang, L. Y., Lin, S. E., & Lee, M. Y. (2010). Exploring the impact of mentoring functions on job satisfaction and organizational commitment of new staff nurses. *BMC Health Services Research, 10*(240), 1–9. https://doi.org/10.1186/1472-6963-10-240

17

Healthy Work Environment: How to Choose One for Your First Job

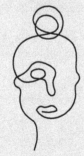

Dorrie K. Fontaine
pronouns: She/Her

Dorrie K. Fontaine, a critical care nurse and teacher, has been an academic leader for four decades. While president of the American Association of Critical-Care Nurses, she observed the joys and struggles of bedside nursing. Meditation, yoga, and daily gratitude practice help her overcome the fears and anxieties of our common human existence.

"Creating a Healthy Work Environment (HWE) enables nurses to provide the highest standards of compassionate care while being fulfilled at work."

–American Association of Critical-Care Nurses

One of the most important decisions you will make is also one of the most difficult:

Where to start your nursing career?

Numerous factors will play into the choice, starting with location, your specialty preference, reputation of the hospital or organization, and most importantly, the overall "feel" of the place and the people in it, especially the nurses who will be your colleagues. That "feel" often has to do with the elements of what we are calling a healthy work environment (HWE), and they can be translated from evidence-based data to information that you can use in your decision. For purposes of this discussion, I will consider a hospital as your primary destination, knowing that public health and community settings are all growing possibilities, and the same HWE standards apply. You likely already have ideas about what constitutes an HWE as you consider all the clinical rotations you have experienced in your training. Here we will sort out what makes one setting stand out as superior to others.

The HWE standards were first promulgated by the American Association of Critical-Care Nurses (AACN) in 2005 and reaffirmed in 2016. While the standards were developed with acute and critical-care nurses in mind, they have proven to be universally accepted in varied hospital units from labor and delivery to the operating room, among others.

This chapter explores how we define HWE, where the standards originated, why a healthy work environment is critical for your career and self-care, and how you can find this kind of workplace when you are looking for your first nursing position.

We spend so much of our life at work, literally 100,000 hours in a full career (Worline & Dutton, 2017). It should be a place that is worthy of your unique passion and dedication. It should be a place where you can grow and develop, using all of your skills and interests. It should have mentors and colleagues across disciplines whom you respect, including your nurse manager. It should recognize you formally and informally for your hard work and contributions. These are the qualities that have defined an HWE in the literature for over 15 years (Ulrich et al., 2006, 2009, 2014, 2019).

Standards for a Healthy Work Environment

In 2005, AACN released the HWE standards, *"AACN Standards for Establishing and Sustaining Healthy Work Environments,"* and they released a second edition in 2016 (AACN, 2016). At the time of a serious nursing shortage, the standards were developed in response to reports of rising medical errors; work environments where poor communication between nurses and physicians, and between nurses themselves, was escalating; reports of staffing inadequacies; and rising moral distress among nurses (AACN, 2016). They developed six standards to underscore the link between the quality of the work environment, excellent nursing practice, and patient care outcomes. The following sidebar outlines these six standards and definitions.

The Six Standards for Establishing and Sustaining a Healthy Work Environment (AACN, 2016):

- **Skilled Communication:** Nurses must be as proficient in communication skills as they are in clinical skills.
- **True Collaboration:** Nurses must be relentless in pursuing and fostering collaboration.
- **Effective Decision-Making:** Nurses must be valued and committed partners in making policy, directing and evaluating clinical care, and leading organizational operations.
- **Appropriate Staffing:** Staffing must ensure the effective match between patient needs and nurse competencies.
- **Meaningful Recognition:** Nurses must be recognized and must recognize others for the value each brings to the work of the organization.
- **Authentic Leadership:** Nurse leaders must fully embrace the imperative of a healthy work environment, authentically live it, and engage others in its achievement.

Healthy Work Environment Standards and Lessons From the Field

There is clear evidence indicating that your work environment will be a significant determinant of both your own and your patients' well-being (Lake et al., 2019). The clear standards outlined in this section deserve your careful consideration as you think about your work environments. As we review these standards, reflect on the units where you have clinical rotations now or, if you are a new nurse, think about your first or current clinical position. Do a mental check of how your clinical settings match the elements and standards of a healthy work environment. How do they measure up?

Skilled Communication

Nurses must be as proficient in communication skills as they are in clinical skills. In education and training programs, nurses spend considerable time learning technical skills such as IV insertion, suctioning a patient on a ventilator, and other competencies. There is much less time and practice spent on how to communicate with patients and families in distress, how to negotiate and advocate for a patient with physicians and team members, and how to deal with ethical issues in care decisions (Dempsey, 2018). This HWE standard emphasizes that nurses should have proficient communication skills to build relationship-centered care, strengthen trust in patients and team members, and prevent miscommunication and errors in care.

Another communication skill is the skill of *speaking up*, of not remaining silent. Even within the intimidating hierarchy of hospital bureaucracies, it is essential to speak up for patients and colleagues when they face discrimination or injustice. Martin Luther King, Jr. put it best: "Our lives begin to end the day we remain silent on things that matter" (Washington, 1992). Does your work environment support, or even punish, speech about things that matter?

Another aspect of communication is respect and its opposite, disrespect. Disrespect is an unfortunate threat to nurses' well-being (Fontaine et al., 2018). Reports of bullying and incivility in clinical settings are increasing with a growing literature on how to handle the disrespect (ANA, 2015; Kisner, 2018). *Incivility* is defined by the American Nurses Association (ANA, 2015, para. 2) as "one or more rude, discourteous, or disrespectful actions that may or may not have negative intent behind them." *Bullying* is defined as "repeated, unwanted, harmful actions intended to humiliate, offend, and cause distress in the recipient" (ANA, 2015, para. 2).

Bullying behaviors occur not only between physicians and nurses, but bullying often occurs nurse-to-nurse as well (Ulrich et al., 2019). Bullying and intimidation can be overt, such as when a nurse criticizes a young colleague in front of a patient, or a more subtle behavior such as eye-rolling in staff meetings. Patients and families are increasingly shown to participate in disrespectful behavior, including violence toward healthcare providers (Ulrich et al., 2019). Increasingly, nurses leave their work setting due to incivility, and this causes vast emotional harm and costs up to $24 billion a year in the costs of nurse replacement (Kisner, 2018). We'll explore incivility a bit more later in this chapter.

In the case of patients and families, discriminatory behaviors are on the increase and reflect society's continued struggle with issues of racism, justice, and respect. Who would wish to work in a racist, hostile environment? Fortunately, there are positive organizations where leaders work to create a respectful culture, making it a priority. Most hospitals recognize these negative communications as a threat to safe and compassionate patient care and to the well-being of their staff. When you interview for a job, ask your interviewer about the policy on incivility and if they follow the ANA position statement. Ask, "What happens when disrespect and incivility occur in this hospital?"

True Collaboration

Nurses must be relentless in pursuing and fostering collaboration. We know that safe patient care relies on teams of multidisciplinary caregivers, but now we also know that effective interprofessional practice improves clinician well-being (Dow et al., 2019; Smith et al., 2018). People need to trust and rely on each other in order to provide the best patient care. "… The nurse can be our greatest ally, but we need to know his/her name first" (Rafelson & Brown, 2014, p. 2502)." Rafelson, a physician, and Brown, a noted nurse-author, write about the magic of relationships forged in the clinical arena and the benefits they bring to quality patient care and improved well-being for all.

History and stereotypes have not always been kind to the nurse-physician relationship, as stories of arrogance, rudeness, and intimidation on both sides are legendary (Siedlicki & Hixson, 2015). We are finally developing an understanding of each discipline's role and how they complement each other with a new training focus on interprofessional practice. Nursing and medical students, as well as other health discipline students, are encouraged to train together so they understand and appreciate each other's roles more clearly. For example, no one discipline owns pain control or end of life care, so why not create scenarios and simulations where we all learn together? Increasingly, advocates recommend the ideal education for health professions students should include pharmacists, chaplains, and social workers along with nurses and physicians in classroom and clinical learning (Dow et al., 2019; Martinussen et al., 2012).

We still face lingering examples of the Nurse Ratched archetype, Ken Kesey's 1962 classic portrait of a cruel nurse in *One Flew Over the Cuckoo's Nest*. We continue to hold onto images of the angry physician in the nursing station with everyone scurrying to get away. But increasingly, the many dimensions of positivity seen in the nurse-physician relationship are better indicators of just how healthy a work environment truly is. Frayed relationships, fear and intimidation, and lack of trust increase the likelihood of errors and decrease clinician well-being (Clark, 2019). When you are deciding where to work, do the team members all know each other's names? Does the team wait for nurses to join in on patient care rounds, or do the doctors start without them? This is respect and collegiality in action, and your opportunities to flourish at work will be greater in this kind of work home.

Effective Decision-Making

The best example of the effective decision-making standard is to look at the hospital's organizational charts and see if nurses are at the top of the organization. Nurses should also be represented on multidisciplinary task forces at the highest levels (Porter-O'Grady, 2019). At the unit level, the nurse manager and physician leader should manage the clinical unit together, and there will be evidence of shared input into key decisions, such as committee participation. Many hospitals are renovating to update or expand. Are nurses involved in these discussions, choosing equipment that is ergonomically safe, beds that do not hurt nurses' and nursing assistants' backs, for example? I recall a hospital that replaced an emergency department and had a beautiful lounge built for physicians and somehow "forgot" to build a nursing staff lounge! Pay attention to how decisions are made. Is there *real* shared governance with nurses on committees throughout the hospital? (Porter-O'Grady, 2019)

Appropriate Staffing

This is usually the number-one question nurses ask about a prospective job. Will there be adequate staff to handle patients safely? Only 39% of nurses in hospitals say they have appropriate staffing (Ulrich et al., 2019). There should be a match between patient needs and nurse competencies. Nursing candidates often choose to shadow a nurse in a unit they are considering (Hargreaves & Pabico, 2020). This creates the opportunity to see if the statements from the nurse manager or interviewers match the reality, from the staff perspective. What does it feel like on a busy shift? How many nurses are on the night shift versus the day shift? What is the staffing model, and is it adjusted for patient acuity? Is ancillary support available?

There is a nursing shortage nationwide, with even more acute needs in specialty areas such as the operating room and critical care (Moss et al., 2016). If an environment is healthy, the turnover rates will be below the national average (Rodriquez-Garcia, M. C. et al., 2020). In 2019, that rate was 17.8% (Nursing Solutions, Inc., 2020). Turnover in hospitals for RNs was 17.2% in 2018 (O'Donnell, 2019).

Meaningful Recognition

While all the healthy work environment standards are important, meaningful recognition stands out for the power it has to inspire confidence in a novice nurse and help to ensure a resilient culture on a unit. In Chapter 20 we will discuss more about how essential it is to feel as though you matter to patients, families, and colleagues. It is important to know that if you were not there, you would be missed. One of the kindest, most caring statements I heard on a clinical unit was when a respected nurse walked in for the start of her shift, and someone said, "Thank goodness Sharon is here. It will be a good day."

One way that the profession recognizes nurses is what is known as the "Daisy Award." The Barnes family (2016) has investigated and supported the power of recognizing nurses for the care they provide in hospitals across the country. Their adult son, Patrick, died of a rare blood disease, leaving behind a 4-month old son. The family vowed to do something significant to recognize the unsung heroes who took such compassionate care of him and the entire family during his eight-week hospitalization. They established the Daisy Award for Extraordinary Nurses in 1999, and the award is now given to hospital nurses all over the US by the Daisy Foundation (Barnes et al., 2016). The Daisy Foundation partners with 4,500 healthcare facilities in all 50 states and 28 countries to celebrate nurses by providing everything a hospital needs to honor an individual nurse every month. (Barnes et al., 2016). Nurses may be nominated by patients, families, or colleagues for their extraordinary compassion. The celebration is a surprise for the nurse, and often the chief nurse executive, nurse manager, nurse and physician colleagues, and the entire unit stage a quick celebration (with cinnamon rolls, Patrick's favorite) during the shift. The nomination letter is read, describing how the nurse went "above and beyond" in compassionate ways. Each awardee receives a certificate, a DAISY award pin for their badge, a hand-carved sculpture called *The Healer's Touch* from Zimbabwe, and a banner to hang in the unit.

It is a memorable and meaningful recognition for the celebrated nurses. As the Barnes state, "Given the stress and demands of today's changing healthcare world, why would an organization not ensure that every nurse has the opportunity to feel these emotions through the work to which they have committed their lives?" (Barnes et al., 2016, p. 166). Qualitative research involving nurses who were nominated for the Daisy award demonstrates multiple benefits for nurses as well as the parents and even the unit culture (Lefton, 2012). In a study involving analysis of 2,000 nominations from 20 institutions, it was noted that the award may increase the value of nursing, enhance team spirit and unit culture, and even reconnect nurses to why they became a nurse (Lefton, 2012).

The culture of a unit determines how nurses experience recognition. In addition to awards, recognition comes through advancement up the clinical ladder, getting a promotion, and achieving clinical certification. Recognition is also exemplified in the everyday moments, such as how people speak to one another. The following scenario was shared with me, and I have never forgotten it.

> A night shift nurse was giving report to the day nurse so she could get home, get the kids up for school, and then try to sleep after an exhausting night. The oncoming shift nurse said to her departing colleague, "I love to follow you. When I follow you on day shift, I know your patient is always well cared for. Drive home safely and sleep well." Isn't this much different than interruptions to ask if this was done, if that drug was given, what lab test results are back? It is often the small compassionate acts that may mean the most and set the tone for a healthy work environment.

Let me share one more example, one of team self-care at its best.

> Another unit at a large, urban hospital has a kind (and potentially lifesaving) culture started by its nightshift nurses. Near the end of their shifts, these night nurses help each other complete their work so they can leave the hospital together. Some of the nurses live close to the hospital, while others drive for up to an hour. When they leave the hospital, nurses pair-off and call each other on their phones. They keep each other on speaker, talking about whatever comes to mind, until they get home safely. Every year, many nurses die from car accidents because they have fallen asleep behind the wheel while driving home after night shift. This unit's culture and buddy system save nurses' lives. As a bonus, they build camaraderie by staying connected outside of work.

Dedicated efforts to create a healthy work environment are the actions that prioritize the well-being of clinicians (Bauer-Wu & Fontaine, 2015). One example is when nurses support fellow nurses with the creation of "resilience rooms." These spaces are on patient units and allow a nurse to take a break and decompress even for a few moments. (We will share more about these rooms in Chapter 19 when discussing Compassionate Care Ambassadors.) In job interviews, feel free to ask people how compassion is displayed on the unit.

Authentic Leadership

As the AACN developed these standards, authentic leadership was almost left off the list. A colleague, Connie Barden, who had been the AACN President in 2003, looked at the five standards and thought something was missing. She wondered who would hold the unit accountable for all of these standards. Of course, the answer was the nurse manager and colleagues. It is not possible to have a healthy work environment if the leaders are not implementing and supporting the standards. How does the manager address and support the staff? Work with colleagues in both good and stressful times? Display trustworthiness and integrity? If you ask nurses about their managers, you will often hear, "They never wear scrubs." This is code for managers who are not really team players and not engaged with their staff. One of my students shares her story of finding a healthy work environment in the following sidebar.

In pursuing the best and healthiest work environment for that first job, it is imperative to get to know the manager. Listen carefully. See if you can determine if their words and actions are congruent; sometimes managers are better at talking the talk than walking the walk. Better yet, speak to the staff who have worked with the manager and discover honest feedback. Managers do have a tough job dealing with turnover, staffing, patient acuity, and changing policies, but it is critical to know how they handle both calm and crisis situations. For example, how do they run staff meetings? Who gets to speak in meetings, and do managers listen when frontline staff share their views?

In repeated studies of healthy work environments, the nurse manager time and again comes up as a major reason clinical nurses stay in their position (Ulrich et al., 2014, 2019). While peer support and a friend at work is important, people leave because they perceive the nurse manager does not care about them or listen to their concerns. It is said that typically nurses do not leave their unit; they leave their manager. When considering a unit, ask for information such as how long the manager has worked in the unit, turnover data, and specific unit quality outcomes, because these will provide insights into authentic leadership.

The Courage to Leave

Interview with Haley Schlottmann, DNP, FNP-BC (she/her)

"As a nurse, I believe I finally found a healthy work environment when I came to work in the NICU after leaving my first RN job."

Haley says finding the courage to recognize that she was not in a healthy work environment was the most important thing she did in her nursing career. After taking the risk and changing jobs, she felt supported and safe, with excellent mentors who wanted her to succeed. She believes that her new managers and preceptors take her seriously, and she feels like she has their constant support.

"To me, a healthy work environment is a place in which I am supported to grow, feel comfortable stepping outside of my comfort zone, and a place where teamwork is apparent...it also means that job expectations match my capabilities as a nurse."

What does she suggest looking for in a healthy work environment?

Haley notes it is important to have supportive physicians and fellow nurses to work beside, but it is especially important to have a manager or leader who works in your best interest and will advocate for your needs. "Leadership styles of managers are important to be aware of, as I know I do not do well under a 'hands off' or alternatively an authoritarian leader. Now I am clear about what I like to see in a manager: thoughtful and clear communication, frequent check-ins, and authenticity."

The important component in deciding on the work environment that will suit you, Haley points out, is to know your own values and learning styles, because each nurse is different.

"Everyone's life would be easier with a healthy work environment."

(Interview with Monika Criman, RN, 2013 BSN and Current Doctor of Nursing Practice in Anesthesia Student, 2nd Lieutenant, Army Reserve, she/her)

Monika recalls that the best nurse managers would come out on the unit, talk to staff, hash out a problem, and not just "get pizza for the staff." They were part of the team and did not separate themselves. Stepping back, she acknowledges that managers who seem disengaged are actually doing a ton, but nurses don't see it, whether hiring staff, ordering supplies, and attending meetings. "Some managers meet metrics but are not in the trenches."

Noting "managers who never wear scrubs" are in every ICU that reports a bad work environment, Monika said that nurses need to feel appreciated and listened to by a manager who then acts on the issues. She shared a good example: A nurse manager announced a new CCRN who was not on the unit that day, and everyone applauded. The manager videotaped it and sent it to the nurse.

In terms of physician and nurse communication, Monika believes it is good sign when the physicians listen and ask to be called by their first name. This is an example of "where the wall is torn down" and sets up the opportunity for respect to develop. She shared other examples of positive interactions with physicians—when they took extra time to explain their rationale for therapies, and in one unit, at noon each day, the attending physician held a huddle with nursing staff to answer their questions.

Incivility in the Workplace

We can't conclude an overview of healthy work environments without a bit more discussion of incivility. Incivility takes various forms, but you definitely know it when you see it. Cindy Clark, the leading nursing expert on incivility, considers it on a continuum from rude behaviors such as eye-rolling and disrespect to more serious instances of intimidation and even physical aggression. She points out that in the pandemic of COVID-19, the extra stress on nurses can lead to more acts of incivility (Clark, 2020). One of my students, Tom, chose to work in a busy emergency department in a large teaching hospital for his first job. For the most part, he enjoyed the pace, his preceptor, and the teamwork of his colleagues. What he was not prepared for was the backbiting and gossip from the nursing staff. He said he would enter the break room and hear them talking about other new graduates in derogatory terms. "Don't they teach them anything in nursing school?" these nurses lamented behind closed doors. He wondered if they talked about him that way as well. It made him wonder if he had made the right choice, choosing to work in this department.

The emotional cost of incivility is harmful and may lead to depression and burnout. And it is not the individual nurse alone who suffers, but patients and families as well. Consider this: A study of teams in a neonatal intensive care unit demonstrated that rudeness alone in this intense clinical environment can negatively influence diagnostic and procedural performance, leaving fragile, premature infants at risk (Riskin et al., 2015).

Nurse managers are essential to "dialing down the drama at work" (Sherman, 2020). Once they notice and see a pattern of abusive behaviors among staff, they have a mandate to stop it early. An effective nurse manager will seek multiple viewpoints to a story, stay reality based, provide coaching to the nurses causing drama, and establish new behavioral expectations and norms (Sherman, 2020).

In these situations, clinical nurses have the responsibility to speak up. Cynthia Clark notes that the keys to stopping incivility also include self-monitoring our behavior and reflecting before acting, speaking, or sending an email that could easily be misinterpreted (Clark, 2020). Schools of Nursing are starting to support these behaviors and become role models for wise actions for students, faculty, and staff, even before a nursing student begins clinical rotations (Fontaine et al., 2012).

Perhaps the best solution is to not hire disrespectful, rude clinicians in the first place. As savvy nurses figure out, hospital units have reputations, and the units that have a reputation for unkind behaviors are the ones to avoid. It is no surprise that these units often have trouble retaining good nurses while others, the units with reputations for supportiveness and positivity, often have waiting lists of nurses wanting to join their team. We have recommended, "Bring into critical care those nurses and physicians with a strong sense of self, who understand self-care, and whose skillful competence is accompanied by sensitivity and warmth" (Fontaine et al., 2018, p. 155). This certainly applies to all clinical settings. We also argued that while being nice to others may be considered a "soft skill," it truly can be hard unless it is practiced repeatedly, and in an authentic way. Kindness cannot be overrated, and we agree with Sharon Salzberg (2005) that kindness is compassion in action.

Personal Perspective

Relationships: The Antidote to Incivility

Interview with Sharon Pappas, PhD, RN, NEA-BC, FAAN (she/her)
Chief Nurse Executive for Emory Healthcare in Atlanta

"I have always believed that relationships are at the core of patient safety. Nurses practicing in positive work environments provide better outcomes for patients and each other. Leaders that create work environments where individuals are safe because they communicate and reinforce positive behaviors have succeeded in giving patients the best opportunity for safe care. In these environments, clinicians know each other, see each other as a source of social support, recognize and regard successes, look forward to seeing each other when they are at work, and celebrate positive patient outcomes."

These positive work environments create *community*—a group of individuals joined by a shared purpose and camaraderie. This sense of community has a tremendous impact on patient care because a respectful team believes patients deserve the best of every discipline and creates every opportunity for effective collaboration. Incivility is rare on these units. This is intentional because the individuals in this type of work environment know how to address incivility when it creeps in.

It is also important to measure clinicians' perception of incivility so that incivility can be addressed. One intervention for incivility is *cognitive rehearsal*—practicing what you would say before it happens (Longo, 2017). Placing educational content on cognitive rehearsal in nursing education and nurse resident programming shows promising results in improving relationships and ultimately the work environment. A work environment where every individual "is treated as a unique, talented, and dedicated professional working in partnership with coworkers to accomplish an aligned and worthy pursuit" is the ultimate goal (Swenson & Shanafelt, 2020, p. 56).

When teams have a shared purpose, they understand the importance of relationships and become vigilant in reinforcing the community they co-created.

A Healthy Work Environment Matters

A healthy work environment can affect all aspects in a unit, from nurse engagement and retention to patient outcomes. An HWE is a foundation for not only patient well-being but the satisfaction of the nursing staff (see Figure 17.1). According to AACN, hospital units that implement the AACN standards outperform those that do not. For example, these units have better nurse staffing and retention, less moral distress, and lower rates of workplace violence (Ulrich et al., 2019).

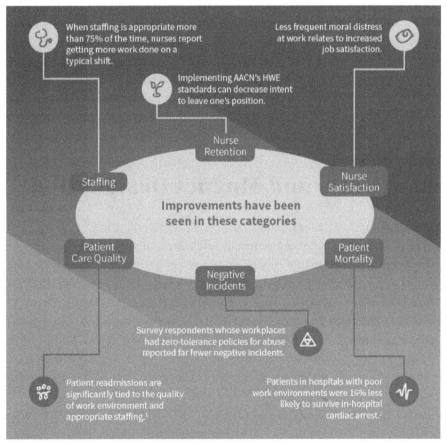

FIGURE 17.1   Nurses and patients benefit from a healthy work environment.

Reprinted with permission. American Association of Critical-Care Nurses. AACN Website. Accessed August 3, 2020. https;//www.aacn.org/nursing-excellence/healthy-work-environments. (c) 2020 by the American Association of Critical Care Nurses. All rights reserved.

In a meta-analysis of 17 studies that identified work environment outcomes, nurses in better work environments had 28–32% lower odds of burnout, job dissatisfaction, and intent to leave. Patient satisfaction was 16% higher as well (Lake et al., 2019).

Four national surveys since 2006 have measured nurses' perception of their work environment across the United States (Ulrich et al., 2006, 2009, 2014, 2019). They have found that healthy work environment standards have been increasingly implemented. Further reporting shows that when units and hospitals adopt the standards as nonnegotiable, significant positive changes in nurse staffing, communication, respect, and leadership result compared to units that have not adopted them. Burnout and retention are also improved. We see that the health of the work environment is improving; however, several areas need to be addressed, including more appropriate staffing and attention to nurses' physical and mental well-being concerns. Nearly one-third of over 8,000 nurses surveyed intend to leave their current position within a year, making retention of skilled nurses a major issue (Ulrich et al., 2019).

Beacon Units and Magnet Designation

The American Nurses Credentialing Center Magnet Recognition Program is considered a mark of excellence because it celebrates nursing autonomy to direct patient care. The Magnet designation is a recognized and sought-after label for hospitals who meet their stringent criteria. Promulgated in the mid-1980s to encourage hospitals to provide a positive nursing culture to prevent high rates of nurse turnover, the term "magnet" was created to denote hospitals who could recruit and retain nurses. Now many hospital executives view it as a mark of overall excellence, and they support nurse leadership to seek the designation with the help of multiple disciplines within an organization. There are over 500 hospitals nationwide with Magnet status, not quite 10% of all hospitals.

The Beacon Award for Excellence is another designation that celebrates hospital units that employ evidence-based practices and the HWE standards to improve patient and family outcomes (www.aacn.org/nursing-excellence/beacon-awards).

Rather than a hospital-wide designation, the Beacon award recognizes individual units, and hospitals may have several awards. You can check on the website by state to see the units in a specific hospital of interest. Both Magnet and Beacon hospitals have nurses who report healthier work environments per the 2018 survey and less intent to leave (Ulrich et al., 2019). Starting your search for an HWE should include checking the hospital's status for Magnet, Beacon, and other awards.

In Real Practice

Stress can be a common phenomenon in all nursing schools, and it affects faculty, staff, and students. Students may bear the brunt of rude and uncivil behaviors resulting from a tense environment. In a pandemic like COVID-19, these stressors can also create other assaults on mental health and well-being. This is to the detriment of successful learning and practice for the student nurse. Clark and Ritter (2018) describe the development of a legally defensible policy for workplace civility that can create a healthy academic work environment. Students will benefit when faculty and staff adopt a policy to foster civility. Do check your own organization for a policy and compare.

Closing Thoughts

Consider your choice of work environment your first act of self-care as a professional nurse. There are thoughtful ways to go about this important decision, and using the healthy work environment standards, as well as Beacon or Magnet designations, is a good starting point. Remember that soon, *you* will be contributing to the health of a clinical environment, whichever one you choose. Your values, integrity, and compassion will give you the opportunity to create an environment that serves the well-being of your patients and fellow healthcare practitioners.

Key Points

- Starting your career in a healthy work environment is one of the most important decisions you will make, and this decision is an act of self-care.

- AACN standards for an HWE include six areas and serve as a benchmark for excellence: skilled communication, true collaboration, effective decision-making, appropriate staffing, meaningful recognition, and authentic leadership.

- HWEs are good for patients and families and ensure better nurse satisfaction, leading to increased nurse retention.

- Your role is to choose a healthy work environment and then strive to maintain and improve it for your patients and colleagues.

References

American Association of Critical-Care Nurses. (2016). *AACN standards for establishing and sustaining healthy work environments: A journey to excellence* (2nd ed.). American Association of Critical Care Nurses. Retrieved from https://www.aacn.org/nursing-excellence/healthy-work-environments

American Nurses Association. (2015). *ANA position statement on incivility, bullying, and workplace violence.* https://www.nursingworld.org/practice-policy/work-environment/violence-incivility-bullying/

Barnes, B., Barnes, M., & Sweeney, C. D. (2016). Supporting recognition of clinical nurses with the Daisy Award. *Journal of Nursing Administration, 46*(4), 164–166. https://doi.org/10.1097/NNA.0000000000000320

Bauer-Wu, S., & Fontaine, D. (2015). Prioritizing clinician wellbeing: The University of Virginia's Compassionate Care Initiative. *Global Advances in Health and Medicine, 5*(4), 16–22.

Clark C. M. (2019). Ending the silence: Antidote to incivility (sigmanursing.org).

Clark, C. M. (2020). The imperative of civility in uncertain times. *Nurse Educator, 45*(4), 173. https://doi.org/10.1097/NNE.0000000000000874

Clark, C. M., & Ritter, K. (2018). Policy to foster civility and support a healthy academic work environment. *Journal of Nursing Education, 57*(6), 325–333.

Dempsey, C. (2018). The antidote to suffering: How compassionate connected care can improve safety, quality, and experience. *Press Ganey Associates.* https://nmonl.wildapricot.org/resources/Documents/NMONL_The%20Antidote%20to%20Suffering%20FINAL.pdf

Dow, A. W., Baernholdt, M., Santen, S. A., Baker, K., & Sessler, C. N. (2019). Practitioner wellbeing as an interprofessional imperative. *Journal of Interprofessional Care, 33*(6), 603–607. https://doi.org/10.1080/13561820.2019.1673705

Fontaine, D. K., Haizlip, J., & Lavandero, R. (2018). No time to be nice in the Intensive Care Unit. *American Journal of Critical Care, 27(2), 153–156.*

Fontaine, D., Koh, E., & Carroll, T. (2012). Promoting a healthy workplace for nursing faculty and staff. *Nursing Clinics of North America, 47*(4), 557–566. https://doi.org/10.1016/j.cnur.2012.07.008

Hargreaves, J., & Pabico, C. (2020). How to choose your first nursing job wisely. *American Nurse Journal, 15*(5), 30–31.

Kisner, T. (2018). Workplace incivility: How do you address it? *Nursing, 48*(6), 36–40. https://doi.org/10.1097/01.NURSE.0000532746.88129.e9

Lake, E. T., Sanders, J., Duan, R., Riman, K. A., Schoenauer, K. M., & Chen, Y. (2019). A meta-analysis of the associations between the nurse work environment in hospitals and 4 sets of outcomes. *Medical Care, 57*(5), 353–361. https://doi.org/10.1097/MLR.0000000000001109

Lefton, C. (2012). Strengthening the workforce through meaningful recognition. *Nursing Economics, 30*(6), 331–338, 355.

Longo, J. (2017). Cognitive rehearsal. *American Nurse Today, 12*(8), 41–42, 51.

Martinussen, M., Adolfsen, F., Lauritzen, C., & Richardsen, A. M. (2012). Improving interprofessional collaboration in a community setting: Relationships with burnout, engagement and service quality, *Journal of Interprofessional Care, 26*(3), 219–225. https://doi.org/10.3109/13561820.2011.647125

Moss, M., Good, V. S., Gozal, D., Kleinpell, R., & Sessler, C. N. (2016). An official critical care societies collaborative statement: Burnout syndrome in critical care healthcare professionals: A call to action. *American Journal of Critical Care 25*(4), 368–376.

Nursing Solutions, Inc. (2020). 2020 NSI National Health Care Retention & RN Staffing Report. Retrieved from https://www.nsinursingsolutions.com/Documents/Library/NSI_National_Health_Care_Retention_Report.pdf

O'Donnell, R. (2019, June 17). Hospital turnover in 2018: The trend continues. Hospital Recruiting.com. Retrieved from https://www.hospitalrecruiting.com/blog/5729/hospital-turnover-in-2018-the-trend-continues/

Porter-O'Grady, T. (2019). Principles for sustaining shared/professional governance in nursing. *Nursing Management, 50*(1), 36–41. https://doi.org/10.1097/01.NUMA.0000550448.17375.28

Rafelson, W., & Brown, T. (2014). The half-wall. *JAMA, 312*(23), 2501–2502. https://doi.org/10.1001/jama.2014.12937

Riskin, A., Erez, A., Foulk, T. A., Kugelman, A., Gover, A., Shoris, I., Riskin, K. S., & Bamberger, P. A. (2015). The impact of rudeness on medical team performance: A randomized trial. *Pediatrics, 136*(3), 487–495. https://doi.org/10.1542/peds.2015-1385

Rodriguez-Garcia, C. M., Marquez-Hernandez, V. V., Belmonte-Garcia, T., Gutierrez-Peurtes, L., & Granados-Gomez, G. (2020) Original research: How magnet hospital status affects nurses, patients, and organizations: A systematic review. *American Journal of Nursing, 120*(7), 28–38.

Salzberg, S. (2005). *The force of kindness: Change your life with love and compassion.* Sounds True.

Seidlicki, S. L., & Hixson, E. D. (2015). Relationships between nurses and physicians matter. *Online Journal of Issues in Nursing, 20*(3).

Sherman, R. O. (2020). Dialing down drama at work. *American Nurse Journal, 15*(6), 24–26.

Smith, C. D., Balatbat, C., Corbridge, S., Dopp, A. L., Fried, J., Harter, R., Landefeld, S., Martin, C. Y., Opelka, F., Sandy, L., Sato, L., & Sinsky, C. (2018). *Implementing optimal team-based care to reduce clinician burnout* [Discussion Paper]. National Academy of Medicine. https://nam.edu/implementing-optimal-team-based-care-to-reduce-clinician-burnout

Swenson, S. J., & Shanafelt, T. D. (2020). *Strategies to reduce burnout: 12 actions to create the ideal workplace.* Oxford University Press.

Ulrich, B., Barden, C., & Varn-Davis, N. (2019). Critical care nurse work environments 2018: Findings and implications. *Critical Care Nurse, 39*(2): 67–84. https://doi.org/10.4037/ccn2019605

Ulrich, B. T., Lavandero, R., Hart, K. A., Woods, D., Leggett, J., Friedman, D., D'Aurizio, P., & Edwards, S. J. (2009). Critical care nurses' work environments 2008: A follow-up report. *Critical Care Nurse, 29*(2), 93–102. https://doi.org/10.4037/ccn2009619

Ulrich, B. T., Lavandero, R., Hart, K. A. Woods, D. Leggett, J., & Taylor, D. (2006). Critical care nurses' work environments: A baseline status report. *Critical Care Nurse, 26*(5), 46–57. https://doi.org/10.4037/ccn2006.26.5.46

Ulrich, B. T., Lavandero, R., Woods, D., & Early, S. (2014). Critical care nurse work environments 2013: A status report. *Critical Care Nurse, 34*(4), 64–79. https://doi.org/10.4037/ccn2014731

Washington, J. M. (1992). *I have a dream: Writings and speeches that changed the world.* HarperOne.

Worline, M. C., & Dutton, J. E. (2017). *Awakening compassion at work: The quiet power that elevates people and organizations.* Berrett-Koehler.

18

Self-Care for Humanitarian Aid Workers

Tim Cunningham
pronouns: He/Him

Tim Cunningham began his professional career as
an actor, then a hospital clown. He began doing
international humanitarian work with Clowns
Without Borders. While a clown, he fell in love with
nurses' ability to connect with patients and families,
even in times of terrible suffering—so he became an
emergency nurse. The rest is history.

"If you have come here to help me you are wasting your time, but if you have come because your liberation is bound with mine, then let us work together."

—Lilla Watson

In his breathtaking novel, *The Plague,* existentialist writer Albert Camus describes a fictional disease outbreak that wreaks havoc in the coastal city, Oran. Though the city in the northern Algeria and the plague that struck that city repeatedly over the course of history were real, the extent to which Camus describes the plague's destruction is exponentially more catastrophic in his novel. First published in 1947, *The Plague* eerily predicts the way our world contracted and responded when a real plague, Ebola virus disease (EVD), later struck countries in West Africa—Guinea, Liberia, and Sierra Leone. The first case of EVD was detected in late 2013, and the last case of what is now known as the West Africa EVD outbreak occurred in March of 2016 (Farmer, 2020). It is important to note that a subsequent outbreak of EVD began in the Democratic Republic of Congo in 2018 and ended in March 2020 (Nsio et al., 2020).

Another pandemic, the novel coronavirus (COVID-19), arose on December 31, 2019 in Wuhan Province, China (Hofmeyer & Taylor, 2020). At the time of this publication, there are more than 118 million cases of COVID-19 around the world. More than 2.6 million people have died (Johns Hopkins, 2021). It is important to note that the spread, manifestations, and case fatality rate of COVID-19 are different from EVD, but the way that the world has responded is similar in many ways.

All outbreaks, epidemics, and pandemics will need frontline healthcare workers to care for the sick. This chapter will give you a taste of what humanitarian healthcare is like so that you will have a better idea how it might fit into your professional plans. We hope this chapter will also present a unique window into the self-care needs and practices of humanitarian health workers.

The Plague's main character, Dr. Bernard Rieux, struggles with the ethics around treating people stricken with the plague. Like Ebola, COVID-19, and most disease outbreaks, the plague was more commonly a disease of the poor. In the case of COVID-19, people from underserved populations who traditionally have less access to healthcare because of racist and inequitable health policies in the United States are more likely to die (van Dorn et al., 2020).

The plague, Ebola, and COVID-19 are all diseases of caretakers. We witness higher proportions of nurses and physicians being infected by and succumbing to these diseases because they experience prolonged exposure at a much higher rate than the general population (Farmer, 2020; Gan et al., 2020). In *The Plague,* Dr. Rieux debates the utility of bringing his poor patients to the hospital where he knows that they will not receive adequate care because of their poverty, and where he knows they are destined to die, no matter what he does.

Throughout the novel, Rieux is constantly exhausted because he gives his all to his patients, day and night, being one of the few doctors willing to care for patients with the plague. You could argue that Rieux practiced little, if any, self-care, because of his dedication to his patients. Although Rieux and the fictional plague are an extreme example, this failure to practice self-care is a real hazard for those who are willing to care for patients during global health crises.

Health for All: The Need for Humanitarian Workers

Around the globe and with increasing numbers, humanitarian crises are erupting, some as critical as the plague that Camus describes, others far worse. The "Global War on Terror," which has been ongoing since 2001 (Wilson, 2005); natural disasters; and other wars fueled by greed for natural resources have led to the forced displacement of more than 65 million people between 2001 and 2018 (Statista, 2020). At the time of this writing, there are 70.8 million people displaced on this planet (UNHCR: The UN Refugee Agency, 2020). The *refugees*, the real people in this incomprehensibly high figure, have been forced to leave their own countries and find a home in another country with the intent to return to their home countries. In addition to refugees, *internally displaced people* are those who are forced to settle in a different, unfamiliar part of their own country or in a camp within their own country. *Asylum seekers* are those who must also flee their country, but because of the situation will never be able to return. They must seek a new permanent home in another country (Human Rights Watch, 2001). As you can imagine, none of these people, while in flight from their homes, have adequate access to healthcare.

Organizations like Médecins Sans Frontières, Partners in Health, International Medical Corps, and International Rescue Committee—to name just a few—work to decrease the suffering of people affected by war, disease, and natural disaster. To do that, they deploy thousands of nurses from around the world to serve in some of the hardest-to-reach regions on this planet as they model a key tenet of the World Health Organization (WHO), which is "Health for All" (WHO, n.d.).

With the onset of the global COVID-19 pandemic, we find what were typically international aid groups now sending nurses to serve within the United States. COVID-19 has made itself a crisis without borders. The Director General of the WHO (2017–2022), Dr. Tedros Adhanom Ghebreyesus, has said, "The right of every individual to basic health services will be my top priority" (World Health Organization, 2020, para. 2). The United Nation's (UN) Sustainable Development Goals echo this charge as the UN aspires to the challenging goal of "Universal Health Coverage" for all people on this planet before 2030 (UNDP: United Nations Development Programme, 2019). None of this will be possible without nurses.

Have you considered working to provide healthcare in humanitarian settings? Have you ever been a part of a short-term or long-term mission? There is great need for nurses like you, if you have the skills and experience to do this kind of work. First, you'll need the nursing skills, of course, and you'll need to develop expertise with them. It is generally recommended that you have *at least* two years of experience working in a hospital setting in your home country, and then add the following skills to your repertoire: language skills, cultural humility, and the ability at all times to remain flexible (Cunningham & Sesay, 2017).

Self-Care in Humanitarian Settings

The remainder of this chapter will focus on ways to practice self-care if you have the opportunity to work in a humanitarian setting. You'll likely experience some tough situations and very high levels of suffering, so what will you do to take care of yourself so that you can be your best self and maintain your own well-being? The following section will focus on the West Africa Ebola outbreak and what we've learned about self-care in that setting for people who traveled from their home countries to treat patients with EVD. The lessons we learned in that setting are applicable to many other humanitarian crises around the world.

Self-Care in the Time of Ebola

During the 2013–2016 West Africa EVD outbreak, more than 28,000 people were infected with EVD and, of those, more than 11,000 people died (Centers for Disease Control and Prevention, n.d.). That infection count includes 898 nurses, physicians, technicians, and other healthcare staff workers who got infected—of those, 518 died (Statista, 2015). That's a 58% case-fatality rate among healthcare professionals infected with EVD. Chances of survival from the disease were grim; however, nurses from around the globe volunteered to leave their homes to support and treat people infected with one of the world's most deadly viruses.

Nurses from countries including Cuba, Nigeria, Canada, the US, Germany, and the UK flooded into West Africa to try to help control the spread of EVD and provide dignified, compassionate care to the sick (Cunningham, 2016). At the time of the West Africa outbreak, there was no known cure for EVD, so the majority of the care our teams gave was made up of nursing care—comfort care, end of life care, cleaning, turning, and most importantly, psychosocial support for our patients. The only treatments available in the worst-hit countries were aggressive hydration therapies, nutrition, and antibiotics for any other opportunistic, or concurrent, bacterial infections (Farmer, 2020). Remember that EVD is a virus, thus no antibiotics would work to treat the disease. Self-care was essential for all of us so that we could remain focused despite very challenging work circumstances.

We faced work challenges that I couldn't have anticipated. We had to do all of our work—starting IVs, drawing labs, feeding, cleaning and playing with (yes, play was a masterful tool for psychosocial support) patients—in cumbersome, hot, and unforgiving personal protective equipment (PPE). Only in situations where there are highly contagious diseases are nurses required to wear such gear, and in most resource-rich settings, like most hospitals in the US, full PPE can be used with Powered Air Purifying Respirators (PAPRs), which circulate air within the suits, helping them keep cool. In West Africa, that technology was not available, so the temperatures inside these suits went well above 38 degrees Celsius (100 Fahrenheit) (Cunningham, 2016).

During the West Africa EVD outbreak, there was technically an abundance of PPE with PAPRs, but they were stockpiled and stored in resource-wealthy countries in case the outbreak spread. That is often the case in humanitarian settings: The places most in need of supplies often cannot get access to them because of governmental laws and policies, lack of transportation, or lack of technology to safely store them (Farmer, 2020). In public health, we use the term "cold-chain" (Ruiz-Garcia & Lunadei, 2010) to describe methods used to transport vaccines, for example, and to make sure they remain at a proper, cooled temperature even if they have to travel thousands of miles and then be stored at a refugee camp with no electricity. The complexities of humanitarian aid make the work even more challenging when supplies are often very hard to come by.

Nursing in Humanitarian Settings

–Valérie Gruhn, RN (she/her)

I always thought that I was strong enough to deal with anything. Working in humanitarian aid, I had seen it all, from the suffering of a war zone to the fear Ebola brings to a community. Taking care of people who lived in these communities—people who had no choice in where they lived and how they lived—meant that I had nothing to complain about. I am privileged. I neglected myself to care for others. I felt guilty. Witnessing the worst of mankind takes a toll on you, and self-care is the only way that allows you to get a sense of normalcy in a world of madness. It does not come naturally to me, but working on my own self-care allows me to better care for others.

Self-Care Practices

The National Academies of Sciences, Engineering, and Medicine report on clinician well-being suggests that clinicians, at baseline, have no more, or no less, resilience than other people (2019). This makes sense, of course. That said, one might opine that nurses, for example, will need to build up more resilience than someone working in say, accounting, because of the nature of the suffering and stress that we face every day. We certainly found that to be the case among nurses who cared for people with Ebola. What tools did nurses use to prepare themselves every day to go back into the "Hot Zone" and care for people with Ebola?

Camaraderie, music, humor, and writing offer opportunities for aid workers to express and care for themselves in different ways. If there is a common theme, it might be that people realize and express their voices as ways to understand the suffering *and* healing they have witnessed. These forms of creative reflection are all encompassed when we think about psychosocial support.

Camaraderie

Overwhelmingly, we learned that nurses reflected on the importance of having a sense of camaraderie with their fellow professional peers. To them, *camaraderie* meant time away from work to be with, hang out with, laugh, and cry with their colleagues. Those times of camaraderie involved talking about work, a lot, but also not talking about the challenges of Ebola and just talking about things like friends, families, relationships, love, and hobbies. These personal conversations helped nurses feel part of a team and that they were not alone during the EVD outbreak. Those who reported that camaraderie was a key factor in self-care also reported that they felt less stress when they were able to have this down-time with their peers. Camaraderie in this sense became synonymous with solidarity (Cunningham et al., 2018).

Camaraderie was not only a common form of self-care in the West Africa EVD epidemic, but also a crucial form of self-care for those professionals serving in the US military (McCormick et al., 2019). What's more, we know that experiencing camaraderie with others has been shown to improve resilience and serve as a form of self-care among our first-responder colleagues—firefighters, emergency medical services, and police (Preyde, 2019).

Camaraderie happens when people share an experience or a series of experiences that they can reflect upon as a way to come together, to feel united. Often, traumatic or challenging experiences bring people together, and from those, a sense of camaraderie is born. The experiences do not have to be traumatic, however—

imagine when a college sports team wins a national championship and entire universities, cities, and even states come together in a joyful way. In its essence, camaraderie can occur when people come together, whether the surrounding circumstances are good or challenging.

Music

"Music gives a soul to the universe, wings to the mind,
flight to the imagination and life to everything."
–Plato

Humanitarian aid workers are either *expatriate*, meaning they have come from another country outside of the country where the humanitarian crisis occurs, or they are considered *national staff*, people who live within the country in crisis. No matter where they are from, a universal language is music, another form of camaraderie and thus self-care. When a person gets out their guitar or another instrument, often a group of people forms around them. Singing together, no matter how talented you are (or aren't), can bring a sense of stress relief. Singing changes the way you breathe; it encourages prolonged and more forceful exhales, which we know can have a calming effect on the body and mind (Austin, 1999; Van Diest et al., 2014). Voluntary and controlled changes in breathing patterns can reduce stress (Everly & Lating, 2019). Aside from the science of respiratory changes when singing, the act of singing is simply fun for many people.

Music is also a key form of storytelling, one that can help preserve and share histories if there are none written down. It is unlikely that the nearly 80 million people on this planet who have been forced to flee their homes would be able to carry family records with them. For many people, narrative storytelling and singing are the only remaining evidence of their family's history. If you are interested in learning more about this, there is an album called *The Calais Sessions*, featuring artists who once lived in the now desiccated Calais Refugee Camp in northern France. (Many people referred to this camp as "The Jungle.") (The Calais Sessions, n.d.)

Humor

Colleagues who treated people dying from Ebola, colleagues living in lockdown situations and treating patients with COVID-19, and my own mentors who treated patients with AIDS in the late 1980s all report that humor has played a vital role in self-care and stress relief. The point is never to laugh *at* someone's suffering, but by finding humor in circumstances or events, caregivers can find relaxation, camaraderie, and group self-care when laughing together. Sometimes that humor can go too far and is called *dark humor*, but maybe that is not always a bad thing either. Humor, in its essence, is contextual. As you have read throughout this book, experiencing positive emotions such as laughter has the power to build your resilience and well-being. Reflecting on the fact that laughter is common in nearly all cultures and a laugh itself can be translated into any language, humor has the power to bring people together, as is seen in crises settings around the globe (Cunningham, 2019). Nurses can use humor both with colleagues and with patients and families to share a sense of lightness and to bring people closer together (Greenberg, 2003).

Writing

Reflective writing, or narrative medicine (see Chapter 8) in many different genres and forms, also was very common among expat caregivers (Catallozzi et al., 2016). The genres included songwriting, poetry, and prose. Some people who wrote for self-care wrote with the intention of sharing what they had written with other people. Others wrote only for themselves with no desire to publish or share with others (Cunningham et al., 2017). Blogging has been helpful for Ebola aid workers as well as humanitarian workers in other international settings (Ager & Iacouvou, 2014). Sometimes practicing self-care through writing, especially blog posts or social media status updates, is an effort to feel heard, to feel empowered, to feel like your voice matters.

Writing your own personal narrative as a nurse does not have to begin when you first begin your work in a humanitarian setting. Consider starting now. Consider how you can begin the practice of reflecting upon your own experiences, in school, in the clinical setting, and in life, and begin to put them down on paper, only for yourself to see. Then, when you find yourself in a stressful setting, or if you find yourself working in a humanitarian setting, this process of writing your nursing narrative will have already become a habit. In essence, you'll be primed to practicing self-care through reflective writing, which will then be another tool in your personal tool kit.

Psychosocial Support for Humanitarian Aid Workers

If you've not realized this already, it should now be clear that self-care is a form of *psychosocial support*, activities and interventions designed to improve the psychological well-being and mental health of people witness to or experiencing suffering (Tol et al., 2011). The Inter-Agency Standing Committee (IASC) is made up of a group of leaders and scholars from across the globe who specialize in psychosocial support for communities affected by war, disease outbreaks, or natural disasters (IASC, 2014). In a report that they published shortly after the COVID-19 pandemic spread from China to neighboring countries, and then the world, they specified two prescient points that are crucial to remember when considering self-care for humanitarian nurses. First, all psychosocial support in response to a humanitarian crisis should begin as soon as the crisis begins. Second, psychosocial support should be culturally sensitive to meet the needs of the people most affected (IASC, 2020).

These two psychosocial support guideposts for nurses who work in humanitarian settings underscore the crucial role of self-care. It should begin when the crisis begins; this book suggests that self-care should begin when you start your nursing studies and never stop. Second, as you've seen in this chapter, the self-care you practice should be self-care that is appropriate to you. Whether it's music, writing, playing games, or just hanging out with your colleagues, the most effective self-care is the practice that is most effective for *you*.

Closing Thoughts

Although self-care practices for nurses working in humanitarian settings may not be very different from self-care practices that you would do in your home setting, the setting often makes the practices more challenging to do. Based on the situation at hand, the crisis, and security issues, you may have to be more creative in how you practice self-care. Because camaraderie is a key element of self-care, if you find yourself working in a humanitarian setting, you should remember the importance of relying on your teammates. They can support you at work and support you "after hours" to mentor, coach, and teach you about self-care. Seeking their help will build your sense of camaraderie, solidarity, and teamwork. Especially in humanitarian and crisis settings, whether they are in your own country or others, the importance of your team and bonding together is perhaps the most important aspect of care for you, your colleagues, and those you are caring for in the crisis.

In Real Practice

To date, there are few publications examining the relationships between self-care practiced in humanitarian settings by nurses and aspects of well-being. For future researchers, your path is wide open if this kind of work inspires you! What is known is that humanitarian work, or working as an expat in a humanitarian (war, natural disaster, refugee camp, etc.) setting, can bring unique stressors.

A meta-analysis by Brooks et al., (2015) includes nurses in its sample of published literature and finds some interprofessional commonalities. Most pressing is the shared idea that poor communication, unclear leadership structures, and ultimately aspects of work requirements that are not clear or unknown cause unnecessary stress on nurses, physicians, and other aid workers. As a counter, this study suggests the importance of teamwork and a sense of camaraderie that can help support wellbeing and, potentially, self-care practices.

Key Points

- Nurses with at least two years of work experience, language skills, cultural humility, and flexibility can provide invaluable care to those facing humanitarian crises.

- Although the rewards can be immeasurable, humanitarian aid work presents unique challenges to nurses' well-being. In addition to witnessing great suffering, nurses face difficult work conditions, limited supplies and resources, and even safety and security concerns.

- Self-care is vitally important for nurses who are in these settings, despite the challenges they may face in practicing them. Experienced humanitarian aid workers have identified camaraderie, music, humor, and writing as effective strategies that cross cultural boundaries and can be practiced in even the most restricted environments.

References

Ager, A., & Iacovou, M. (2014). The co-construction of medical humanitarianism: Analysis of personal, organizationally condoned narratives from an agency website. *Social Science & Medicine, 120,* 430–438. https://doi.org/10.1016/j.socscimed.2014.05.053

Austin, J. H. (1999). *Zen and the brain: Toward an understanding of meditation and consciousness.* MIT Press.

Brooks, S. K., Dunn, R., Sage, C. A., Amlôt, R., Greenberg, N., & Rubin, G. J. (2015). Risk and resilience factors affecting the psychological wellbeing of individuals deployed in humanitarian relief roles after a disaster. *Journal of Mental Health, 24*(6), 385–413. https://doi.org/10.3109/09638237.2015.1057334

The Calais Sessions. (n.d.). *Recording the talented musicians of the Calais 'Jungle.'* https://www.thecalaissessions.com/

Camus, A. (2012). *The plague.* Vintage.

Catallozzi, M., Cunningham, T., Striplin, M. (2016). The use of narrative practices by expatriate health care providers treating Ebola patients in Western Africa from 2013–2016. *The Intima: A Journal of Narrative Medicine.* Fall, 2016. Retrieved from http://www.theintima.org/academic-mz?rq=striplin%20cunningham

Centers for Disease Control and Prevention. (n.d.). *Ebola (Ebola virus disease).* https://www.cdc.gov/vhf/ebola/history/2014-2016-outbreak/index.html

Cunningham, T. (2016). *The use and role of narrative practices to mitigate compassion fatigue among expatriate health workers during the Ebola outbreak of 2013–2016* (Doctoral dissertation, Mailman School of Public Health, Columbia University).

Cunningham, T. (2019). Clowns in crisis zones: The evolution of Clowns without Borders International. In *The Cultural Turn in International Aid* (pp. 224–240). Routledge.

Cunningham, T., Catallozzi, M., & Rosenthal, D. (2018). Camaraderie and community: Buffers against compassion fatigue among expatriate healthcare workers during the Ebola epidemic of 2013–16. *Health Emergency and Disaster Nursing, 5*(1), 2–11. https://doi.org/10.24298/hedn.2016-0014

Cunningham, T., Rosenthal, D., & Catallozzi, M. (2017). Narrative medicine practices as a potential therapeutic tool used by expatriate Ebola caregivers. *Intervention: Journal of Mental Health Psychosocial Support in Conflict Affected Areas, 15*(2), 106–119. https://doi.org/10.1097/WTF.0000000000000138

Cunningham, T., & Sesay, A. (2017). The triple menace in volunteer international aid work: Three harmful pitfalls. *Journal of Emergency Nursing, 43*(5), 478–481. https://doi.org/10.1016/j.jen.2017.05.016

Everly, G. S., & Lating, J. M. (2019). Voluntary control of respiration patterns. In G. S. Everly Jr. & J. M. Lating, *A clinical guide to the treatment of the human stress response* (pp. 315–329). Springer.

Farmer, P. (2020). *Fevers, Feuds, and Diamonds: Ebola and the Ravages of History*. Farrar, Strauss and Giroux.

Gan, W. H., Lim, J. W., & David, K. O. H. (2020). Preventing intra-hospital infection and transmission of COVID-19 in healthcare workers. *Safety and Health at Work.*

Greenberg, M. (2003). Therapeutic play: developing humor in the nurse-patient relationship. *Journal-New York State Nurses Association, 34*(1), 25–31.

Hofmeyer, A., & Taylor, R. (2020). Strategies and resources for nurse leaders to use to lead with empathy and prudence so they understand and address sources of anxiety among nurses practising in the era of COVID 19. *Journal of Clinical Nursing.* doi:10.1111/jocn.15520

Human Rights Watch. (2001). Refugees, asylum seekers, and internally displaced persons. *Human Rights Watch World Report, 2001.* Retrieved from http://www.hrw.org/wr2k1/

Inter-Agency Standing Committee. (2014). Strategic Response Plan Guidance. Geneva: Interagency Standing Committee. https://www. humanitarianresponse. info/en/programme-cycle/space/strategicresponse-planning-guidance-templates, accessed February 19, 2016.

Inter-Agency Standing Committee. (2020, March 17). *Interim briefing note addressing mental health and psychosocial aspects of COVID-10 Outbreak.* IASC. https://interagencystandingcommittee.org/iasc-reference-group-mental-health-and-psychosocial-support-emergency-settings/interim-briefing

Johns Hopkins University & Medicine. (2020). Coronavirus resource center. Retrieved from https://coronavirus.jhu.edu/

McCormick, W. H., Currier, J., Isaak, S. L., Sims, B. M., Slagel, B. A., Carroll, T. D., Hamner, K., & Albright, D. (2019). Military culture and post-military transitioning among veterans: A qualitative analysis. *Journal of Veterans Studies, 4*(2), 228. https://doi.org/10.21061/jvs.v4i2.121

National Academies of Sciences, Engineering, and Medicine. (2019). *Taking action against clinician burnout: a systems approach to professional well-being.* National Academies Press.

Nsio, J., Kapetshi, J., Makiala, S., Raymond, F., Tshapenda, G., Boucher, N., Corbeil, J., Okitandjate, A., Mbuyi, G., Kiyele, M., Mondonge, V., Kikoo, M. J., Van Herp, M., Barboza, P., Petrucci, R., Benedetti, G., Formenty, P., Muyembe Muzinga, B. M., Kalenga, O., I., ... & Muyembe, J.-J. T. (2020). 2017 Outbreak of ebola virus disease in northern democratic republic of Congo. *Journal of Infectious Diseases, 221*(5), 701–706.

Preyde, M. (2019). Evaluation and feasibility of a comprehensive program for post-traumatic stress disorder in military, veterans, and first responders. *International Archives of Nursing and Health Care*, *5*, 128. https://doi.org/10.23937/2469-5823/1510128

Ruiz-Garcia, L., & Lunadei, L. (2010). Monitoring cold chain logistics by means of RFID. *Sustainable radio frequency identification solutions* (pp. 37–50). https://doi.org/10.5772/8006

Statista. (2015). *Ebola cases and deaths among health care workers due to the outbreaks in West African countries as of November 4, 2015.* http://www.statista.com/statistics/325347/west-africa-ebola-cases-and-deaths-among-health-care-workers/

Statista. (2020). *Number of refugees worldwide from 2001 to 2019, by type.* https://www.statista.com/statistics/268719/number-of-refugees-worldwide/

Tol, W. A., Barbui, C., Galappatti, A., Silove, D., Betancourt, T. S., Souza, R., Golaz, A. & van Ommeren, M. (2011). Mental health and psychosocial support in humanitarian settings: Linking practice and research. *The Lancet*, *378*(9802), 1581–1591. https://doi.org/10.1016/S0140-6736(11)61094-5

UNDP: United Nations Development Programme (2019, September 20). *Universal health coverage for sustainable development – Issue brief.* UNDP. https://www.undp.org/content/undp/en/home/librarypage/hiv-aids/universal-health-coverage-for-sustainable-development---issue-br.html

UNHCR: The UN Refugee Agency. (2020). *Philippines: Figures at a glance.* https://www.unhcr.org/ph/figures-at-a-glance

Van Diest, I., Verstappen, K., Aubert, A. E., Widjaja, D., Vansteenwegen, D., & Vlemincx, E. (2014). Inhalation/exhalation ratio modulates the effect of slow breathing on heart rate variability and relaxation. *Applied Psychophysiology and Biofeedback*, *39*(3/4), 171–180. https://doi.org/10.1007/s10484-014-9253-x

van Dorn, A., Cooney, R. E., & Sabin, M. L. (2020). COVID-19 exacerbating inequalities in the US. *The Lancet*, *395*(10232), 1243–1244. https://doi.org/10.1016/S0140-6736(20)30893-X

Wilson, R. A. (Ed.). (2005). *Human rights in the 'War on Terror.'* Cambridge University Press.

World Health Organization. (n.d.) *Priorities: Health for all.* https://www.who.int/dg/priorities/health-for-all/en/

World Health Organization. (2020). Vision statement by WHO Director-General. Retrieved from https://www.who.int/director-general/vision

19
Sowing Seeds of Resilience: Compassionate Care Ambassadors

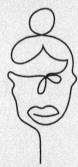

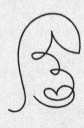

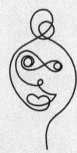

K. Jane Muir
pronouns: She/Her

K. Jane Muir, an emergency department nurse and doctoral student, is passionate about the mind-body connection, clinician well-being, and compassionate, high-quality patient care. During her undergraduate studies, she was fortunate to learn about contemplative practices and apply them in her personal and professional life.

Hannah R. Crosby
pronouns: She/Her

Throughout her life, Hannah R. Crosby's experiences as a patient have run the gamut from excellent to poor. The impact of those encounters has drawn her to collaborating with and supporting healthcare workers during the course of her career. For personal nourishment, Hannah teaches and practices yoga, hikes with her family, and bakes.

Susan Bauer-Wu
pronouns: She/Her

From an early age, Susan Bauer-Wu was drawn to the mind-body-spirit connection through caring for family members with serious illness—and also through early clinical experiences in oncology and palliative care. This perspective provided a guidepost for her to explore different contemplative practices, including meditation, personally and professionally over several decades.

"Never doubt that a small group of thoughtful, committed citizens can change the world; indeed, it's the only thing that ever has."

—Margaret Mead

Resilient nurses are primed to provide high-quality, compassionate care for patients and families. As a nurse, you are exposed to many stressors and competing demands in your everyday work. How can you be resilient—in other words, be your best self—to skillfully navigate the challenges in the clinical setting? Taking good care of yourself is only part of what fosters resilience. Equally important are organizational and peer support systems and resources that promote nurses' well-being and healthy work environments. The cultivation of healthy work environments in the clinical setting is critical in promoting patient care delivery that is compassionate for patients and fulfilling for nurses (American Association of Critical-Care Nurses, 2016).

In this chapter, we share an example of a program that can contribute to a healthy work environment by promoting self-care and compassionate care. We describe how to create and sustain a Compassionate Care Ambassador program based on our experience at the University of Virginia Compassionate Care Initiative (Bauer-Wu & Fontaine, 2015). Our aim is to provide practical information to help you successfully implement an ambassador program at your workplace, whether on an individual clinical unit or throughout a medical center or health system.

The Compassionate Care Initiative at the University of Virginia

The Compassionate Care Initiative (CCI) at the University of Virginia (UVA) was founded in 2009 by former dean Dorrie Fontaine. CCI promotes clinician (and student-clinician) wellness and high-quality, compassionate clinical care through a variety of educational offerings and by supporting Compassionate Care Ambassadors to be role models and champions in their respective settings (Bauer-Wu & Fontaine, 2015). CCI's guiding vision is to have a resilient healthcare workforce with happy and healthy nurses, physicians, and other professionals who work together in high-functioning clinical teams where heart and humanness are valued and embodied.

CCI is guided by four central concepts and values (Bauer-Wu & Fontaine, 2015):

1. **Resilience:** Resilience is fundamental to being an engaged and effective clinician.

2. **Mindfulness:** Mindfulness is a key to fostering resilience and connection with others (colleagues, patients, and families) and finding meaning in work.

3. **Interprofessional collaboration:** Resilient clinicians are more likely to be team players who work collaboratively with interprofessional colleagues.

4. **Healthy work environment:** Resilient clinicians who are less stressed and more present and collegial can co-create healthy work environments where every member of the team can thrive.

A Compassionate Care Ambassador is a clinician who is a champion of resilience and whole-person care. Compassionate Care Ambassadors catalyze or implement changes or interventions in their respective clinical areas with the goal to positively influence the well-being and morale of their colleagues as well as patient care (CCI, 2019). They serve as role models within their healthcare workplace by promoting activities and educational opportunities that support clinician wellness, compassion, stress management, and interprofessional collaboration, thereby contributing to healthy work environments (Harmon et al., 2018). Ultimately, that is the charge of the Compassionate Care Ambassadors—to help build a healthy clinical community by fostering a work culture and environment that supports and prioritizes self-care, resilience, and collaboration.

This chapter serves as a guide for you to form and sustain an ambassador program in your work setting. We will discuss the following:

- How to garner organizational and leadership support for a Compassionate Care Ambassador program

- How to organize your ambassador program

- Ideal qualities of Compassionate Care Ambassadors and ambassador recruitment

- Strategies to sustain an ambassador program

- Sample projects and activities to offer
- How to maintain resilience as a leader of an ambassador program

Because each work setting is unique, we encourage you to experiment and adapt any of the methods and ideas to your specific organization and circumstances. As we will discuss in the following sections, developing a Compassionate Care Ambassador program requires assessing the needs and interests of your colleagues, securing buy-in from institutional leaders, and developing a plan to carry out the program.

Assessing the Need for a Compassionate Care Ambassador Program

Conducting a needs assessment will help you understand the interests and priorities of the nurses (as well as other clinicians and staff) in your work environment and to determine if developing a Compassionate Care Ambassador program is feasible. A needs assessment can be through a survey, discussion during a staff meeting, or informal conversations during breaks or meals. Questions to consider in such an assessment include (Bauer-Wu & Fontaine, 2015; Germer & Neff, 2013):

- Are staff members interested in engaging in resilience-promoting activities?
- Are they receptive to a collective effort to promote staff resiliency?
- What kinds of activities or unit/hospital-wide projects interest them? Would they help in creating these activities?

Assessing the priorities, challenges, and experiences within the context of your work setting will allow you to gather firsthand support and "evidence" from your colleagues for the need to develop such a program. Results from the needs assessment can also facilitate discussions with healthcare leaders and decision-makers at your institution—part of making the case for an ambassador program.

Getting Started: Gaining Support for the Ambassador Program

After conducting a needs assessment, the next step in developing an ambassador program is to gain support from leadership within your unit or broader healthcare work setting. It is important to first identify the key leaders you will approach about your idea (Twigg & McCullough, 2014). Who are the decision-makers to contact to initiate a new program like this? For example, a nurse manager, supervisor, or committee chair may be the key leader who can make a decision (or offer advice) to start an ambassador program. If you're looking to propose an institution-wide ambassador program, then approaching department leaders, the Chief Nursing Officer, or the Chief Nurse Executive may be appropriate as well.

It is important to consider key details the leaders would be interested to know about the potential ambassador program. For example, most unit leaders are interested in identifying the benefit (i.e., to staff and patients) of a new program and how it aligns with their priorities (Twigg & McCullough, 2014; Weberg, 2010). Given that hospitals are centers of patient care delivery, clinician leaders are highly interested in improving patient outcomes, especially those linked to nursing care. Therefore, it may be beneficial to present a nurse leader with peer-reviewed evidence on the need for nurse retention and resiliency strategies. The associations among nurse stress, job dissatisfaction, and patient outcomes are well established (Aiken et al., 2002; Choi et al., 2012; McHugh et al., 2011).

An ambassador program not only promotes nurse resiliency but also fulfills an important mission by the American Nurses Association and several national healthcare organizations to deliver safe and high-quality healthcare to patients and communities (McMenamin et al., 2015; National Academies of Sciences, Engineering, and Medicine, 2019). Understanding the evidence to support clinician resiliency is crucial to gain support for an ambassador program. Medical errors and other adverse clinical events compromise cultures of healthcare safety within hospitals (Cimiotti et al., 2012; Tubbs-Cooley et al., 2019). Increased nurse turnover exacerbates nursing shortages and subsequently exacerbates unsafe patient-to-nurse staffing ratios resorted to out of necessity (McMenamin et al., 2015). Literature evaluating healthy work environments in healthcare suggests that developing clinician resiliency committees on healthcare units can contribute to necessary cultural shifts in hospital unit culture (Hersch et al., 2016; Muir & Keim-Malpass, 2019; Trail & Cunningham, 2018).

The benefits of developing an ambassador program are not only linked to clinician resiliency, but also may be associated with decreased turnover and improved patient care, thereby possibly leading to cost reductions as well (Han et al., 2019; Moran et al., 2020). Given that healthcare affordability and spending reduction is a national priority, it will be beneficial to provide supporting documentation, with peer-reviewed publications that describe the theory, evidence, and case examples of the benefits of such clinician resiliency programs (McMenamin et al., 2015).

Additionally, for unit- or hospital-wide programs, you should be prepared to present to the leadership a prospective budget necessary to start and maintain your ambassador program. This budget should consider any supplies or equipment needed to recruit participants, facilitate meetings, and implement events or activities on your unit. Outline one or two potential projects or events that the ambassador program would implement with relevant timelines and associated costs. Finally, it is helpful to outline a clear schedule for ambassador recruitment, event brainstorming and implementation, and routine check-ins with managers over the course of the first year of your program. The following sidebar outlines a sample budget associated with an ambassador program project, a Compassionate Care Cart.

Compassionate Care Cart

Individual Item Costs

Notebooks (10) = $33.80

Lavender sachets (10) = $40

Charms (10) = $30

Smartfood Popcorn (1 bag of 12): $4.48

Dove dark chocolates (3 pack x 7.61 oz = ~22 oz) = $11.35

Assorted tea bags (1 pack) = $3.18

Burlap gift bags (1 pack of 10) = $13.99

Water (1 pack of 12) =$1.98

Total cost for 10 staff members: $138.78

Metric Development

Your unit or hospital leadership may be interested in developing metrics around your program to ensure that the program is serving the identified need and purpose of the group. In collaboration with individuals in your work setting, consider these questions:

- What does a successful program look like in your designated setting?

- How can we best measure this success? (e.g., ambassador recruitment and retention, number of events/activities, number and roles of participants)

- How frequently will we check in with our goals and perform new needs assessments?

The answers to the above questions may come to light once you reflect on the purpose of your ambassador program, as discussed in subsequent paragraphs. The following paragraphs detail the development and expansion of an ambassador program within a designated healthcare setting context.

Creating the Ambassador Program

An ambassador program can be composed of clinical nurses, or a mix of interprofessional clinicians who share a common desire to cultivate healthy, resilient work environments (CCI, 2019). Consider whether your ambassador program will be embedded within one clinical unit, multiple units, or various settings within your health system (CCI, 2019). You may decide to initially pilot your ambassador program on one clinical unit and expand over time to other clinical units and settings (Bauer-Wu & Fontaine, 2015). Across all settings, it is important to identify individuals who share similar motivations and who can commit to the time and effort to participate in the ambassador program (Bauer-Wu & Fontaine, 2015; Harmon et al., 2018).

As you develop your own program, it will be important to seek out necessary support and resources. It may be helpful for the lead organizer of the ambassador program (you or another identified individual) to work with a mentor or fellow colleague to distribute the efforts. Initial program development may include identifying ambassador candidates and potential funding sources. Depending on your clinical setting (unit- or hospital-wide, academic or community hospital, health system or single hospital), you may consider expanding your ambassador program to include students (if at an academic medical center) or members of community organizations (Bauer-Wu & Fontaine, 2015). If your clinical setting is situated within a larger health system, there may exist personnel support and financial mechanisms that can support building your ambassador program (Harmon et al., 2018). For example, your hospital may have a volunteer office with personnel who can advise on program development or offer grants for initiating an ambassador program. If affiliated with a university, your hospital may have resources in place within the health professional schools that can provide funding, advice, and mentoring on group organizing, and potential individuals to help lead the ambassador program.

Choosing Ambassadors

Once you have identified the appropriate collaborators to begin an ambassador program, take time to consider the ideal qualities of potential ambassadors. The qualities should include being purpose-driven, dedicated to include a diverse group of individuals within the program, and accountable with behaviors that align with the program's values. Characteristics of potential ambassadors should include:

- Role model of self-care, resilience, and mentoring

- Passionate and excited about the purpose of the ambassador program

- Inclusive and welcomes different experiences and perspectives

- Exemplifies work-life integration

- Embodies compassion and kindness for others and self

- Has time and energy to commit to being an ambassador

- Communicates well and can inspire others

- Exemplifies timeliness and professionalism with communication and follow-through with projects

- Insightful and creative

- Supports sustainability of the ambassador program through identification and recruitment of new ambassadors

- Speaks up and addresses systemic challenges

- Advocates for the well-being of peers and colleagues

The qualities will vary by program purpose, setting, organizational culture, and more. The support systems you've identified in your healthcare setting can assist you in conceptualizing the ideal qualities of an ambassador. In identifying the key attributes of an ambassador and understanding the direction of your program (discussed below), you are well situated to recruit a team of ambassadors.

Defining the Purpose of the Ambassador Program

To identify ideal qualities of an ambassador, it is important to determine the direction of the ambassador program early on. Developing a firm understanding of the ambassador program's direction and purpose facilitates member recruitment. Such purpose development will also aid in designing projects and events by the group. You may choose to collaborate with your unit leadership, mentors, and other support systems in developing the ambassador program's purpose.

Questions that can guide development of the purpose include:

- What is the targeted setting where the program will take place?

- Who is the targeted audience the group will serve (e.g., nurses only vs. interprofessional, unit-based vs. multiple units or across medical center)?

- What is the identified objective of the ambassador program within our setting?

- What types of activities are needed to fulfill our mission in our setting?

Once developed, the mission can be communicated on your unit, at nursing leadership meetings across the hospital, at ambassador recruitment events within your hospital, at ambassador events, and on relevant social media sites to advertise the group. Below is an example of a Compassionate Care Ambassador program mission:

> The goal of the "Nurse Undergraduate Resiliency Engagement (NURSE)" group is to cultivate a culture of inquiry and practice around evidenced-based resilience practices that can be translated into the clinical practice sphere to support nurse well-being and compassionate patient care delivery.

Recruitment and Sustainability

> "The foundation of every great team is a direction that energizes, orients, and engages its members" (Haas & Mortensen, 2016, para. 5).

Word-of-mouth promotion is a highly effective strategy to recruit new ambassadors, especially if the spokesperson is inspiring and articulate. As a nurse, sharing your passion and experience with peers will be the most effective way to spark interest in your program. While recruiting, be ever mindful of sustainability; try to engage new ambassadors from different backgrounds and years of experience. Cultivating a vibrant Compassionate Care Ambassador program requires aligning interests between the leaders and potential ambassadors. Planning a recruitment or interest meeting is an ideal place to identify future members of the program. Other recruitment ideas include doing a brief presentation at the following venues:

- New employee orientation
- Shared/clinical governance meeting
- Beginning of a staff meeting
- Interest meetings

Interest meetings can be held by the initial ambassadors or in conjunction with activity fairs that are already taking place on the unit or within the larger institution. An interest meeting allows for communication about the purpose and activities of the ambassador program. Potential members can also ask questions. You should be ready to clearly communicate your group's direction and needs when people ask how they can be involved.

In preparation for an interest meeting where recruitment for the ambassador program takes place, it is important to have answers to the following questions (example answers italicized):

- What is the time commitment required of an ambassador in this program?

    An ambassador should be prepared to attend 50% of group meetings and can attend at least 50% of planned ambassador events.

- What types of activities should an ambassador be expected to do?

    The ideal ambassador is excited to brainstorm or plan self-care and resilience activities for clinicians on their unit. They will co-plan at least one event per year. They should attend at least half of all events planned each year to support other ambassador projects.

The Work of Ambassador Programs

The identified direction (purpose) and setting of your ambassador program will inform the type of activities the group pursues and delivers. Each ambassador program will look different in terms of the amount and type of events planned; there is not a prescription for success in every case. For example, your ambassador program may decide to limit activities to educational brown bag lunches or journal club meetings where clinician resiliency literature is discussed. Conversely, you may decide to focus your programming on resiliency practices and activities for staff. An example of such activities is a "check-in" meditation during nurse huddle at the beginning or end of each shift. You may decide to gradually increase the number of events you plan over time as you identify what events work well in your identified setting.

Thus, projects and activities can vary greatly with countless possibilities. Decisions of what to pursue are determined by the ambassadors' interests, what is most feasible to implement, the needs of those they serve, and available resources. Consider collaborating with committees, institutions, and organizations within your hospital and community. If you are part of an academic medical center, collaborating with the academic side (e.g., Schools of Nursing, Medicine, Health Sciences) may offer opportunities for ambassador recruitment and mentorship. If you are part of a community hospital, collaborations with local businesses such as yoga, meditation, or wellness studios may offer rich, creative programming opportunities.

Suggested Ambassador Projects

- Resiliency cart for clinicians
- Self-care "sampler" events offering drop-in yoga, meditation, art, or exercise
- Group creativity breaks (painting, poetry, music)
- Mini retreats offsite at nature settings
- Resource sharing, such as podcasts, meditation apps, and classes to promote resilience at health system or community
- Social media
- Inspiring quotes and photos
- Promotion of resilience-related events
- Sharing of ambassador projects
- Speaker series/panels (to talk about self-care and stress-reduction practices)
- "Mindfulness moment" or "pause" at nursing huddle before a shift
- Chair massage (local therapists may volunteer or do at reduced rate)
- Therapy dogs during high-stress periods (see Figure 19.1)
- Monthly "teas"—tea and treats for team camaraderie
- Create dedicated resilience spaces (transform cluttered unused closet)

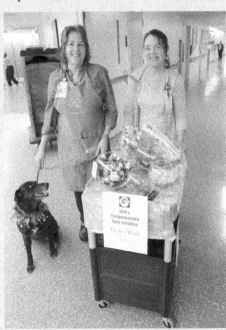

FIGURE 19.1 Therapy dogs at UVA.

Note: Ambassador projects can be tailored to specific clinical units and academic settings. Group collaboration on ambassador projects is encouraged.

Program development takes thoughtfulness, time, patience, and constant evaluation by the ambassadors and the clinicians they are serving. It may be valuable to create and distribute simple surveys after each of your events for specific feedback or periodically to solicit general feedback. Input from colleagues is essential to ensure that your programming is serving a valuable purpose and meeting identified needs. Some examples of ambassador activities that have been successful at the University of Virginia:

- **Compassionate Care Cart:** The Compassionate Care Cart (refer to Figure 19.1) is "resiliency on wheels" for students in the UVA School of Nursing and clinicians within UVA hospital. The cart offers students and clinicians self-care items such as lavender sachets, touch stones, mindfulness meditation resources, booklets, and snacks. The cart frequently travels with a therapy dog as well. Given that clinicians do not always have time for a break, the cart brings a restful and recharging experience to the clinical unit. The cart has one to two key leaders who oversee cart planning, feedback, and improvement. Several ambassadors volunteer to bring the cart around in the School of Nursing and in the hospital. The cart integrates the clinical and student ambassador groups to provide students and clinicians with a resilience break in their busy days. This initiative is an example of cross-departmental collaboration between hospital and academic entities for ambassador event planning.

- **Tea Time:** The "tea time" project was initiated by a pediatric palliative care physician. She purchased ceramic teacups and prepares tea and homemade goodies for the staff on the different units she works. She does this periodically, often in response to a distressing period on the unit. After hearing about these teas at an ambassador meeting, another ambassador from a different clinical area initiated something similar, adapting for her team. Tea is a simple way to show appreciation, gather colleagues together, and support one another.

- **Interdisciplinary Team Check-Ins:** The interdisciplinary team check-in is also a simple yet profound practice. Initiated by a pediatric palliative care nurse practitioner, she recognized the need for all members of the team to connect before difficult family meetings. These check-ins involve taking the pulse of the team by simply asking each person to share one word or phrase that describes how they are feeling at that moment. The simple check-in practice allows each individual to give voice to their thoughts and feelings and provides space for the team to support each other and be on the same page before meeting with the family. The check-in can also inform the roles and flow of the meeting; depending on what is shared, responsibilities may need to shift. The check-in could be adapted for team huddles at shift change as well as to understand how to support colleagues. The team benefits, as do the patients and families.

- **Resilience Spaces:** Space is a precious commodity in hospitals. In some clinical settings, even staff break rooms are nonexistent. A few nurses decided to take the initiative to change that. They noticed that their colleagues were going to the bathroom to take a moment to catch their breath or clear their mind. They identified a space on the unit, not much bigger than a closet, that wasn't being used. They created a lovely "resilience room" by painting the walls an inviting color, adding a comfortable chair and a few yoga mats, and providing some reading materials and resources. The staff on that unit now have a place where they can pause and recharge during their shift. Since sharing their story in an ambassador meeting, other units across the health system have claimed similar spaces for their own "resilience rooms." They are generally not big spaces, but they always have a big impact.

It may be valuable to identify specific ambassadors who are dedicated to working on projects, ideas, or events. For example, two ambassadors may dedicate the year to planning a self-care sampler or designing a survey to receive feedback from their peers. Be mindful of projects taking place throughout the year to ensure that the number of events scheduled is realistic for the ambassadors and of the greatest need for the group you are serving.

Structuring Ambassador Meetings

Meetings among the ambassadors are necessary to develop ideas for new activities and foster a community of support among the group. Meetings ought to take place on a regular basis and last as long as feasible. Flexibility with meeting length is crucial given schedule variations among individual group members and competing demands that may exist on clinical units. Therefore, it is beneficial to prioritize scheduling ambassador program meetings while maintaining flexibility with meeting durations and necessary cancellations. An example of scheduling that has worked for our organization is at least monthly meetings lasting 60 to 90 minutes to ensure meaningful engagement with one another and to address timely issues.

Specific meeting times and locations should consider ambassadors' varied schedules and locations, which may require regular time and location changes to facilitate participation. Scheduling meetings is a unique challenge that clinician leaders face while operating an organization situated within a healthcare context. You may consider hosting virtual and online meetings in order to expand access to individuals with competing schedule demands, physical distance challenges, and personal life responsibilities. Creativity and flexibility with meeting formats can further extend inclusivity in ambassador program participation.

The success of the ambassador program is in part determined by the effectiveness of the meetings. Therefore, thoughtful planning to create fruitful meetings is recommended. Important considerations when planning an ambassador meeting include the following:

- Have a clear meeting intention (e.g., program development, peer support, or social).

- Set and send the meeting agenda ahead of time. Request input in creating the agenda.

- Begin with a brief grounding practice (see "Script for Grounding Practice" sidebar that comes later).

- Brainstorm new ideas for activities.

- Share successes and challenges in implementing projects. Celebrate and support one another.

- Include a poem or reflection at the beginning or the end of the meeting. Invite different people to do this.

Consider structuring ambassador meetings with a beginning intention practice followed by introductions of new members and current updates on projects. Allow sufficient time for dialogue and sharing, while keeping in mind remaining agenda items.

Encourage ambassadors to contribute topics to meeting agendas. Allocate time to review if scheduled meeting dates, times, and locations are appropriate for the group.

Such a brief guided practice at the start of ambassador group meetings helps everyone be more focused and feel less stressed. An option is to use a bell to signal the beginning and the end of the practice.

Script for Grounding Practice

Settle into a comfortable sitting posture. Your back is relatively straight, but not rigid. Both feet are flat on the floor, and hands placed on the lap or folded together. Head and neck are balanced. If you'd like, close your eyes or lower your eyes with a soft gaze.

Feel your body supported by the chair, and feel your feet on the floor.

Take three, full slow breaths in and out. Be sure to exhale fully.

Check in and notice how you feel right now.

For the next minute, breathe normally and gently bring awareness to the experience of breathing. Notice the sensations of the air entering your body and then releasing, leaving your body.

Consider saying to yourself, "Breathing in, I notice what it feels like to breathe in; breathing out, I notice what it feels like to breathe out."

Notice any resistance you may have to doing this practice. Try not to judge this resistance. Note where the resistance is felt the most, perhaps in your stomach, your head, your hands.

Settle back now with the breath, noticing the belly rising and falling, or perhaps noticing air entering and leaving your nostrils. Notice the pause between the inhale and the exhale of each breath.

Check in now with an intention you may have for yourself, for this day, or for this next meeting. What would you like to let go of? What would you like to be grounded in today?

Sit with this intention now, using the breath as an anchor with each inhale and exhale.

Gently wiggle your toes and fingers. When you are ready, gently open your eyes, gradually taking in the light in the room.

Adapted from Bauer-Wu (2011)

Sustainability

When undertaking any new program in a clinical setting with inherent turnover, it is important to think about its sustainability beyond your involvement. Though some strategies may work better than others, there are a few conditions that are fundamental to successful group collaboration—compelling direction, strong structure, supportive context, and shared mindset (Haas & Mortensen, 2016)—that are applicable here. As mentioned previously, identifying a shared mission and goals that support the aim of the ambassador group is critical to both sustainability and recruitment. Inspiration and creativity will be squandered if members do not know the direction of the ambassador program or their role. Additionally, it is important to understand that ambassador group sustainability is not a stagnant process, and you should return to the mission and goals often, especially as the program grows and membership turns over.

For example, with the Compassionate Care Initiative's Ambassador program at UVA, we have a plenary session at the beginning of each semester to review our mission and develop our objectives for the coming months. We have found that this meeting gives our ambassadors the opportunity to help shape the program's direction and communicate a shared mindset. A few approaches to consider relevant to engagement and sustainability, which may or may not be available at your institution, include:

- Having an application process for membership
- Structuring your group in a way that mimics nursing shared governance or Magnet® hospital accreditation practices within your institution
- Offering clinical ladder advancement for engaged participation
- Providing a stipend for specific responsibilities
- Getting paid to attend ambassador meetings and activities, if done during off hours

Though our ambassador program has largely been a grassroots effort, with individuals self-selecting to be involved, it is important to provide a membership engagement and sustainability structure. Your program can have a plethora of individuals who consider themselves "members," yet are they contributing to the shared objectives? If your program lacks ambassador engagement and sustainability structure, ambassador accountability will most likely be lacking as well. Invest the time to create a sustainability and ambassador engagement plan to achieve the mission of the ambassador program in the long run.

Maintaining Resilience as an Ambassador

Compassionate Care Ambassadors must balance fulfilling the mission of the program in conjunction with fulfilling clinician and personal life duties—this is no small feat! The success of a Compassionate Care Ambassador program requires a significant amount of commitment from all ambassadors, especially for those who are the initial organizers of a group in its beginning stages. Leadership in an ambassador program can be challenging regardless of the program's stage of development.

Ambassador Leadership Self-Care Challenges

Compassionate Care Ambassadors face challenging leadership tasks as described above, plus often face challenges associated with changing the workplace culture. If a work environment is not accustomed to a clinician resilience program, ambassador leaders can face administrative and peer resistance. Developing a new ambassador program in a setting that is not accustomed to such a concept can be challenging as new perspectives challenge traditional activities in a hospital or clinic setting. Lead ambassadors should allocate time to routinely reflect on not only the progress of the program's development, but also their own self-care and energy levels. It is crucial to identify support groups or "allies" such as researchers, clinicians, and peers who support the identified mission of the group and can offer leadership guidance. On an individual leader level, it is important to allocate time for self-reflection and restoration. One strategy for such reflection can take place through a variety of writing prompts.

Suggested questions can serve as a guide for one's reflective writing:

- Is the time I am allocating to the ambassador program's development reasonable?

- What areas of leading the program's development are the most challenging at this time?

- What domains of program work should be reduced to facilitate my self-care?

- Which resources can I use for programmatic tasks, mission development, or recruitment delegation?

- Which resources can I reach out to for general leadership support?

- What areas of communication must be strengthened between individuals or groups assisting with the development of this program?

- What activities are most needed for me to feel balance between developing this program and balancing my personal, professional life?

- What recent experiences are especially meaningful and most impactful?

- What aspects of program development bring me joy?

- Who or what am I grateful for in this journey of developing a compassion program?

Ambassador Burnout

You know the common airline expression, "place the oxygen mask on yourself before helping others." Within the nursing profession, this phrase refers to cultivating well-being and self-care practices in order to adequately provide high-quality care, presence, and kindness to patients (Bakhamis et al., 2019). In a similar manner, Compassionate Care Ambassadors must strive to "talk the talk" and "walk the walk" in practicing self-care and resilience while encouraging others to do so. As a leader in the clinical community disseminating information about self-care and resilience, it is crucial to allocate time for personal self-care, resilience, and reflection often.

Clinician burnout, as discussed in prior chapters, is characterized by emotional exhaustion, depersonalization, and feelings of low personal accomplishment (Maslach, 1999). Burnout as a leader of an extracurricular group is commonly overlooked and seemingly invisible, yet can contribute to significant stress for individuals. In order to remain balanced and resilient in all settings, it helps to identify self-care practices that allow you to feel restored. The following sidebar highlights some potential self-care practices, and of course, there are many included in this book. It's important to identify which practices are most beneficial that can be implemented at times of the day that best restore you. For example, exercise or gentle stretching may be a valuable restorative activity you perform at the end of your shift. Alternatively, you may prefer to conduct a brief meditation, or "The Pause," during certain times in the work day (Bartels, 2014; Cunningham et al., 2019; Muir & Keim-Malpass, 2019). Remember, self-care is unique to each individual. Be kind to yourself as you identify which restorative resiliency practices work best for your schedule and overall needs.

Examples of Self-Care Activities to Foster Ambassador Resilience

- Reflective writing
- Movement practices (exercise, gentle stretching/yoga, T'ai Chi)
- Time in the outdoors
- Creating/consuming artwork
- Listening to/creating music
- Time with friends and family
- Counseling or therapy
- Reading
- Time with animals
- Travel
- Meditation/quiet time
- Drinking tea/coffee
- Taking a bubble bath

Note: Such practices will look different for each individual; these examples may help you determine a self-care plan that works for you.

Ambassador resilience is an essential step toward success within a Compassionate Care Ambassador program. The resilience of the ambassadors should be prioritized and reevaluated on a scheduled basis (at least twice a year). Consider allocating time for ambassador group resilience by planning group retreats or resilience-based activities. There is no "right way" to practice self-care and build resilience; do whatever resonates and seems the most appropriate for you. Retreats, social gatherings, and collaborations on a collective reflective art project are just a few ideas of resilience-based activities an ambassador group can participate in.

Closing Thoughts

A Compassionate Care Ambassador program can be instrumental in fostering resilience and creating healthy work environments. We have offered practical advice on how to create and sustain an ambassador program as well as examples of successful projects. You can apply the many strategies, tips, and guidance points from this chapter to begin such an ambassador program within your healthcare setting. Whether your unit or hospital is already supportive of clinician well-being or you are starting entirely from scratch, if you have the passion, you have the power to make a difference in your clinical setting; even small steps can create positive change and can be especially rewarding. Developing a Compassionate Care Ambassador program will have many benefits: ripples extending far beyond helping one individual nurse, to positively

In Real Practice

If you choose to start or participate in an ambassador program at your hospital or in your health system, consider how you can document and track your progress. There is a need for publications in this area so that other nurses and nurse leaders can learn about the powerful impacts that ambassador programs—focusing on well-being, self-care, and resilience—can have on a health system.

One paper by Cunningham and Çayir (2021) describes a resilience retreat intervention that was inspired and supported by a Compassionate Care Ambassador program. This paper provides a pre-test/post-test study using a modified anxiety scale and measurements to assess intention of continuing self-care practices. It finds that resilience retreats can reduce a sense of state anxiety while inspiring people to continue practicing self-care after the retreat is over. This is a very small study, and its findings are not generalizable; however, it may inspire others to replicate similar research at a more robust level and, most importantly, it may inspire leaders to listen to their ambassadors in order to build more compassionate and resilient work settings.

transforming organizational culture and leading to higher quality and more compassionate care of patients and families.

Key Points

- Compassionate Care Ambassador programs foster healthy work environments.

- Clarity on the program purpose and qualities of the ambassadors helps to ensure impact and sustainability.

- Regular, well-organized ambassador meetings can facilitate new ideas and provide opportunities for peer support and celebration.

- Ambassadors' projects and activities vary greatly and are derived largely from the setting, resources, individuals you are serving, and interest of the ambassadors.

- Systems to support self-care, like an ambassador program, foster compassionate care.

References

Aiken, L. H., Clarke, S. P., Sloane, D. M., Sochalski, J., & Silber, J. H. (2002). Hospital nurse staffing and patient mortality, nurse burnout, and job dissatisfaction. *JAMA, 288*(16), 1987–1993. https://doi.org/10.1001/jama.288.16.1987

American Association of Critical-Care Nurses. (2016). AACN standards for establishing and sustaining healthy work environments. *A journey to excellence*, 2nd edition. Executive summary. https://www.aacn.org/~/media/aacn-website/nursing-excellence/healthy-work-environment/execsum.pdf

Bakhamis, L., Paul, D. P., Smith, H., & Coustasse, A. (2019). Still an epidemic: The burnout syndrome in hospital registered nurses. *Health Care Manager, 38*(1), 3–10. https://doi.org/10.1097/HCM.0000000000000243

Bartels, J. B. (2014). The pause. *Critical Care Nurse, 34*(1), 74–75. https://doi.org/10.4037/ccn2014962

Bauer-Wu, S. (2011). *Leaves falling gently: Living fully with serious and life-limiting illness through mindfulness, compassion, and connectedness.* New Harbinger Publications.

Bauer-Wu, S., & Fontaine, D. (2015). Prioritizing clinician wellbeing: The University of Virginia's Compassionate Care Initiative. *Global Advances in Health and Medicine, 4*(5), 16–22. https://doi.org/10.7453/gahmj.2015.042

Choi, J., Flynn, L., & Aiken, L. H. (2012). Nursing practice environment and registered nurses' job satisfaction in nursing homes. *The Gerontologist, 52*(4), 484–492. https://doi.org/10.1093/geront/gnr101

Cimiotti, J. P., Aiken, L. H., Sloane, D. M., & Wu, E. S. (2012). Nurse staffing, burnout, and health care–associated infection. *American Journal of Infection Control, 40*(6), 486–490. https://doi.org/10.1016/j.ajic.2012.02.029

Compassionate Care Initiative. (2019, December 11). Compassionate care initiative ambassadors. https://cci.nursing.virginia.edu/team/ambassadors/

Cunningham, T., & Çayir, E. (2021). Nurse leaders employ contemplative practices to promote healthcare professional well-being and decrease anxiety. *JONA: Journal of Nursing Administration, 51*(3).

Cunningham, T., Ducar, D. M., & Keim-Malpass, J. (2019). "The Pause": A Delphi methodology examining an end-of-life practice. *Western Journal of Nursing Research, 41*(10), 1481–1498. https://doi.org/10.1177/0193945919826314

Germer, C. K., & Neff, K. D. (2013). Self-compassion in clinical practice. *Journal of Clinical Psychology, 69*(8), 856–867. https://doi.org/10.1002/jclp.22021

Haas, M., & Mortensen, M. (2016, June). The secrets of great teamwork. *Harvard Business Review,* 70–76. https://hbr.org/2016/06/the-secrets-of-great-teamwork

Han, S., Shanafelt, T. D., Sinsky, C. A., Awad, K. M., Dyrbye, L. N., Fiscus, L. C., Trockel, M., & Goh, J. (2019). Estimating the attributable cost of physician burnout in the United States. *Annals of Internal Medicine, 170*(11), 784–790.

Harmon, R. B., DeGennaro, R., Norling, M., Kennedy, C., & Fontaine, D. (2018). Implementing healthy work environment standards in an academic workplace: An update. *Journal of Professional Nursing, 34*(1), 20–24. https://doi.org/10.1016/j.profnurs.2017.06.001

Hersch, R. K., Cook, R. F., Deitz, D. K., Kaplan, S., Hughes, D., Friesen, M. A., & Vezina, M. (2016). Reducing nurses' stress: A randomized controlled trial of a web-based stress management program for nurses. *Applied Nursing Research, 32,* 18–25. https://doi.org/10.1016/j.apnr.2016.04.003

Maslach, C. (1999, August). A multidimensional theory of burnout. *Theories of Organizational Stress,* 68–85.

McHugh, M. D., Kutney-Lee, A., Cimiotti, J. P., Sloane, D. M., & Aiken, L. H. (2011). Nurses' widespread job dissatisfaction, burnout, and frustration with health benefits signal problems for patient care. *Health Affairs, 30*(2), 202–210. https://doi.org/10.1377/hlthaff.2010.0100

McMenamin, P. D., Peterson, C. M., McHugh, M., & Sochalski, J. A. (2015). Optimal nurse staffing to improve quality of care and patient outcomes. [Executive Summary.] Avalere. https://www.nursingworld.org/~4ae116/globalassets/practiceandpolicy/advocacy/ana_optimal-nurse-staffing_white-paper-es_2015sep.pdf

Moran, D., Wu, A. W., Connors, C., Chappidi, M. R., Sreedhara, S. K., Selter, J. H., & Padula, W. V. (2020). Cost-benefit analysis of a support program for nursing staff. *Journal of Patient Safety, 16*(4), e250–e254.

Muir, K. J., & Keim-Malpass, J. (2019). The emergency resiliency initiative: A pilot mindfulness intervention program. *Journal of Holistic Nursing, 38*(2), 205–220. https://doi.org/10.1177/0898010119874971

National Academies of Sciences, Engineering, and Medicine. (2019). *Taking action against clinician burnout: A systems approach to professional well-being.* Author.

Trail, J., & Cunningham, T. (2018). The compassionate university: How University of Virginia is changing the culture of compassion at a large, American public university. *Journal of Perspectives in Applied Academic Practice, 6*(3), 49–56. https://doi.org/10.14297/jpaap.v6i3.358

Tubbs-Cooley, H. L., Mara, C. A., Carle, A. C., Mark, B. A., & Pickler, R. H. (2019). Association of nurse workload with missed nursing care in the neonatal intensive care unit. *JAMA Pediatrics, 173*(1), 44–51. https://doi.org/10.1001/jamapediatrics.2018.3619

Twigg, D., & McCullough, K. (2014). Nurse retention: A review of strategies to create and enhance positive practice environments in clinical settings. *International Journal of Nursing Studies, 51*(1), 85–92.

Weberg, D. (2010). Transformational leadership and staff retention: an evidence review with implications for healthcare systems. *Nursing Administration Quarterly, 34*(3), 246–258.

section V
The Heart of a Nurse

20

Mattering: Creating a Rich Work Life

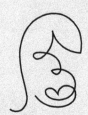

Julie Haizlip
pronouns: She/Her

Julie Haizlip, a pediatric critical-care physician, recognized that she feels most like she matters when she is teaching and personally connected with students. Now teaching at a school of nursing, she is committed to interprofessional education and collaborative practice. She and her family are on a quest to attend a hockey game in all 31 NHL venues.

"Every one of us is looking
for the same thing—we want
to know we matter."

—Oprah Winfrey

Why do you want to be a nurse?

You must have been asked this question many times—by friends, family, professors, or perhaps on your college applications. The question of why you want to be a nurse points to the meaning of your work. What is your internal motivation? The response is unique for each student, but some common answers include:

- I want to help people.

- There will always be jobs in nursing.

- A nurse was important in the care of my loved one, and I want to do that for someone else.

- Nurses care for people holistically.

Whatever the meaning is for you, it is the right one. That meaning has driven you to pursue the profession of nursing and to commit to a career of serving others.

A question you may not have been asked is, "How will you know that what you are doing as a nurse matters?"

There is more to this question than what might immediately meet the eye. To *matter* means to be of importance or to have significance (Oxford English Dictionary, n.d.). So, this question could mean, "How will you know your work is important or significant?" It could be measured by discrete outcomes, like my patient isn't getting bedsores because I turned him appropriately, or my patient is getting better because I safely administered her medications and attended to her condition. Or perhaps it could be that my patient is less nervous because I explained what would happen in the procedure that she is about to have done, or my patient's family was at peace when he died because the team provided time and information that allowed them to have closure. For you, the answer to this question likely reflects the aspects of the job that you find most satisfying and significant.

Another important aspect of the question "How will you know that what you are doing as a nurse matters?" is the "how will you know" component. What is the source of the feedback? What form does it take? For some, simply knowing that you have done something meaningful is enough. For others, it is important to receive validation from others. Take a moment to think about a time when you felt like you mattered. What was the situation? Did it involve someone else? What were your actions? Did you accomplish something? How did you contribute? How did you know that you mattered in that moment? As you reflect back, how do you now know that you mattered? Hold on to this reflection from the past and your hopes for your future as a nurse as we consider the concept of *mattering*.

Introduction to Mattering

To understand mattering and how it applies to you as a nurse, let's start at the beginning. *Mattering* was first described by Rosenberg and McCullough (1981) when looking at relationships in families. When the term "significant other" was coined, it suggested that there are some who are significant to an individual, and that there must be others who are not. To matter is to be significant. It means that someone notices you and wants you around. It means that what you want or need is important to them. If you matter, others rely on you. You bring something to the relationship, and others value your unique contribution.

While mattering originated in work done with families, it is clearly applicable to other relationships as well. Consider people who matter to you. This list undoubtedly includes not only family members, but also many others such as friends, teachers, coaches, teammates, members of your faith community, and pets. Perhaps it includes a boss or a coworker. The connections you have made in all realms of your life contribute to mattering.

It is not surprising to find that when you feel like you matter, it affects your well-being. Researchers in the social sciences have linked mattering to a number of essential elements of well-being such as self-efficacy, personal growth, relatedness, social belonging, and life satisfaction (Flett, 2018; Prilleltensky, 2014; Prilleltensky & Prilleltensky, in press; Reece et al., 2019). When you feel like you matter, you lead a richer and more connected life.

Mattering as a Construct

Mattering was first defined in the realm of interpersonal relationships (Rosenberg & McCullough, 1981). This construct, now known as *interpersonal mattering*, encompasses four domains: awareness, importance, reliance, and ego-extension (Elliot et al., 2004; France & Finney, 2009; Rosenberg, 1985; Rosenberg & Mc-Cullough, 1981):

- *Awareness* represents the simple idea that others are cognizant of your presence and would miss you if you were not there.

- *Importance* to others is their genuine expressed care and concern.

- *Reliance* suggests that others depend on you or that your actions influence the lives of those around you.

- *Ego-extension* represents the notion that others feel a sense of pride in your successes or disappointment in your failures, as though your performance reflects not only on yourself, but also on them.

Each of the four domains of mattering speaks to important contributors to psychological well-being. The need for others to be aware of your presence relates to the need for social belonging. In their landmark work, Baumeister and Leary (1995) determined that the need to belong and form secure interpersonal attachments is a fundamental human motivation. Growing from an evolutionary need to be part of a group to ensure survival, humans are compelled to connect with others and to be a valued part of a community (Baumeister & Leary, 1995). As sure as the threat of being ostracized or forgotten strikes fear in our hearts, knowing that others accept and desire having you as part of their lives creates a sense of contentment, joy, and security that is unrivaled.

The desire to feel important is similar to the need to be noticed, but importance incorporates the element of perceived social support (Elliott et al., 2004). If you are significant enough to someone that they would go out of their way to attend to your wants or needs, that is a true indication that you matter. Perceived social support contributes to well-being by bolstering feelings of self-esteem (Baumeister & Leary, 1995; Cohen & Wills, 1985). *Self-esteem* describes an overall assessment of one's intrinsic worthiness and competence (Prilleltensky & Prilleltensky, in press). While self-esteem is a personal appraisal, it is clearly affected by the actions of others and is understandably enhanced when you see that others are willing to invest in you.

Reliance suggests that your actions have an impact and can positively influence the lives of others (Elliott et al., 2004). Your friends, family, and coworkers know that they can count on you. When others rely on you, it suggests you are effective, dependable, and trustworthy. Reliance contributes to mattering by enhancing self-efficacy. *Self-efficacy* describes the knowledge that you are capable of creating desired outcomes through your own actions (Bandura, 1977). It means that you have the ability to contribute and that others value your contribution.

Hive psychology describes the need of individuals to be a part of something larger than oneself (Haidt et al., 2008). Haidt suggests that blurring the boundaries between oneself and others allows for a sense of community that promotes lasting happiness. The fourth component of mattering, ego-extension, invokes the idea of this kind of bond. Ego-extension (as described earlier in the chapter) represents the notion that others feel a sense of pride in your successes or disappointment in your failures, as though your performance reflects not only on yourself, but also on them (France & Finney, 2009). It is hard to imagine a stronger bond with another person than being seen as an extension of their being. Imagine your parents' pride when you were accepted to nursing school, your coach's excitement when you made the play that won the game, or your music teacher glowing after your performance. Remember how it felt to see how your achievement affected them.

418 Self-Care for New and Student Nurses

Scholars agree that self-esteem, self-efficacy, the experience of social belonging, and being part of something larger than yourself (i.e., your hive) are essential elements of well-being (Diener et al., 2018; Dutton et al., 2016; Flett, 2018; Prilleltensky, 2020, Prilleltensky & Prilleltensky, in press; Seligman, 2012), and all are incorporated in interpersonal mattering. However, practically, you don't need scholars to explain the association of mattering with well-being. If you simply recall a time when you mattered and see how your body reacts, it is self-evident. The experience of mattering likely brings a smile to your face. It may evoke a sense of pride or satisfaction. Knowing that you have positively impacted someone, that you mattered, is reward in itself.

But mattering is not limited to relationships between individuals. Isaac Prilleltensky (2020) suggests that we strive to *matter*, which he defines as adding value and feeling valued, in each of four domains: the self, interpersonally, at work, and in communities. Since we are focusing on mattering in the context of you and your role as a nursing student, let's turn next to the role of mattering in the well-being of students in colleges and universities.

Mattering in Education

The schools we attend and the communities within them are crucial to our sense of mattering. For many of us, the time we have spent in classes and extracurricular activities with our teachers, coaches, and peers may equal or surpass the waking hours we have spent with our families, jobs, and other aspects of our lives. Accordingly, it is important to consider how our experiences in our academic environments affect our sense of mattering.

Mattering in the Classroom

In his book *The Psychology of Mattering: Understanding the Human Need to Be Significant*, Gordon Flett (2018) emphasizes that schools, colleges, and universities are not just physical environments; they are also powerful and complicated psychological environments. Our perception of mattering as a person and a student are molded by our senses of fit and belonging in those environments. Flett (2018) states that "going to school is a very different experience for the student who feels like he or she matters compared to the student who feels uncared for and invisible" (p. 225). It is crucial for us to reflect on this sentiment because the psychological environment of the school has a tremendous impact on student learning. Schlossberg (1989) first approached this topic when considering adults who were returning to school. She was concerned that students, especially those who do not fit the norm, who are not made to feel like they belong, quickly become marginalized. Her work has inspired educators to consider how best to promote connections for and among students.

Flett (2018) states that students tend to be "motivated and engaged to the extent that they perceive that people at the school actually care about them" (p. 226). Caring in an academic setting can come from myriad sources: a professor who takes the time to get to know you not only as a student but as a person, a teaching assistant who is invested in helping you grasp a concept, peers who meet you to study or for a cup of coffee, or a counselor who reaches out at a time when you are struggling. The key is in knowing that you have been seen and valued as an individual and in feeling that someone is invested in your success. Mattering also arises from having an opportunity to have a voice at your school and a chance to contribute. Take a moment to think about your experience as a nursing student. Who or what has made you feel like you matter? When have you felt seen or heard? How have you or could you have added value?

For many students, the answers to the questions will come easily, but for individuals who may not fit the traditional stereotype of a nurse or a student at your college or university, it may be a bit more complicated. Anyone who identifies as being outside the norm may not readily feel as comfortable or as welcomed (Flett, 2018). A male student may feel out of place in a female-dominated profession. Someone whose class schedule conflicts with important religious observances might be hesitant to approach the topic. A student who cannot afford the class textbook might be uncomfortable explaining why they did not complete the assigned reading. Shy or depressed students may have trouble establishing new friendships or reaching out to borrow notes if they miss a class. In such cases, it could be easy to become marginalized and to struggle to find mattering in this new environment. This vulnerability presents an opportunity for you as a student to engage with others who are at risk of becoming marginalized. In helping them feel like they matter, chances are it will do the same for you.

Mattering in Clinicals

Entering the clinical environment for the first time is both exciting and intimidating. It is a student nurse's first opportunity to begin to apply all of the knowledge they have accrued, an opportunity to observe and learn from experienced nurses at the bedside, and a chance to interact with patients. In my experience as a medical student, it was also the time when I realized how much I still had to learn. As a student in the fast-paced environment of a hospital or clinic, you could feel like you are in the way or that asking questions identifies to your preceptor what you do not know. Or, you can enter the clinical environment seeking an opportunity to add value.

Clinical instructors and preceptors choose to work with student nurses because they are invested in your education. In addition to learning about physical assessment, medications, and the art of caring for another person, take a moment to learn something about your preceptor. Why did they choose nursing? What do they enjoy most about working with students? What is the most important thing they do in a day's work? Can your preceptor tell you about a time when they felt like they mattered? The answers to these questions will provide you with valuable insight into the profession of nursing and may provide a much-needed boost for your preceptor.

Clinicals also provide an opportunity to spend a few extra minutes with a patient. What can you learn about that patient as a person? Perhaps they could share with you what their experience has been with the illness or issue that brought them to the hospital or clinic. How is this experience affecting their life? What do they value most about the care their nurses provide? What advice would they have for you as a future nurse? Asking questions and taking the time to listen to the answers provides a valuable service to anyone, but is particularly important if a person is alone, confused, scared, or uncomfortable. You have the potential to make that person feel seen and heard and to show them that they matter. You can add value by helping that individual feel valued. You may also learn something that has been overlooked or not considered by the team caring for that person and can serve everyone involved by bringing that something to light.

As you participate in your clinicals, there will likely be times when you are the least experienced person in the room, but there are so many ways you can contribute. Your interest can inspire and energize your teacher. Your caring and compassion can make the difference for a distressed individual. As you learn, you can share your new knowledge with your classmates and listen to their experiences. There are many ways you can add value, and when you do, you will end the day with the knowledge that you mattered.

Mattering at Work

Before you know it, you will graduate from nursing school and find a position in a hospital, clinic, or office. You will again be building new relationships, this time with other nurses, interprofessional colleagues, and patients. This new job will be the first step in your career as a nurse, and this will be a new environment where you will strive to matter. Mattering at work is a relatively recent area of investigation, but the principles are similar. Each of us wants to add value and feel valued (Prilleltensky, 2020) in our profession.

The idea of mattering at work has been approached from a few different perspectives. Jung and Heppner (2017) suggested that mattering at work included two distinct components: interpersonal mattering and societal mattering. The interpersonal domain is based on the work that has already been discussed (Elliott et al., 2014, France & Finney 2009; Rosenberg & McCullough, 1981) but focuses specifically on relationships with coworkers and supervisors. *Societal mattering* represents one's sense of the value of their work as it contributes to society or meets a societal need.

Jane Dutton and her colleagues (2016) focused on a sense of social-valuing at work. In a very interesting study, they interviewed hospital custodians about their daily work and interactions with others (Dutton et al., 2016). The participants in their study discussed how the actions of others influenced their sense of whether or not their work was valued. In one discouraging case, a janitor discussed how a group of physicians consistently stood in his way each day as he tried to clean the floor despite the fact that he asked them several times to move so that he could complete his work. On the other hand, a different janitor spoke of a time that he was doubled over in pain and one of the doctors came over, addressed him by name, and asked about his symptoms and made some recommendations (Dutton et al., 2016). It is not difficult to guess which of these individuals felt as though he mattered and which one did not.

Reece et al. (2019) approached mattering at work from a different, action-oriented perspective. This group of researchers focused on achievement and recognition as the drivers of mattering at work. Based on previous work that demonstrated a strong correlation between self-efficacy and job satisfaction (Judge & Bono, 2001; Parker, 1998), they proposed that mattering at work occurs when your actions produce desired results. Reece et al.'s (2019) *achievement* is analogous to Prilleltensky's (2020) *adding value*. Similarly, the *recognition* component aligns with *feeling valued*. One critical difference between this work (Reece et al., 2019) and Jung's work (Jung, 2015; Jung & Heppner, 2017) is that it focuses on the impact of one's work at the organization level only and on recognition from peers and one's organization. Reece et al.'s (2019) assessment intentionally does not emphasize the affective contribution of relationships to mattering, nor does it consider the influence of one's work and its value to society.

Mattering in Nursing

How does mattering apply to your career in nursing?

My colleagues (Morela Hernandez, Natalie May, Courtney McCluney, Beth Quatrara, Valentina Brashers, and Sarah Ware) and I have been asking that question (Haizlip et al., 2020). Our work focuses on mattering in healthcare professionals: What does it mean, what creates it, how does it affect us? We believe that mattering at work may be particularly important for healthcare professionals, because this desire to positively influence others' lives is at the heart of our professional identity. Furthermore, if our hypothesis is true, not-mattering at work could lead to disengagement and burnout.

When we surveyed 324 nurses across the United States, we found that nurses who experienced higher levels of mattering reported that they also found more meaning in work; felt more supported by their peers, their manager, and their organization; and were more engaged (Haizlip et al., 2020). The nurses who had a higher sense of mattering also reported less burnout in their jobs. Unfortunately, a small number of nurses reported that they "can't remember the last time" they felt they mattered. This is what we hope to prevent.

We asked the nurses to share stories about when they felt like they mattered and heard a wonderful variety of answers. Most often, they described experiences with patients, but we also heard about pride in their professional expertise, the value of relationships with colleagues, the impact of being recognized by peers or the organization, and there were some stories when a nurse simply knew she had made a difference (Haizlip et al., 2020). Some examples include:

Experiences with Patients

> "When I have helped a child have fun and laugh so they forget they are in the hospital for a little bit." (R. 1218)

> "I had a patient thank me for getting her through a really rough time when she was very sick and thought she wouldn't make it. She told me what I had said to her stuck with her and it meant a lot to her. It makes all of the hard times I deal with worth it." (R. 1009)

> "When I brought a plate of Christmas dinner to a patient who didn't have any family and she cried." (R. 1214)

Professional Expertise

"A child for whom I was caring was restless, irritable and although her physical condition showed no overt signs of deterioration, both her mother & I felt that she was getting worse. I called the physician and he trusted me enough to come and see the patient even though I could not give him a specific reason for my concern. By the time he arrived, which was only a few minutes, the patient's blood pressure was dropping and she was going into cardiac failure. By that time, I had the crash cart in her room and had called the charge nurse so we were able to immediately initiate treatment and prevent an actual arrest. ... it could have gotten much worse if I had not been paying such close attention and called when I did. It mattered that I had been the one taking care of that patient at that moment in time and was able make a difference in her care." (R. 1227)

"I had a new mom who was scared to take care of her preemie baby. I worked with this mom every day to learn how to handle, bathe, and feed her baby. She turned into a confident, capable caretaker for her baby. It was so rewarding to see her grow and become the mom she needed and hoped to be for her baby." (R. 1132)

Relationships with Colleagues

"When I started noticing that the more experienced nurses were accepting me and had started including me as one of their own." (R. 1316)

"One day my coworkers said how happy they were to see me that day. They told me how much they enjoyed working with me and thanked me for all my help that day." (R. 1146)

"When my daughter passed and so many of my coworkers and supervisors showed lots of love and support." (R. 1258)

Recognition

"Every day the doctors thank me for my help with the patients."
(R.1123)

"I was asked to speak to the Joint Commission for my department's process and procedures. I was praised by my immediate supervisor and later received a personal handwritten note from the company's CEO thanking me for an outstanding job. I later found out the Joint Commission representative used me, saying my name, as an example of excellence when speaking to the CEO about her findings." (R. 1234)

Simply Knowing I Made a Difference

"Thankfully, I feel like I matter every day at work. I am here and do my job well, I am always willing and able to assist other nurses when needed and I go the extra mile for each of my patients"
(R. 1041)

"I have had many opportunities to help people cope with emergency situations. Any time that I can help with either physical or emotional help is meaningful to the patients." (R. 1004)

Regardless of their years in practice, their practice environment, the shift they worked, or the amount on their paycheck, almost all of the nurses we surveyed were able to identify a moment or some aspect of their work that made them proud, touched them, and was rewarding and memorable to them (Haizlip et al., 2020). These nurses know that they matter. As you read through these quotes, what stuck out to you? Did one of them, in particular, strike a chord? Or did many of them appeal to you for different reasons?

Pay particular attention for a moment to the quotes where a nurse just knew that he or she mattered. I encourage you to think about what might make you feel proud and valued in your work. How can you know you matter even in the absence of feedback from patients, colleagues, or the organization? While recognition or gratitude from someone else is always nice, being able to identify and appreciate your own mattering is an important skill that will help you find fulfillment in your work.

Closing Thoughts

Throughout a career in nursing, you will undoubtedly witness the broad expanse of the human experience. You will sit with individuals in pain and witness terrible suffering. You will temper anxieties and join in people's great joys and reliefs. You will experience awe in the strength of others. Nursing provides a unique window into the lives of others, and it is a privilege to be invited into those lives as a healer, an expert, and a companion. However, nursing is also a profession where you pay significant attention to what is or could possibly go wrong. There will be times you will face challenges with patients and with systems that leave you feeling defeated. If you are not careful, it is possible for the negativity to permeate into more realms of your life (Haizlip et al., 2012). It takes deliberate practice to focus on the positive aspects of your professional life.

When you experience moments of mattering, take note. Think about what

In Real Practice

In Woodley and Lewallen's (2020) qualitative study, the authors continue their previous work exploring and describing the lived experience of Hispanic/Latinx BSN students in the United States. They identify challenges these students face, in addition to the academic rigors of nursing school: simultaneously living in the two worlds of school and family, and the cross-cultural tension and stress they encountered in school. One of the students' "adjustment responses" found in this particular study was a deep sense of connection to their patients and families. One student said about a distressed maternity patient, "She wanted someone to hear her and...I was there to listen to her." With language and cultural knowledge, the students knew that they mattered in profound ways in their chosen profession.

occurred. Notice who was involved. Focus on your accomplishments. Consider your contributions and the value you added. Acknowledge what made you feel valued. Was it feedback from someone else? Can you appreciate what you did based simply on your experience? Savor those moments. Because as the respondent in our survey said, it is those moments that make all the challenging ones worth it.

Key Points

- Mattering is the product of adding value and feeling valued.

- A sense of mattering can result from and contribute to elements of well-being such as self-efficacy and perceived social support.

- Mattering manifests in all aspects of one's life—self, interpersonal relationships, communities, and at work.

References

Bandura, A. (1977). Self-efficacy: Toward a unifying theory of behavioral change. *Psychological Review, 84*(2), 191–215. https://doi.org/10.1037/0033-295X.84.2.191

Baumeister, R. F., & Leary, M. R. (1995). The need to belong: Desire for interpersonal attachments as a fundamental human motivation. *Psychological Bulletin, 117*(3), 497–529. https://doi.org/10.1037/0033-2909.117.3.497

Cohen, S., & Wills, T. A. (1985). Stress, social support, and the buffering hypothesis. *Psychological Bulletin, 98*(2), 310–357. https://doi.org/10.1037/0033-2909.98.2.310

Diener, E., Lucas, R. E., & Oishi, S. (2018). Advances and open questions in the science of subjective well-being. *Collabra: Psychology, 4*(1), 15. https://doi.org/10.1525/collabra.115

Dutton, J. E., Debebe, G., & Wrzesniewski, A. (2016). Being valued and devalued at work: A social valuing perspective. In B. A. Bechky & K. D. Elsbach (Eds.), *Qualitative organizational research: Best papers from the Davis Conference on Qualitative Research* (Vol. 3, pp. 9–52). Information Age.

Elliott, G., Kao, S., & Grant, A.-M. (2004). Mattering: Empirical validation of a social-psychological concept. *Self and Identity, 3*(4), 339–354. https://doi.org/10.1080/13576500444000119

Flett, G. L. (2018). *The psychology of mattering: Understanding the human need to be significant.* Academic Press/Elsevier.

France, M. K., & Finney, S. J. (2009). What matters in the measurement of mattering? A construct validity study. *Measurement and Evaluation in Counseling and Development, 42*(2), 104–120.

Haidt, J., Patrick Seder, J., & Kesebir, S. (2008). Hive psychology, happiness, and public policy. *Journal of Legal Studies, 37*(S2), S133–S156. https://doi.org/10.1086/529447

Haizlip, J., May, N., Schorling, J., Williams, A., & Plews-Ogan, M. (2012). Perspective: The negativity bias, medical education, and the culture of academic medicine: Why culture change is hard. *Academic Medicine, 87*(9), 1205–1209. https://doi.org/10.1097/ACM.0b013e3182628f03

Haizlip, J., McCluney, C. Hernandez, M., Quatrara, B., & Brashers, V. (2020). Mattering: How organizations, patients, and peers can affect nurse burnout and engagement. *JONA: The Journal of Nursing Administration, 50*(5), 267–273. https://doi.org/10.1097/NNA.0000000000000882

Judge, T. A., & Bono, J. E. (2001). Relationship of core self-evaluations traits—self-esteem, generalized self-efficacy, locus of control, and emotional stability—with job satisfaction and job performance: A meta-analysis. *Journal of Applied Psychology, 86*(1), 80–92. https://doi.org/10.1037/0021-9010.86.1.80

Jung, A.-K. (2015). Interpersonal and societal mattering in work: A review and critique. *The Career Development Quarterly, 63*(3), 194–208. https://doi.org/10.1002/cdq.12013

Jung, A. K., & Heppner, M. J. (2017). Development and validation of a Work Mattering Scale (WMS). *Journal of Career Assessment, 25*(3), 467–483. https://doi.org/10.1177/1069072715599412

Oxford English Dictionary. (n.d.). Matter. In *Oxford English dictionary*. Retrieved 2020 from https://www-oed-com.proxy01.its.virginia.edu/view/Entry/115085?rskey=aw05tS&result=3#eid

Parker, S. K. (1998). Enhancing role breadth self-efficacy: The roles of job enrichment and other organizational interventions. *Journal of Applied Psychology, 83*(6), 835–852. https://doi.org/10.1037/0021-9010.83.6.835

Prilleltensky, I. (2014). Meaning-making, mattering and thriving in community psychology: From co-optation to amelioration and transformation. *Psychosocial Intervention, 23*, 151–154. https://doi.org/10.1016/j.psi.2014.07.008

Prilleltensky, I. (2020). Mattering at the intersection of psychology, philosophy, and politics. *American Journal of Community Psychology, 65*(1–2), 16–34. https://doi.org/10.1002/ajcp.12368

Prilleltensky, I., & Prilleltensky, O. (2021). *How people matter: Why it affects health, happiness, love, work, and society.* Cambridge University Press.

Reece, A., Yaden, D., Kellerman, G., Robichaux, A., Goldstein, R., Schwartz, B., Seligman, M., & Baumeister, R. (2019). Mattering is an indicator of organizational health and employee success. *Journal of Positive Psychology*, 1–21. https://doi.org/10.1080/17439760.2019.1689416

Rosenberg, M. (1985). Self-concept and psychological well-being in adolescence. In R. Leahy (Ed.), *The development of the self* (pp. 205–246). Academic Press.

Rosenberg, M., & McCullough, B. C. (1981). Mattering: Inferred significance and mental health among adolescents. *Research in Community & Mental Health, 2*, 163–182.

Schlossberg, N. K. (1989). Marginality and mattering: Key issues in building community. *New Directions for Student Services, 48*, 5–15. https://doi.org/10.1002/ss.37119894803

Seligman, M. E. (2012). *Flourish: A visionary new understanding of happiness and well-being.* Simon & Schuster.

Woodley, L., & Lewallen, L. (2020). Acculturating into nursing for Hispanic/Latinx Baccalaureate nursing students: A secondary data analysis. *Nursing Education Perspectives, 41*, 235–240. https://doi.org/10.1097/01.NEP.0000000000000627

The Power of Purpose in Restoring Our Well-Being: A Conversation With Erik Pérez, OTD, OTR

Erik Pérez is a pediatric occupational therapist at the University of St. Augustine in Austin, Texas. He was drawn to the profession as a young man; his cousin was a certified occupational therapy assistant who "spent his career playing with kids!" As he learned more, Erik realized that this work could tap into "the creative aspect that I recognized was a strength of mine, but I could use that in a way that helped others."

When asked to describe exactly what an occupational therapist (OT) does, Erik quickly said, "We're problem solvers. It is about connecting people with things they want to do but that they think they can't." He explained that the term "occupation" refers to anything that people do, and our occupations fall into two categories—activities that serve a purpose, and activities that provide meaning. Purposeful occupations can include eating, drinking, sleeping, dressing, bathing, and exercise. These are activities that keep us alive and well, what OTs refer to as "activities of daily living."

The other bucket of activities, those that provide meaning, may include traveling, spending time with family and friends, and hobbies. For many of us in health professions, our work provides meaning. Some activities fall into both purposeful and meaningful categories. Erik said that for him, cooking for his family is one of these occupations. "I love to cook. Cooking is a way to nourish my family, to express my creativity, to show my love, and to connect with my ancestors."

Meaningful activities (or occupations) vary and are unique to each individual. One person may find hiking or rock climbing meaningful, and another may feel connected to the world through photography. From a self-care standpoint, Erik encourages us to identify those meaningful activities and make time and space for them in our lives. This is so important for our well-being. For those of us with demanding careers and multiple roles (nurse, parent, child, friend, spouse), it can be helpful to find ways to make purposeful occupations meaningful. In other words, if you have to do something anyway, find a way to make it meaningful.

This is where the problem-solver aspect of occupational therapists comes into play. Erik shared that because his work involved playing with children all day, it was often difficult to come home and play with his own children. This made him feel as though he was failing in his most important role of father. His solution was to recognize his own need to decompress before fully stepping into dad mode, and after work each day, he tries to spend about 30 minutes quietly alone before engaging with his family. This allows him to bring his best self to his wife and children.

Sometimes the problem of *how* to bring meaning to purposeful activities entails a bit of reframing, or cognitive reappraisal. For example, unlike Erik, you may consider cooking to be a chore. But if you can reframe the activity as a way to express your love for someone (including yourself), to bring people together at a meal, to express your creativity, or to learn a new skill, you have the ability to infuse a purposeful activity with meaning.

Another example could be your commute to work. If you have to walk quite a distance from where you park, you could reframe that journey as an opportunity to listen to music, connect with the world around you, or strengthen your body. Erik knows colleagues who use their commuting time to meditate and reflect. A palliative medicine colleague prays for his patients while he walks to his clinic. Erik also recommends that when you struggle to find meaning in your nursing work, take some time to reflect on why you chose nursing in the first place. Reconnect with your sense of meaning.

This underscores one of the core foundations of occupational therapy, a profession that came about when thousands of injured veterans returned home from war: a sense of purpose and meaning has the power to restore our well-being. As nurses and healthcare professionals, we help our patients do this all of the time, and Erik reminds us to be intentional about how we "reconnect to meaning" for ourselves.

21

Integrating a Life That Works With a Life That Counts

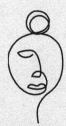

Dorrie K. Fontaine
pronouns: She/Her

Dorrie K. Fontaine, a critical-care nurse and teacher, has been an academic leader for four decades. While president of the American Association of Critical-Care Nurses, she observed the joys and struggles of bedside nursing. Meditation, yoga, and daily gratitude practice help her overcome the fears and anxieties of our common human existence.

"...what is it you plan to do with your
one wild and precious life?"

—Mary Oliver

There is a reason that nursing has been considered the most honest and ethical profession for 18 years in a row (Reinert, 2020). Consider this from the former dean of the Yale University School of Nursing, Donna Diers (2004):

> Nursing puts us in touch with being human. Nurses are invited into the inner spaces of other people's existence without even asking, for where there is suffering, loneliness, the tolerable pain of cure, or the solitary pain of permanent change, there is a need for the kind of human service we call nursing. (p. 143)

We have truly chosen a profession that puts service, often the care of vulnerable strangers, as a top priority in creating a life that counts.

As the continuing cycle of nursing shortages and burnout (National Academy of Medicine, 2019) demonstrate, nurses are a precious, if vulnerable, resource. During the COVID-19 pandemic, while nursing shortages existed in some geographic areas and specialties, other nursing positions were temporarily eliminated. Health systems furloughed some nurses and overworked others (Karlamanga & Mason, 2020). We have yet to fully grasp the impact of the pandemic (and other simultaneously occurring healthcare trends) on nursing attrition, retention, and recruitment into nursing education programs.

But this is what we know for sure: Society has a tremendous stake in not only educating nurses but in retaining them in the profession. As a nurse educator for most of my working life, I am well aware that societal issues have an impact on a nurse's well-being. But I also know that many nurses succeed in weathering many of these external forces by creating meaningful, purposeful lives that strengthen them. The strength comes from integration—the integration of their work, career, home, family, and personal pursuits (Whyte, 2009). In this chapter, I'd like to explore this process with you to help you find fulfillment and joy amid the many challenges of being a nurse.

Many business and organizational leaders have recommended employees strive to maintain a "work-life balance" in order to increase their well-being and satisfaction. They suggested that by keeping work and life in completely separate boxes we could improve our focus and productivity while protecting our personal time away from work. In fact, separation is nearly impossible. It's hard not to think about a patient you're worried about when you're falling asleep at night. It's hard not to worry about your sister who is struggling while you're entering information into a patient's chart. Sometimes work schedules and life's demands are not consistent or convenient. The notion of a work-life balance seemed like an almost cruelly impossible standard. Fortunately, a newer idea, that of integration, is taking hold because it can lead to synergy and authenticity without fostering a fractured lifestyle (Friedman, 2014). An integrated life may be attractive to nurses who desire a full life where multiple roles support each other, not compete, and lead to greater joy and happiness.

This chapter offers several ways to consider an integrated life where work and home, plus what we refer to as the life of the self, are intertwined to synergize, not compete, and lead to human flourishing. Salzberg (2014) refers to this as *real happiness* at work. Strategies that can lead to an integrated life are highlighted with examples and specific steps. The idea of composing a life, your life as a nurse, can be an intentional process to improve confidence in your chosen career, inspire optimism in all pursuits, and create an improved sense of well-being.

Choosing Nursing and Composing a Life

We chose nursing for a variety of reasons, including perhaps personal stories of survival or maybe receiving or observing exquisite compassion and caring from a nurse. Many of us have role models and family members in the healthcare professions. We may want to join a helping profession at a time of great healthcare need, like the COVID-19 pandemic, or we may hope for a career that will be sustainable physically, emotionally, and economically. Nurses, like others starting out in a new profession, imagine their life enriched by the work they will do, and most are also interested in having a full life. For those who chose nursing as a second career, bringing skills and experiences from another field, they too can enrich our profession and offer their valuable insight on composing a life. As we know, it is sometimes "messy" and not a straight path, but it can surely be rewarding in the end.

Making an Impact

–Reanna Panagides, BSN 2020 (she/her)

"It's been exciting to be part of this history, to be on the front lines. It's humbled me. It's a scary time and people are afraid, but also a time where people are coming together, and we are supporting one another. I'm honored to be playing a part. I think a lot about what I want to get out of life, and it relates to having an impact in a positive way on the world. I'm thankful to have found my way in nursing; it's one way I can impact the world. It's also a reminder that clinicians must keep full their own reservoir of resilience and well-being."

In composing a life, we often make choices that reflect our passion. By choosing the label, "I am a nurse," you make a statement to the wider world about the kind of person you are and want to be. Just announce to any stranger in the seat next to you on a plane that you are a nurse (or student nurse), and you will often hear very personal stories and be asked many questions. Even strangers, in only hearing the label "nurse," can understand that you must be a caring person and that you have probably developed wisdom in your training and experience.

Nurse is a label to be proud of, but it is not the sum total of your life. Anna Quindlen noted in a *Short Guide to a Happy Life*, "You cannot be really first-rate at your work if your work is all you are" (2000, p. 16). This may be why some brand nursing as a calling, not a job. Your decision to become a nurse will afford you endless opportunities to experience meaning and purpose in your work, but this choice can also have a tremendous positive impact on all aspects of your life. My own path into nursing began with a love of science, then a desire to work closely with people in need. I thought I might enjoy the intense interpersonal aspects that come with a nursing career. A high school friend applied to colleges for nursing, so I did, too. It was the best decision for me, the right match, and I am continually struck by the wonderful effect this decision has had on other areas of my life.

Being a nurse does have a profound impact on how we view the world. Several years ago, a nursing student at the University of Virginia, Monika Criman, received a University Award for Projects in the Arts to write a book compiling stories of the clinical experiences of third year (junior) nursing students. She asked the students to reflect on an experience that shocked them, touched them, changed their perspective, or reminded them why they chose nursing. As Monika points out in her introduction to the book, *This Journal Belongs to a Nursing Student*, these stories and poems will make you smile, cry, laugh, cringe, and maybe even make you want to become a nurse (2013).

It is no surprise that so many students shared an experience of birth and death in their stories for the book. Many also looked inward in search of the meaning of these natural processes and their own understanding of a nurse's role in these events. Why am I here? How do I best serve? How does this profound experience affect all areas of my life? That so many students recorded these moments of life and death meant that nursing, as Donna Diers noted, "puts us in touch with being human" (Diers, 2004, p. 143). As Dean of the school, I ordered a copy for every new nursing student each year. Their day one assignment was to read it and reflect on the journey ahead.

Choices in Composing a Nursing Life

Our lives in nursing are unique and complicated, or one could say, graced by multiple choices. They include many decisions, such as:

- First job: Do I want to work in a small community hospital or an academic healthcare center? Do I want a specialty of pediatrics, critical care, public health, or something else?

- Career: Do I want to be a nurse practitioner, or should I stay at the bedside and consider research or teaching later?

- Family: How far away are my parents, what is my commuting time, and what are my caregiving responsibilities?

- Friends/relationships: How do I find a committed relationship and partner, and should I have children, if at all?

- Personal interests or hobbies: How do I start and maintain an exercise program/yoga, join a community group and professional organization, and prioritize alone time?

Bateson (1990) refers to this envisioning process as composing a life, where life is seen as a work in progress and a creative one that engages us all at some point. Her stories about five women and their challenges in "composing a life" highlight the tradeoffs that occur. Bateson's message is a realistic but hopeful one that competing demands can somehow be enhancing. This is the beginning of viewing life in an integrated way.

There are as many ways to make these decisions as there are nurses, probably. We all know individuals who careen from one pursuit to another—college majors, jobs, relationships, or new hobbies—as their way of exploring and finding their way. Others very intentionally plot a path to a chosen career and life. Everyone relies on reflection about their experiences to greater or lesser degrees. Yes, life can throw us a curveball, upset our plans, and set us planning anew. This is what happened to Anna Quindlen in her sophomore year of college when her mother was diagnosed with cancer at age 41. Anna left college for a year to care for her mother until she died, and the experience changed her perspective on so many aspects of life, and therefore her path. Serendipity also plays a role in surprising and positive ways. But in general, most nurses give major thought to these key questions and decisions outlined above.

The Three Marriages

While the term work-life balance continues to be used frequently, it is considered a misnomer by those who advocate against this binary choice for an assumed ideal lifestyle (Friedman, 2014; Whyte, 2009). The hallmark of an integrated life is satisfaction with the various dimensions of how we typically evaluate and celebrate success in our lives. Nurses often envision and compose their lives hoping for a smooth integration of a work life, a home life, and what we may call a life of the self. We should give up the pretense of work-life balance as too simplistic. David Whyte, a poet and organizational development coach, suggests we focus on what he calls the "three marriages," a metaphor for the intense commitment embodied in each. He outlines the first as the real marriage of finding a partner or a significant relationship; next comes the work commitment; and finally, the self, including the bigger questions of meaning and purpose. These three engage each other and necessarily evolve and grow. Neglecting any one can lead to erosion of integrity and cause unhappiness. A central concept in this integration is the importance of belonging in all the intertwined "marriages" (work and home and self) and having a life you perceive as worth living.

Personal Perspective

Integration and Synergy Are Better Than Balance
—Haley Schlottmann, DNP, FNP-BC (she/her)

I have learned to adapt to job stresses as best as I can, and I like the word "integration" much better than work-life balance because work-life balance assumes they each operate in a silo irrespective of each other. Work-life balance assumes you either "have it" or you don't, but work-life synergy means there's a give and take, a reciprocity. Synergy means an ebb and flow, showing how increasing demands in one domain can lead to a reprioritization in the other domain, and that is OK, and should always be OK.

As a self-admitted perfectionist, synergy between work and home demands are difficult to grapple with, as it is nearly impossible to achieve truly perfect synergy at all times. I have slowly developed synergy in my life by accepting the things I cannot change and always focusing on a goal professionally (seeking clinical advancement, participating in a quality improvement project, or even setting a goal to search for jobs that *do* match my definition of a healthy work environment), and most importantly taking time away from work!

In order to bridge the "work silo" with the "life silo," self-care is important to allow room to feel vulnerability when one of these domains does not feel "right" and letting myself prioritize one over the other without guilt. Finding ways in which I begin to feel synergy again is useful to take inventory of, like practicing yoga, journaling, deep breathing, or even going for a walk. Even just intentionally putting a name to my feelings helps when feeling out of balance. Lastly, I achieve synergy by setting boundaries—when work demands feel too high, intentionally limiting time spent doing work at home, or when home life feels too stressful, intentionally working on ways to improve my professional self. Good friends and an impartial/unbiased mentor help more than anything!

In Whyte's Three Marriage model, the first "marriage" is the committed partnership, a relationship to be sought, nurtured, and celebrated. This forms a safe, protected place to be your authentic self and provides you with the confidence to venture out in the world each day to complete the second "marriage" goal of a committed work life. Using the empathy and compassion learned in nursing can make this work commitment a reciprocal one when an organization, for example a hospital, treats all staff with respect, kindness, and gratitude. The third "marriage" requires delving deeply into the self, coming to acknowledge wants, desires, and core values. Nursing is a commitment, both physically and emotionally; it also centers our entire being and identity.

One Hundred Thousand Hours at Work

We spend at least one hundred thousand hours at work during our lifetime, according to researchers Worline and Dutton (2017), who study work and organizational compassion. That is a pretty long "marriage"! After reading this statistic, I calculated my "life at work hours" as a startling 95,880 hours, working as a clinical nurse and professor, and that does not even include working as a nursing assistant through college. With these numbers, it is hard to imagine that your life at work can ever be completely separated from life at home.

Nurses are rewarded with a profession that gives meaning and great satisfaction. Even after a busy 12-hour shift, a nurse driving home can think back to the family member who was so grateful for the care they provided to a critically ill child, and it can cause a smile despite tiredness. As you have read in other chapters of this book, some nurses even briefly journal at the end of each shift to reflect on these moments. No matter how they transition from work to home, nurses tend to be perfectionists who often struggle with an internal critic who says, "You are not enough, you did not do enough, you did not respond quickly enough…" That's a lot of "not enough" rattling around in our heads.

Brené Brown (2010) writes of what she calls "imperfections as vulnerabilities" that we need to confront. Difficult to do, they can make us examine our intention and purpose and thus help us become our more authentic self.

According to Brown, choosing authenticity means what she calls wholehearted living by (2010, p. 50):

- Cultivating the courage to be imperfect, to set boundaries, and to allow ourselves to be vulnerable

- Exercising the compassion that comes from knowing that we are all made of strength and struggle

- Nurturing the connection and sense of belonging that can only happen when we believe we are enough

These important reflections on courage, vulnerability, compassion, and connection are some of the benefits of an integrated life and the synergy we seek.

Benefits of Integration

There are several reasons I encourage you to seek an integrated life. First, an integrated life reflects your authentic self by fostering clarity, meaning, and purpose. Second, this view of life invites an assessment, or self-evaluation, across multiple roles, giving you an opportunity to have many paths to achievement and success. Finally, integration fosters well-being, joy, and happiness (Achor, 2010).

Integration Reflects the Authentic Self

Being yourself and letting others see you as you truly are will help you build a keen sense of belonging and confidence. When you view your life as integrated, it invites others to see your strengths *and* the struggles that make you more human and approachable. This requires humility, even vulnerability. But all nurses wish to feel a sense of belonging, whether in relationships, a clinical unit, or in other social groups.

Imagine hearing as you walk on the clinical unit, "I'm so glad you're here today. Now I know we're going to have a good day." This remark, coming from an authentic place, makes you feel valued, respected, and engenders reciprocal feelings. It's easier to feel kindly toward someone who is kind to you, and this is one reason why kindness and the vulnerability inherent in it can make for better work environments. People who can reveal themselves, who they really are, are helping to create a more humane workplace.

We crave workplaces where kindness is visible, not just signs on the walls that tout a workplace is a compassionate one (Worline & Dutton, 2017). We have the capacity to create compassionate workplaces by being open and responsive with our colleagues, beginning with our own honest and authentic reflections. If a colleague speaks sharply to you, you might reflect on how that made you feel, but also what may have caused it to happen in the first place. Is your colleague having a bad day? Has something happened at home? Leveraging our capacity to reflect, be curious, and offer grace creates compassion in our work "marriage."

We can create synergy by bringing, in a good way, our home life and pursuits to work through authentic conversations. Just as we yearn to get to know our patients as people, not just as a diagnosis or medical record number, so we can enrich our relationships with our peers. Nurses who value compassionate collegiality will go out of their way to learn about their fellow team members, not in a gossipy way, but in a supportive one. Who has a special needs child, or an ailing mother in another state? Who is getting married in a few months? Who plays in a bluegrass band on Saturday night, and who wants to go with us to hear them?

These conversations open up all sorts of possibilities for connection and belonging. It is delightful to learn that a nurse colleague is also a marathon runner, animal shelter volunteer, or a published poet. The "slash" career professional is a wonderful identifier—think of nurse/clown (one of our editors is a leader in the Clowns Without Borders organization), nurse/singer, nurse/rower, and others (Brown, 2010). Friendships form and strengthen as colleagues rely on each other in difficult clinical situations but with this added bond, knowing you see and care about their authentic selves.

Similarly, speaking at home to your friends, family, or partner about your work and work colleagues will allow these members of your life a chance to better understand the intensity and demands of your other "marriage." Of course, it is important to never violate patient privacy, but reflecting aloud about the joys and challenges you are experiencing at work is an act of vulnerability that reveals who you are as a nurse and professional. By being authentic in *all* of your relationships, you will bring work, relationships, and your true self together in synergy, allowing each "marriage" to enhance the other.

Integration Offers Multiple Ways to Achieve Success

In this integrated approach, you are not "grading" yourself only on how you perform as a clinical nurse, a friend or partner, parent, or whatever other roles you embody. You have multiple ways to view success and achievement. When life in one area is trending downward, like friends moving away or a relationship changing, you may be energized at work by being given challenging assignments, being promoted up the clinical ladder, or attending a motivating conference. Integration leads to many ways to chart progress toward your own varied goals. Being upset by disappointment in any role is normal but can be temporary and offset by the other aspects of life that bring solace, perspective, and enjoyment.

Integration Fosters Well-Being, Joy, and Happiness

Because we spend so much time at work—recall that figure of 100,000 hours—it is natural to look for ways to enhance well-being, joy, and happiness there. The Institute for Healthcare Improvement's (IHI) project on creating more joy at work has seen positive results (Feeley & Swenson, 2016; Perlo et al., 2017). I believe well-being, joy, and happiness can flow naturally into all aspects of our life.

I found this to be true when the University of Virginia School of Nursing joined an IHI Joy in Work Prototype pilot project in 2017 (Feeley & Swenson, 2016; Perlo et al., 2017). In an eight-week rapid cycle improvement project, six nursing faculty and staff, who were also members of the standing Healthy Work Environment committee at our school, voluntarily came together weekly and followed a set process along with 13 other hospitals and organizations. IHI provided a coach and weekly sessions. The commitment involved choosing a problem to fix, something they called, "What is a pebble in your shoe?"

The IHI framework for improving joy in work consists of these four steps (Feeley & Swenson, 2016; Perlo et al., 2017):

Step 1: Ask staff, "What matters to you?"

Step 2: Identify the unique impediments to joy in work in the local context.

Step 3: Commit to making joy in work a shared responsibility at all levels.

Step 4: Use improvement science to test validated approaches in your organization.

The pebble in our shoe, which is step one above, was too many emails. The surprise intervention was to simply stop them on weekends and after 5 p.m. during the work week. As Dean, I was the skeptical one, but after encouraging faculty and staff to keep their emailing traffic within work hours, the results showed a record 80% satisfaction for faculty and staff after a few short weeks. There were still emails flowing after hours, but there was no expectation for us to view them and respond until we returned to our desks. Even in my retirement, I still receive feedback about the joy of email-free weekends from my former faculty and staff.

Limiting email may not work in a busy clinical setting, but it taught me that small changes can have a tremendous impact, demonstrate respect and caring, and even translate into other aspects of our lives. What simple change can you consider making at home, for example, that might seem impossible but could greatly improve your happiness and joy? There are many strategies to strengthen integration and create synergy in life.

Strategies for an Integrated Life

There are many ways to begin paving the way for an integrated, joyful, meaningful life as a nurse. I will close this chapter with a few suggestions, but I encourage you to keep your eyes and ears open for new ideas. There are more and more resources available to you in books, podcasts, mindfulness apps, professional conferences, free online courses, and more. Seeking and constructing the life you desire will be a lifetime pursuit for you, I hope.

Know Yourself

The first step to an authentic, integrated life is self-assessment, or paying attention and noticing those qualities and beliefs that make you uniquely you. In his book, *The Happiness Advantage*, Shawn Achor (2010) defines *self-assessment* as being honest, facing facts, knowing what you are good at, and boldly claiming your signature strength. Self-reflection and making time for introspection can come from a mindfulness practice and possibly a retreat, slowing down to be fully present, and journaling to understand your own values. What is nonnegotiable for you? How would you like to be remembered? If you overheard someone talking about you, what would you want them to say? Being free to reveal yourself to others comes from surety that you deeply know and accept your true self. The importance of self-awareness is a common theme throughout this book and is essential to developing an integrated life (Worline & Dutton, 2017).

Seek Support

Nursing offers the opportunity to join groups outside of the routine support you strive for and hopefully receive from family, friends, and social groups like a book club or church choir. Because nurses specialize right away in their first job, they have the opportunity to investigate and become a member of that nursing specialty organization. Joining can have the benefit of not only creating a sense of belonging, but offering education and support for nurses like you. As you will read in the following sidebar, I joined a professional organization four decades ago that became my "professional home."

American Association of Critical-Care Nurses (AACN) as My Professional Home

–Dorrie K. Fontaine, PhD, RN, FAAN

I joined AACN four decades ago as a new nurse in critical care. A nurse in my ICU said she was going to a meeting at a local hospital and I should come along. That began a long relationship with AACN from attending local and regional meetings, becoming certified, joining and leading chapters, speaking for the first time on a clinical topic (scary), and eventually being elected to the board of directors and then becoming the national president. AACN is the largest specialty nursing organization in the world. I went from giving small talks in local hospitals to speaking in front of 10,000 nurses and exhibitors at the National Teaching Institute. Most importantly, the nurses I met have become lifelong friends. My entire family knows many of these nurses because they visit regularly, and we are in each other's lives as mentors and friends.

Offer Support to Others

To receive support, you first must give it to others. Nurses at work who maintain an awareness of all their team members and their needs and stressors are ones who foster respect and a sense of belonging. In their book *Awakening Compassion at Work,* Worline and Dutton (2017) revealed the importance of this to hospital housekeeping staff who often felt invisible and ignored. It has been a strange "benefit" of the COVID-19 pandemic that we now appreciate hospital housekeeping staff more acutely. We all should feel like we matter at work, as we discussed in the previous chapter of this book.

In my years as a professor and Dean, I was always so pleased to observe the kindness and support nursing students offer to one another, their friends, and their families. Continue to make this effort and maintain relationships with family and friends, even long-distance. Maintaining relationships near and far can keep you feeling socially connected and supported when you need to belong to something besides your job. I'm a big fan of handwritten cards, which may be old fashioned now, but they do provide tangible joy to the loved ones in your circle. Saying yes to volunteer groups in the community is another way to support others while simultaneously widening your own social circle.

Offer Gratitude to Yourself and Others

Gratitude practices have been discussed in this book, and they are so important in creating an integrated, authentic life. Begin with loving-kindness for yourself, and then widen that gratitude circle to include your work, family, and friends. This practice is paramount as you strive to create a meaningful life (Salzberg, 2014). Each night or morning, simply write down three things you are grateful for. As you read in Chapter 3, a gratitude can be as simple as a hot cup of coffee or a walk with a friend. J. Bryan Sexton, a psychiatrist and researcher at Duke University, is just one scientist studying this idea with patients as well as clinicians (Sexton & Adair, 2019). His findings lend support to the effectiveness of this simple intervention; he has found that in as few as 15 days, the practice can generate a "wow" factor of gratitude and hope. And as we have discussed throughout this chapter, taking the time to verbally thank someone for their hard work, a specific kindness, or support is one way to reveal your authentic self.

Use Kindness as Your Default Response

This is not always easy, but it gets easier with practice. Begin by paying attention and noticing what those around you may need. You probably already do this well for your patients, so it may simply involve flexing this muscle a bit more broadly. It is difficult sometimes to listen to others' opinions and then pause before reacting or speaking. It is not easy to assume positive intent or consider a more generous interpretation when someone hurts or offends us. And I must add that not all "intents" are positive, as in the case of racism, sexism, or homophobia, for example. We must still respond to these behaviors in ways that align with our values and integrity and in ways that do not further harm the victims of these remarks.

George Saunders (2014), in a convocation speech at Syracuse University years ago, spoke of regrets in his life. His number one regret: failures of kindness. He tells a story from third grade, when classmates bullied a little girl every day and he stood by and did nothing. Saunders suggests that throughout our lives, we have periods of high kindness and low kindness. His advice: Increase the periods of high kindness.

Develop a Spiritual Discipline

This does not mean religion in a strict or traditional sense but rather a habit of deep reflection on meaning and purpose that is truly at the heart of why we chose nursing. Examination of the self and having a frequent connection to your deepest heart can be accomplished with mindfulness, meditation retreats, or time in nature. Some choose yoga or other methods like keeping a journal to connect to their inner lives. As a basis for an integrated life, there is no substitute for staying in touch with our spiritual essence, our core beliefs, and the ways we make sense of the often random and seemingly senseless world around us.

Cultivate a Healthy Work Environment

Finally, just as we wish and plan for a loving home and family environment, we should strive to have this in our work setting as well. In Chapter 17 we explored the importance of choosing a first nursing job in a place that embodies the qualities of a healthy work environment. We spend so much time at work, and our experiences in that space have an impact on *our lives* as well as those of our patients and families.

Once you find yourself in a supportive clinical setting, then it is important for you to cultivate practices that will help sustain this positive environment. Practice kindness, notice the needs of others, be curious about your coworkers, be grateful, express vulnerability, and be authentic in your interactions. The benefits will be reaped beyond the boundaries of your work life—they will flow to your home and social lives as well.

In Real Practice

Twenty nurses and physicians in pediatric critical care were interviewed about their personal self-care strategies (Wei et al., 2020). Results demonstrated that finding meaning in work, being positive, and nurturing connections with others were among key strategies. Having a life well integrated suggests that work that inspires you and strong relationships can help prevent burnout. Nursing students can use this data to remind themselves why they went into nursing and to continue to find ways to focus on friends and family despite the pressures of school.

Closing Thoughts

An integrated life does not mean that you design a life made up of neat, tidy compartments cut off from one another. Instead, use the interconnectedness of your three marriages—work, home, and self—to complement and support one another. A bad day at work can be balanced by joy at home. Experiencing compassion at work is a gift you can bring home to the ones you love. Gratitude and kindness are ingredients that can be sprinkled throughout.

An integrated life is an authentic life. Knowing yourself and being vulnerable enough to share your authentic self with others will lead to improved well-being, more joy at home and work, and greater meaning in your life.

"Get a life, a real one," Quindlen (2000, p. 16) encourages us. A real life is one filled with love, generosity, and paying attention to small things and savoring the joy they bring. Could this not be an antidote for perennial nursing shortages? Could it lead the way to stemming the tide of burnout? Could it lead to a stronger nursing workforce and a healthier citizenry? I hope that you will try to find out.

Key Points

- The concept of an integrated life is more realistic and attainable than the previously used goal of work-life balance. The metaphor of the "three marriages"—work, home, and self—underscores the importance and sacred nature of each part of our lives.

- The goal of an integrated life is to improve and sustain your well-being, foster more joy at home and work, and enhance your meaning and purpose in life.

- The key to an authentic life is your own authenticity and being able to share your authentic self with those around you. Often sharing who we truly are requires courage and vulnerability. One benefit of sharing your true self with others is stronger, more meaningful relationships.

- Strategies to create an integrated life include knowing yourself, giving and receiving support, practicing gratitude and kindness, developing a spiritual discipline that is appropriate for you, and cultivating a healthy work environment.

References

Achor, S. (2010). *The happiness advantage.* Crown Business.

Bateson, M. C. (1990). *Composing a life.* Plume.

Brown, B. (2010). *The gift of imperfection.* Hazelden.

Criman, M. (2013). *This journal book belongs to a nursing student: A collection of reflective writings.* University of Virginia School of Nursing.

Diers, D. (2004). *Speaking of nursing...Narratives of practice, research, policy, and the profession.* Jones & Bartlett.

Feeley, D., & Swenson, S. J. (2016). Restoring joy in work for the healthcare workforce. *Healthcare Executive, 31*(5), 70–71.

Friedman, S. D. (2014). *Leading the life you want: Skills for integrating work and life.* Boston: Harvard Business School Publishing.

Karlamangla, S., & Mason, M. (2020). Thousands of healthcare workers are laid off or furloughed as coronavirus spreads. *Los Angeles Times.* Retrieved November 2020 from https://www.latimes.com/california/story/2020-05-02/coronavirus-california-healthcare-workers-layoffs-furloughs#:~:text=In%20California%2C%20thousands%20of%20nurses%2C%20doctors%20and%20other,Care%20to%20tiny%20rural%20hospitals%20to%20private%20practitioners

National Academy of Medicine. (2019). *Taking action against clinician burnout: A systems approach to professional well-being report release event.* https://nam.edu/event/taking-action-against-clinician-burnout-a-systems-approach-to-professional-well-being-report-release-event/

Perlo, J., Balik, B., Swenson, S., Kabcenell, A., Landsman, J., & Feeley, D. (2017). *IHI framework for improving joy in work.* http://www.ihi.org/resources/Pages/IHIWhitePapers/Framework-Improving-Joy-in-Work.aspx

Quindlen, A. (2000). *A short guide to a happy life.* Random House.

Reinert, R. J. (2020, January 6). Nurses continue to rate highest in honesty and ethics. *Gallup.* https://news.gallup.com/poll/274673/nurses-continue-rate-highest-honesty-ethics.aspx

Salzberg, S. (2014). *Real happiness at work: Meditations for accomplishment, achievement, and peace.* Workman Publishing.

Saunders, G. (2014). *Congratulations, by the way: Some thoughts on kindness.* Random House.

Sexton, J. B., & Adair, K. C. (2019). Forty-five good things: A prospective pilot study of the Three Good Things well-being intervention in the USA for healthcare worker emotional exhaustion, depression, work-life balance and happiness. *BMJ Open, 9*(3), e022695. https://doi.org/10.1136/bmjopen-2018-022695

Wei, H., Kifner, H., Dawes, M. E., Wei, T. L., & Boyd, J. M. (2020). Self-care strategies to combat professional burnout among pediatric critical care nurses and physicians. *Critical Care Nursing, 40*(2), 44–53.

Whyte, D. (2009). *The three marriages: Reimagining work, self, and relationship*. Riverhead Books.

Worline, M. C., & Dutton, J. E. (2017). *Awakening compassion at work: The quiet power that elevates people and organizations*. Berrett-Koehler.

Second-Career Nursing: "I Wanted to Be a Happy Nurse"

A Conversation with Susan Goins-Eplee, MSN

When Susan Goins-Eplee tells you that her career as a hospital chaplain was the best preparation for nursing, it makes perfect sense. As a chaplain-turned-nurse, Susan has wisdom to share with all nurses, but especially older ones. Accelerated programs for second-career or second-degree nurses have become an effective means of addressing the nursing workforce shortage, and factors that ensure their work success and satisfaction is another facet of self-care.

The chaplaincy taught Susan about the importance of boundaries. "I grew up in the South," she says. "I was a good Southern woman. I had a lot of progressiveness in my life, my family, and my church, but the idea of limits and boundaries is very difficult for women of my generation. I grew up trying to please everyone, not wanting to upset anyone or make anyone angry. My chaplaincy training challenged me to my core. A supervisor said to me at one point, 'There is nothing that is unspeakable.' I grew up in a world where *everything* is unspeakable! I eventually learned that there's a way to be compassionate, caring, empathetic, *and* honest, and that has been so important in my nursing. I think honesty in the healthcare setting is so refreshing. With our patients, we want so many things to be unspeakable, but hard things need to be spoken."

As a chaplain, Susan honed her boundary-setting skills and even modelled those behaviors for her patients. Despite possession of these newfound skills that included the fine art of saying "no" and going home when her shift ended, she experienced a devastating episode of burnout during her chaplaincy. In addition to her work and the distress of caring for cancer patients, she was also a wife, a mother to two girls, and her parents' daughter. It was during this crisis that she learned the importance of having a supervisor who kept her best interest at heart. Her supervisor sent her to employee assistance and wholeheartedly supported her leave of absence.

The idea of becoming a nurse had nagged at Susan for nearly three years. When she finally told her boss, she said, "'I am thinking about it, but I want to be a happy nurse.' He knew exactly what I was talking about. Because I knew happy nurses, and I knew miserable nurses. I made up my mind that I was only going to do this if I was the kind of nurse who loves her work and gets a lot of satisfaction out of it."

Susan has managed to find satisfaction in her work, but she admits it's not always easy. One thing she learned in the chaplaincy was to "separate the person from their behavior." She explains, "Patients are in pain. They're scared. After I had my own cancer diagnosis a couple years ago, I learned that most of our bad behavior comes from fear and being afraid. Everyone we take care of is afraid, and they act out in pretty horrible ways. And I think a lot of nurses take that personally. Because I had some pretty specific training that went all the way back to clinical pastoral education, I recognize how that's about *them*, not about *me*. That seemed to really help."

She underscores the importance of self-care. "We always rise to the occasion better if we're rested, well-fed, balanced, happy. These are the days when we can be our best selves. When we don't react out of our best selves, we get caught up in that little dance we do with our patients, and we take things personally. We get wounded when we're not at our best. I still have to work on this quite a bit, but when I find myself getting impatient or frustrated, I know to sit with a manager or a trusted friend. Just talking it out helps a lot."

Susan confesses that sometimes it's harder to deal with her physician colleagues, and she uses the same mindset. "I have to remember that an intern or a resident is scared, and sometimes they are coming across all puffy and arrogant, and the truth is that on the other side of that arrogance is a scared person. Just like I'm scared when I'm in a situation where I don't know what to do."

She has also found some assets, even gifts, that as an older nurse, she can bring to her work. When patients are making end-of-life decisions, for example, she can name what others are feeling. She can say to her nurse colleagues and the resident, "This is really bothering me, too." There may be something comforting, she thinks, in hearing the emotions named and spoken by a woman old enough to be their mother. "That's when I'm a happy nurse," she says, "when at the end of the day I realize I didn't just get frustrated. Who knows what everyone is carrying in their backpack? This is hard for me, too. This creates a bridge, not a wall."

Susan has also learned the value of asking for help, especially as a new nurse. She observes that new nurses now go through a three-month orientation period, but she says, "The first thing I'd want new nurses to know, it's not like when you come off orientation there's a magic switch and you know everything you're supposed to know!"

"I know this happened to me," she continues. "I came off my first day of orientation, and maybe they were hazing me a bit, but I had patients spread out all over the unit. One patient had a brand new trache, just out of the ICU, and blood was all over the place. I didn't know what to do, but I tried to figure it out on my own. By the end of the day, I was crying, and my preceptor saw me and said, 'Why didn't you tell me you needed help?' Well, I didn't know I could do that!" Susan laughs when she tells this story, but it's not hard to imagine what a horrible day that was.

"Ask for help. Absolutely."

Susan is 55 years old. She's been a nurse for 12 years, and she says, "I still have to ask for help. Maybe that's one of the things that happens along the way, you realize there's never a time you don't need help. You're never going to know everything. Ever. But we have so many people we can turn to for help—doctors, our nurse colleagues, managers, chaplains, ethics consult services— they are all here because they want to help. It is OK to ask these people to help us."

Reflecting on her position as an older, second-career nurse, Susan acknowledges that she is in many ways different from her younger colleagues. "I'm slower with technology," she says. "And I'm not as quick on the uptake. Those young whippersnappers can hold so much new information, but we older people already have so much in our brains! So sometimes they see us as moving slower and making more work for them." She sees that a lot of older nurses leave the bedside, and respects that each older nurse should trust their instincts and make the decision that is right for them. "But we really do need to keep older nurses at the bedside. You lose all that learned experience when they're not there."

Her other advice for her older peers is to be sure to rest on your days off. "If you do 12-hour shifts, you're not going to last if you're not using those four days off a week to really care for yourself. If I work two 12-hour days in a row, I just have to know I'm taking the next morning off. I sit there with a cup of coffee and stare at stuff. I need to know that next morning will be free. As 'doers,' which most of us are when we're in the medical profession, it's hard to give ourselves permission to do nothing, but it's so important."

Susan's best advice? Find a manager or leader who has your best interest at heart. Ask for help. Trust your instincts. Rest. Choose a job that you can manage; be honest about your limitations. Take deep breaths.

"When I was growing up, I was always very sincere about wanting to help people. I never ever have a doubt that I'm making a difference in someone's life. It is an opportunity to care for people in an incredibly profound and intimate way, and if that's what you value, then I don't know of any better way to do it than nursing. I never walk away from a day at work thinking, 'I wonder if I helped somebody today?' Sometimes it's such a tiny thing, it's remembering to get their diet order in on time so they get their dinner that night. There are big ones, too. Like someone who says, 'I'm tired. I don't want to do this anymore. Would you help me talk to the doctors? I'm ready to stop this treatment.' That's a huge moment. You get that moment not because you've been there for 20 minutes. You've been there for 12 hours and maybe even the day before, or the week before. I never have any doubt in my mind that I have the opportunity to make a profound difference in the lives of people. If that's what's important, and it is for me, that's what makes me a happy nurse."

22

Providing Compassionate Care and Addressing Unmet Social Needs Can Reduce Your Burnout

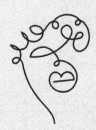

Susan B. Hassmiller
pronouns: She/Her

Sue Hassmiller speaks before national audiences about the future of nursing, nursing leadership, and health equity. After spending the last 10 days of her husband's life with him in the intensive care unit, Sue advocated for better patient care and published a memoir, *Resetting: An Unplanned Journey of Love, Loss, and Living Again.* She found love again with Lewis Sandy and takes great joy in hiking, the theatre, and her grandchildren, Abby and John.

"If you want others to be happy,
practice compassion.

If you want to be happy,
practice compassion."

—Dalai Lama

Florence Nightingale, the founder of modern nursing, believed that nursing was a calling and that nurses should be attuned to the needs of patients (American Association of Critical-Care Nurses, 2019). Many choose the nursing profession out of a deep desire to help others. Yet, with the passage of time, many nurses become overworked, exhausted and unhappy—and they may no longer feel connected to the passion to serve that initially led them to become caregivers (Dempsey, 2018). According to the RN Work Project, a Robert Wood Johnson Foundation–funded study that followed nurses for 10 years, nearly 18% of nurses left their first job after one year (Brewer & Kovner, 2012). The loss of purpose and passion is distressing for nurses who no longer feel as fulfilled in their profession. It also negatively affects the patients and families for whom they care: Patient satisfaction levels are worse in hospitals with more nurses who are dissatisfied and burned out (McHugh et al., 2011). It is imperative, therefore, to prevent and address nurse burnout.

The Virtuous Cycle of Compassionate Care

One important way to prevent nurse burnout is for clinicians (with facilitation from their healthcare organizations) to be able to provide compassionate care to patients and their families, including opportunities for nurses to address their patients' unmet social needs. *Compassionate care* means "sensitivity to suffering in self and others with a commitment to try to alleviate and prevent it" (Gilbert & Choden, 2013). Compassion is a virtuous cycle: The more you understand about patients and their families and the context in which they live, the more you will be able to care for them—and the more satisfied you will feel for helping them (Dempsey, 2018). To underscore the importance of compassion, Christina Dempsey, the chief nursing officer at Press Ganey, developed a compassionate connected care model. The model teaches nurses to acknowledge the suffering of patients and their families and use nonverbal and verbal communication to express compassion, to reduce anxiety, to facilitate patient and family autonomy, and to help coordinate and anticipate care (Pittman, 2019). After all, it only takes a clinician about 56 seconds to develop a connection with a patient or family member and make them feel valued (Dempsey, 2018).

How to Establish a Connection in 56 Seconds

Start by introducing yourself and asking the patient what they prefer to be called. Make sure it is a good time for the patient. Let them know that you are up to date on their care. Then ask them what they like to do when they aren't in the hospital. Listen to their response for an aspect you can connect with: perhaps they'll mention a hobby, pets, or loved ones. Once you have established a small personal connection, you can explain to them what you plan to do (perform an assessment, get their medications, speak with the medical team).

Research shows that patient and caregiver satisfaction are connected. When workplaces reward compassionate acts and support staff during tough times, more patients rate the care they experience highly (McClelland & Vogus, 2014). Similarly, when nurses recommend their place of work, patients are also more likely to recommend the organization to others (Dempsey, 2018). Clinicians who feel compassionately treated by their organization and each other say that they are more robust, creative, and open (Cole-King & Gilbert, 2014). When caregivers are engaged, they feel that they belong, that they provide good care, and that they contribute meaningfully (Dempsey, 2018). In other words, nurses who give to others receive benefits in terms of their own resiliency and job satisfaction.

Compassionate care includes understanding the context in which the patient and family members live. We know that medical care alone is not enough to improve health; meeting people's nonmedical needs is equally important. Health is greatly influenced by nonmedical factors that affect communities, such as access to jobs that pay a living wage, safe housing, reliable transportation, walkable neighborhoods, good schools, fresh food, and adequate green spaces (Braveman & Gottlieb, 2014).

Nurses should consider the following questions: Does the patient have enough food to eat? Do they live in an apartment with good ventilation? Is it safe for them to exercise outside? If falling is a risk, does the patient have to climb stairs on a regular basis? A growing number of health organizations recognize that medical care alone is not enough to improve people's health. In fact, where people live and work, their income, their education level, and other factors have as much, or more, influence on their physical, mental, and emotional well-being as their access to healthcare. Evidence shows that 80% of health outcomes are due to behavioral, social, economic, and environmental factors in a person's life, while actual medical care impacts just 20% (University of Wisconsin Population Health Institute, 2014).

Nurses, who spend the most time with patients and their family members, are well-positioned to help (Reinhart, 2020). In fact, nurses across the United States already help individuals tackle nonmedical needs every day—from assisting with housing, to arranging ride-shares so patients can get to appointments, to advocating for other patient needs (Robert Wood Johnson Foundation, 2019). Interviews with more than 500 US nurses conducted in 2018 by the Robert Wood Johnson Foundation showed that most nurses say they want to help people meet unmet needs, but they don't necessarily have the time or institutional buy-in to do so. Giving nurses the tools to be able to help patients and their families meet unmet social needs could help patients and their families live healthier lives and to experience greater well-being *while also* reinvigorating nurses' sense of purpose and calling.

Compassionate Care Above and Beyond

Examples abound of nurses providing compassionate care and addressing unmet social needs. Darris Bohman, BSN, CEN, for example, noticed that many of the emergency department patients at TriHealth Bethesda Butler Hospital in Cincinnati returned repeatedly for care, and she suspected a high rate of unmet social needs. Many of the patients were eligible for Medicaid, and the area had a known lack of primary care—one way through which patients could connect with needed social services (Werrlein, 2019).

She and a colleague, Jennifer Williams, BSN, RN, CEN, established the Community Connection Center, where nurses and other students from Miami University of Ohio screened emergency department patients using a questionnaire from the Centers for Medicare and Medicaid Services. They found that nearly 30% of patients did not have enough to eat, and up to 43% of patients reported at least one unmet social need (Werrlein, 2019).

A "Win Moment"

–Danielle (Dani) Giaritelli, BSN, RN (she/her)

I work in the Acute Respiratory Intensive Care Unit (ARICU) and was encouraged by my colleagues to write about this "Win Moment."

A really special experience I had was a patient experience with a mom and her son, both suffering from COVID. Both were patients in our unit at the same time, three rooms apart. The mother, near death, was on a heart-lung machine called extracorporeal membrane oxygenation (ECMO), chemically paralyzed, and in liver failure. Her son, who had been near death at one time, had also been chemically paralyzed and proned (positioned onto his stomach). But he began to recover and was now near discharge to acute rehab. I got the privilege to care for both of these patients on separate occasions, as well as getting to know the family. The day of the plan to remove the mother from life support, I was able to ask the son if he wanted to see his mom one last time. We placed him in a converter chair and were able to bring him to be with his mother before she passed.

This experience was overwhelmingly emotionally, but also so incredible. As I wheeled the son back to his room, I couldn't help but stand in his room as I cried. As difficult as that moment was, it also reminded me why I became a nurse. For these moments, one life passed, but another just had a miraculous recovery. And how incredible it was to be able to bring him to his mother to see her one last time. As I sat there, overwhelmed with mixed emotions, my eyes filled with tears, I told the son that recoveries and moments like this are the reason I became a nurse. And even in the most difficult days, this is why we keep showing up, no matter the circumstance, to make differences such as this one.

The son was set to go to acute rehab. Because he needed long-term ventilation support, he had a treacheostomy, but he was able to speak with a special valve and I got to know him more, now that we could talk back and forth. A week after his discharge the most special thing happened. The son (the patient) called the unit and had asked to speak with me (Dani, as my peers know me). I was not on the unit, but received a text from the charge nurse that said the patient had called and asked for me and said to thank me for the care and "make sure Dani knows I walked 100 feet in rehab."

I read this text and began to find myself with tears again, as I was so touched by this. It was another reminder that in the midst of chaos or uncertainty, what we are doing makes a difference and is the reason we are able to continue providing patient- and family-centered care.

Bohman and Williams reached out to several local social service organizations, including the Supplemental Nutrition Assistance Program office and the Butler County Homeless Coalition, to share information, develop relationships, and spread the word that the emergency department could serve as an access point for social services. Patients who reported an unmet social need received a list of local organizations that included the hours of operation, contact information, services provided, and documents needed to qualify. Noting that staff are excited about having more tools to support patients, Bohman says, "We have better interactions with the population we serve, so patient and provider satisfaction are both up" (Werrlein, 2019, para. 13).

Helping Patients With Many Unmet Social Needs

Megan Williams, MSN, RN, CNL, offers another example. Williams helps patients with complex care needs improve their health and reduce healthcare costs as the program manager of ONE Health, a partnership between Regional One Health, a hospital in Memphis, and the Camden Coalition, a nationally recognized care intervention for individuals with complex health and social needs. ONE Health works with a network of 250 community groups across the region to enable chronically ill, uninsured patients to navigate the health system and connect with social services (Vaida, 2019). The goal is for patients to get healthier and visit the hospital less. As of mid-July 2019, ONE Health had aided more than 200 uninsured patients after illness and socioeconomic problems led them to repeatedly seek help in the emergency department or hospital bed. In its first eight months, ONE Health resulted in 69 fewer inpatient admissions and 156 fewer emergency visits and had a total benefit to Regional One Health's bottom line of $1.95 million (Vaida, 2019).

Williams finds the work rewarding: "This work is a calling for me," she says. "I just want to love on people that haven't had enough love in their lives. Everyone needs an advocate who understands the complexity of the systems and has the heart to help them" (Vaida, 2019, para. 11).

Rush Medical Center and Food Insecurity

Rush Medical Center in Chicago makes it easy for nurses to screen for food insecurity and other needs through its Food Is Medicine program. When a patient is admitted, a nurse asks a standardized set of screening questions about housing insecurity and access to food, primary care, and transportation that appear on the electronic medical record system that the hospital uses (Rush Medical Center personal communication, February 7, 2020). If the patient demonstrates a need, the nurse can click twice in the computer system to refer the patient to programs that can assist with unmet social needs. The programs reach out to patients after they return home to connect them to services in their community. Patients with demonstrated food insecurity also receive a grocery bag packed by volunteers to take home once they are discharged (Rush Medical Center personal communication, February 7, 2020).

Questions That Rush Medical Center Nurses Ask Patients About Their Unmet Social Needs

When a patient is admitted to Rush Medical Center, a nurse asks the following questions as part of the patient's initial assessment. If the patient indicates a need for help, the nurse can click a button on the electronic health record to refer the patient to social services.

1. Do you have a doctor (primary care physician) or nurse that you see regularly?

2. Do you have health insurance or a medical card?

3. Are you worried that your food will run out before you have money to buy more?

4. In the last 12 months, have you run out of food that you bought and didn't have money to get more?

5. In the last two months, have you had difficulty paying your electric, gas, or water bill?

6. Do you have a hard time finding transportation to and from your medical appointments?

7. Do your currently have a place to stay/live?

8. In the next two months, will you have a place to stay/live?

Source: Rush Medical Center, Personal Communication, February 7, 2020).

Profile of Laurie Ouding

RN, LNC (she/her)

Laurie Ouding, RN, LNC, a pediatric staff nurse at Rush Medical Center, believes that asking patients and their families about their unmet social needs has helped to address the systemic reasons why patients are in the hospital (L. Ouding, personal communication, February 14, 2020). In the following passage, she explains how that has contributed to a greater feeling of satisfaction in her work.

Why did you become a nurse?

There were several nurses in my family, including my aunt and grandma. I saw how nurturing and compassionate they were. I've always wanted to help others, and nursing was a good fit.

What are some of the challenges related to unmet social needs that you see as a nurse?

I work on the pediatric floor at Rush Medical in Chicago. Every day, I see nutrition-related illnesses. There's been an increase in the number of kids admitted with obesity and malnutrition, diabetes at a younger age, and kids so chronically constipated they are hospitalized for invasive treatment—all related to poor nutrition and a more sedentary lifestyle than ever before. Treating the results of food inequity and a lack of nutrition knowledge in the hospital or doctor's office is not working, as evidenced by these kids suffering on a daily basis.

How are you helping to meet unmet social needs?

Our floor participates in the Food Is Medicine program. We ask eight questions when kids are admitted to our floor as part of our initial assessment (see sidebar above). If patients and their families answer that they are worried their food will run out before they have a chance to buy more, our electronic medical record will automatically refer them to a food pantry in their neighborhood and contact social service organizations to follow up with them when they return home. Hospital volunteers also give them a grocery bag filled with food to take home with them.

How do you fit this into your work?

Nurses are busy, but our admission assessment takes five extra minutes, and we are addressing issues that improve health. Before, we were only putting a bandage on the problem of hunger. Am I willing to take five extra minutes to help someone? Absolutely.

How does asking about unmet social needs and addressing these issues make you feel in terms of overall job satisfaction and well-being?

It's given me the tools to actually do something to address a problem rather than a symptom. My job satisfaction and well-being are higher.

My Experience With Compassionate Care

I believe that nurses can provide two types of compassionate care—meeting unmet social needs and understanding the patient and family on a personal level. Both are important. You can ask, "What matters to the patient?" rather than, "What is the matter with the patient?" I speak from personal experience. In September 2016, my husband and soulmate, Bob, was in a serious bike accident. I spent the next ten days by his side—the tubes and machines separating us—as his condition steadily deteriorated and his systems failed one by one. My family and I made the heart-wrenching decision to remove him from life support and let him go.

Two nurses, Abby and Kathy, stood out for their compassion. They held me up when I could not stand, and they provided the empathy I desperately needed. Abby, the receiving trauma nurse anesthetist, told me how devastated she felt by what had happened. She hugged me and said she wished that she could take my pain away. Afterward, she reached out to me. She described what an extraordinary person my husband was in the face of a life-threatening accident and how the two of them communicated with one another—and how the event changed her own life by causing her to question her own priorities and to be more passionate. To know what transpired between her and Bob would never bring Bob back, but it gave me a sense of peace that there was a human being whose spirit and touch connected in a very profound way at a very important time.

Kathy was one of the ICU nurses who cared for Bob. She paid attention to our pictures on the bedside stand, asked about our personal lives, and shared some of hers. She offered to drive me home one evening during a rainstorm after her shift ended. Kathy placed her CD player next to Bob and inquired what kind of music he liked after touching his upper shoulder and face—the only places where he still had feeling. She moved his paralyzed body to one side so that I could lie next to him. When the time came to turn off Bob's machines, Kathy stayed way beyond her shift's end until Bob's heart stopped beating. She made me feel that it was her honor and privilege to stay with me. She hugged me and touched me, and I will never forget her.

Abby told me later that caring for Bob reinvigorated her own life. "There was no box to check off afterward, no deadline to meet, but the personal reward was well worth the effort," she said. "I am blessed to work in a position where I can be acutely reminded of how precious life is, and how powerful small acts of kindness are." Seeing our relationship made her question whether she was living without regret and holding back in important ways. Abby says she made radical life changes, including meeting and marrying her husband, whom she met while traveling in Iceland with "an awakened soul." She says that she is "committed to delivering competent, compassionate care and forging meaningful, beneficial relationships with patients and their loved ones" (A. Karlsson, personal communication, September 2019). She and Kathy share their wisdom about providing compassionate care in the following section.

Our Tips for Providing Compassionate Care

Wisdom from Abby Karlsson, CRNA, and Kathy McLernan, RN, the two nurses who cared for my husband, Bob. Abby states:

"As healthcare professionals, we are so fortunate to have careers that offer the most important kind of job and soul satisfaction by allowing us to connect with others and help our fellow man in times of need—take advantage of this and do the little things!"

1. Find something that connects you to the patient to develop trust.

2. Communicate to the patient's family with compassion and empathy.

3. Treat your patients like you would your own family members.

4. Include as a measure of your success whether you can make your patients smile.

5. Take care of the whole patient.

6. Hold the patient's hand, speak the reassuring words, and get the granola bar.

7. Stay in touch with someone you have bonded with and let this relationship continue to be a healing one.

Interview with Elizabeth Métraux:
Nurses as Catalysts for Change
(she/her)

Elizabeth Métraux is a writer, researcher, and founder of Women Writers in Medicine. Formerly at the helm of communications for the National Institutes of Health's Office of Workforce Diversity, Elizabeth has spent the last decade traveling throughout the country studying how to create a more fulfilled, inclusive, and purpose-driven clinical workforce. She currently leads clinician-centered community building efforts for Optum, the nation's largest employer of healthcare professionals.

Q: In this chapter, readers learned about nurses who have taken the initiative to address social determinants of health among their patients. These nurses have established food pantries for their patients and linked them to social services in the community, for example. You have conducted research and listened to nurses' and other clinicians' stories for years. How do you see social and structural determinants of health affecting their well-being?

A: I've traveled to nearly every state in the nation studying the experiences of clinicians. I've cried with providers after mass shootings. School nurses have shared the impact of hunger, addiction, and domestic violence on students in their classrooms. I've seen providers take a knee for Black victims of police brutality and stand arm-in-arm with mothers at the US-Mexico border as they beg for their children to be released from detention facilities. There aren't prescriptions for the kind of trauma that nurses and their patients absorb on a daily basis.

When the public refuses to act on policies that would mitigate human suffering, clinicians assume responsibility for addressing the consequences of that inaction. Truth is, it's impossible to separate the well-being of providers from the pain endured by patients. Research shows that the conditions that show up in the clinic are driven by issues that have nothing to do with medicine; they're social, rooted in economic and educational disparities, racism, and health behaviors (Artiga & Hinton, 2018). If we're serious, then, about healing our communities, we need to get serious about addressing the social causes that lead individuals to hospitals and lead healthcare workers to despair.

Q: This is a book about self-care for student and early-career nurses. What advice would you give an early career nurse encountering patients who are literally the faces of these social and systemic national failures? Are they doomed to experience burnout as they valiantly care for these vulnerable patients?

A: This is what I would tell them: You've found your calling, now find your voice—and your people. Author David Kessler (2019) has posited that following the five stages of grief, there's a sixth: meaning-making. It's imperative that wellness practices go beyond

continues

continued

individually focused exercises like journaling and exercise and extend to include agency-building efforts like advocacy and legislative action. If you enjoy journaling, consider turning an entry into a letter to the editor. If you have a knack for oration, lend your time to municipal and Congressional testimony. Share your expertise by engaging with community structures such as school boards, city councils, task forces, and nonprofits. Join professional organizations that engage in advocacy and policy change, such as the American Nurses Association or Partners in Health. There are many examples of clinicians launching campaigns like White Coats For Black Lives, VoteHealth 2020, social media messages like #thisismylane, and countless movements that aim to influence policy that has a direct effect on health.

To start, it's a great idea to find a few colleagues that share your passion and just start getting together. Small affinity groups can go a long way to cultivating the relationships that are essential to collective action and personal wellness. Consider monthly dinners, a book club around topics of social justice, or periodic storytelling nights that give clinicians a space to share their concerns. Invite expert speakers who are knowledgeable about social issues or who are experienced changemakers. In time, your cohorts will become your allies in advocacy.

Maya Angelou said, "There is no greater agony than bearing the untold story." As we grieve the preventable hardship experienced by our patients and about which medicine offers few avenues for recourse, we have an opportunity to turn those stories into powerful calls to action. In doing so, we can transform our moral distress into a catalyst for change.

In Real Practice

Compassion is always at the heart of what we do, but we know there are countless ways that compassionate care can be diminished. The COVID-19 pandemic has certainly shown us the power of compassion, but also its fragility when nurses and others face threats on multiple levels. Hofmeyer et al. (2020) present nine strategies for organizations to embrace in order to foster and strengthen their healthcare workers' ability to provide compassionate care, even under the most challenging circumstances. The strategies, which include harnessing effective leadership and cultivating community at work, might best serve as the gold standard of support at all times, not just during global crises.

Closing Thoughts

Over the course of our careers, most of us will need to be reminded periodically of the calling we felt to choose nursing and to impact others. After I began speaking publicly about the importance of compassion, several nurses approached me after my talks and said, "You can't give what you don't have." But as St. Francis so aptly notes, "It is in giving that we receive." The more that you understand about patients and their families and the context in which they live, the more you will be able to care for them, and the more satisfied you will feel. My hope is that you will provide exceptional clinical and compassionate care, including addressing the unmet needs of patients and their families.

Key Points

- An important way to prevent nurse burnout is for healthcare organizations to facilitate clinicians in being able to provide compassionate care to patients and their families, including opportunities for nurses to address their patients' unmet social needs.

- Compassion is a virtuous cycle: The more you understand about patients and their families and the context in which they live, the more you will be able to care for them—and the more satisfied you will feel for being able to help them.

- Patient and provider satisfaction are likely to increase when clinicians provide compassionate care and address unmet social needs.

References

American Association of Critical-Care Nurses. (2019, April 24). *A conversation with Florence Nightingale*. https://www.aacn.org/nursing-excellence/nurse-stories/a-conversation-with-florence-nightingale

Artiga, S., & Hinton, E. (2018, May 10). *Beyond health care: The role of social determinants in promoting health and health equity* [Issue brief]. Henry J. Kaiser Family Foundation. https://www.kff.org/disparities-policy/issue-brief/beyond-health-care-the-role-of-social-determinants-in-promoting-health-and-health-equity/

Braveman, P., & Gottlieb, L. (2014). The social determinants of health: It's time to consider the causes of the causes. *Public health reports*, *129*(1_suppl2), 19–31. Available at https://journals.sagepub.com/doi/abs/10.1177/00333549141291S206

Brewer, C. S., Kovner, C. T., Greene, W., Tukov Shuser, M., & Djukic, M. (2012). Predictors of actual turnover in a national sample of newly licensed registered nurses employed in hospitals. *Journal of Advanced Nursing, 68*(3), 521–538. https://doi.org/10.1111/j.1365-2648.2011.05753.x

Cole-King, A., & Gilbert, P. (2014). Compassionate care: The theory and the reality. In S. Shea, R. Wynyard, & C. Lionis (Eds.), *Providing compassionate healthcare: Challenges in policy and practice* (pp. 68–84). Routledge.

Dempsey, C. (2018). The antidote to suffering: How compassionate connected care can improve safety, quality, and experience. *Press Ganey Associates.* https://nmonl.wildapricot.org/resources/Documents/NMONL_The%20Antidote%20to%20Suffering%20FINAL.pdf

Gilbert, P., & Choden, K. (2013). *Mindful compassion: Using the power of mindfulness and compassion to transform our lives.* Constable-Robinson.

Hofmeyer, A., Taylor, R., & Kennedy, K. (2020). Fostering compassion and reducing burnout: How can health system leaders respond in the Covid-19 pandemic and beyond? *Nurse Education Today, 94,* 104502. doi:10.1016/j.nedt.2020.104502

Kessler, D. (2019). *Finding meaning: The sixth stage of grief.* Scribner.

McClelland, L. E., & Vogus, T. J. (2014). Compassion practices and HCAHPS: Does rewarding and supporting workplace compassion influence patient perceptions? *Health Services Research, 49*(5), 1670–1683. https://doi.org/10.1111/1475-6773.12186

McHugh, M. D., Kutney-Lee, A., Cimiotti, J. P., Sloane, D. M., & Aiken, L. H. (2011). Nurses' widespread job dissatisfaction, burnout, and frustration with health benefits signal problems for patient care. *Health Affairs (Project Hope), 30*(2), 202–210. https://doi.org/10.1377/hlthaff.2010.0100

Pittman, P. (2019, March 12). *Activating nursing to address the unmet needs of the 21st century: Background paper for the NAM Committee on Nursing 2030.* Robert Wood Johnson Foundation. https://publichealth.gwu.edu/sites/default/files/downloads/HPM/Activating%20Nursing%20To%20Address%20Unmet%20Needs%20In%20The%2021st%20Century.pdf

Reinhart, R. J. (2020). Nurses continue to rate highest in honesty, ethics. *Gallup.* https://news.gallup.com/poll/274673/nurses-continue-rate-highest-honesty-ethics.aspx

Robert Wood Johnson Foundation. (2019). Unpublished audience research. "In Their Own Words: Nurse Insights on the Unmet Needs of Patients." Princeton: RWJF.

University of Wisconsin Population Health Institute. (2014). *County health rankings key findings.* Robert Wood Johnson Foundation. https://www.countyhealthrankings.org/sites/default/files/2014%20County%20Health%20Rankings%20Key%20Findings.pdf

Vaida, B. L. (2019, September). For the uninsured in Memphis, a stronger safety net. *Health Affairs, 38*(9), 1420–1424. https://www.healthaffairs.org/doi/full/10.1377/hlthaff.2019.00999

Werrlein, D. (2019, January 23). *By asking questions, nurses see beyond emergencies.* Campaign for Action. https://campaignforaction.org/by-asking-questions-nurses-see-beyond-emergencies/

23

Showing Up With Grit and Grace: How to Lead Under Pressure as a Nurse Clinician and Leader

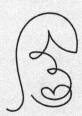

Elizabeth A. (Lili) Powell
pronouns: She/Her

Throughout her career, Elizabeth A. (Lili) Powell has been fascinated by the ways human beings make meaning, influence others, and accomplish worthy goals together. Resilience, communication, and leadership thread through her academic travels—from rhetorical and performance studies to business education and now to nursing, focusing on compassionate care. To replenish her own grit and grace, Lili meditates and runs, reads and writes, practices and teaches yoga, and ponders the curiosities of life with others.

"You gotta have a servant's heart to be a good nurse; and you've got to be able to see the world as having the potential to be better than it really is to lead forward and up."

—Megan Tribble

Learning the ropes. Cutting your teeth. Paying your dues. Earning your stripes.

Embedded in these idioms are truths about the experience. Let's face it. Traveling the path from a student nurse into a fully minted professional marks an arduous and significant transition. Although each skill is different, the experiences of learning, nursing, and leading have at least one thing in common: performing well under pressure.

As you have read in this book, self-care can take many forms, and by now you understand self-care isn't all bubble baths and chocolates. In this chapter, self-care takes the form of cultivating two inner resources that are especially well suited to showing up and leading well—grit and grace.

In all fairness, you won't learn these skills in an instant, for they are truly a lifetime's work. But today you can get started, or start again. In this chapter, you will learn how to:

- Envision leading with grit and grace

- Understand the challenges of managing yourself while leading under pressure

- Picture the inner and outer dimensions of showing up

- Learn from Manny's leading mindfully story

- Try specific practices that grow grit and grace

What Are Grit and Grace?

You may have heard expressions like "she exemplifies grit and grace" or "he leads with grace under pressure." But what are grit and grace, and where do they come from? And what difference do they make for showing up?

Leadership coach Cari Coats sees a leader's capacity for grit and grace as essential. Citing Merriam-Webster, she explains that "grit can be defined as 'firmness of mind or spirit; unyielding courage in the face of hardship or danger.' The definitions of grace include ease of bearing and 'disposition to or an act or instance of kindness, courtesy, or clemency'" (Coats, 2019, para. 3). She also asserts that the synthesis of grit and grace sets leaders—especially women leaders—apart. Coats acknowledges that like leadership presence, leading with grit and grace is enigmatic, but we know it when we see it.

> It's the [leader] who commands the room simply with her presence. She's poised under pressure and able to handle strong-willed people in an author-itative, yet respectful way. She's confident, self-aware and very comfortable in her own skin. Her strength of character and humility drive her actions. She's a woman who knows who she is and is able to exercise authority with the appropriate warmth and empathy (Coats, 2019, para. 9).

For budding nurse clinicians and leaders, the good news is that both grit and grace can be cultivated through practice. For example, as you read in Chapter 2, grit involves working passionately and consistently over time toward a long-term goal (Duckworth, 2016). Though grit may be associated with grand accomplishments, it can also come from small everyday actions that help you feel a greater sense of agency, determination, and vitality (Hanson, 2018). Think of grit as both the prac-tice and the result of renewing your passion and perseverance.

For example, suppose you hit a stumbling block on a project at school or work. You feel stuck and want to relieve your frustration. At that point you have a choice: 1) pull out your phone and check social media and get sidetracked for the rest of the day or 2) take a deep breath or a brief walk and then try a different approach to overcoming the obstacle. The latter is more likely to build grit because it builds your ability to delay instant gratification, take constructive action, stick with your focus and goal, and actually figure things out (Clear, 2018). Over time, practicing grit tends to bring a greater sense of happiness and well-being (Duck-worth, 2016).

Spiritual and contemplative teachers have long maintained that grace may be culti-vated through prayer and meditation. In psychology, grace has been studied under other terms such as kindness, giving, generosity, altruism, and compassion, all of which imply an expression of care. Caring, of course, is central to nurses' calling to comfort patients; however, nursing and positive organizational studies scholars find that expressions of care also benefit leadership and organizations in work settings (Watson, 2006; Worline and Dutton, 2017). In the context of leading under pressure, kindness is a capacity that needs to be replenished to prevent or skillfully manage fatigue and burnout (Fontaine et al., 2018). Compassion with self-awareness and equanimity also prevents one's ego from taking over and turning into "toxic altruism" (Halifax, 2018).

Imagine grace then as grounded altruism, or care with calm and composure. While you may adopt a formal practice such as prayer or meditation, grace can also be practiced in small everyday ways. One of my favorites is to approach small daily courtesies as an opportunity. For example, adopting an attitude of goodwill while holding the door for a mom struggling with a stroller or striking up a genuine conversation with a cashier about her cat earrings can transform an otherwise empty gesture or transaction into a real human connection that brightens someone else's day, and mine too. Note that a practice like this takes no additional time. It only requires a different conscious mindset and an openness to receive a momentary gift of humanity.

Grit and grace become even more powerful when combined. Though they sound paradoxical, gritty grace and graceful grit have a certain feel. For instance, a colleague who works as a palliative care liaison refers to the "fierce compassion" needed in his work. He calls on the strength of his commitment to grace to continue to treat a patient as a human being and not the machines attached to them, and he calls on grit with compassion to help families and patients make difficult decisions such as withdrawing life support (J. Bartels, personal communication, 2017).

Grit helps you shift from fog into focus and determination. Grace helps you shift from overwhelm into calm and care. Combined and cultivated through mindful practices, grit and grace can grow in you over time so you can use them at a moment's notice. The result is surfing the highs and lows of performing well under pressure. By doing this inner work, you can then translate your gains into helping your team grow their grit and grace too, as you'll see in a story later in this chapter.

The Challenges of Managing Yourself While Leading Under Pressure

Crises bring leadership moments into high relief. During the COVID-19 pandemic of 2020, nurses and other healthcare workers responded under daunting conditions. Amplified by extreme risks to caregivers' own physical, emotional, mental, and spiritual health, nurses showed up to do the seemingly impossible. "The Wounds Are Still Fresh," a short video documentary published through *The New York Times,* vividly illustrated the toll on clinicians (Hapangama et al., 2020), while commentaries such as "Stigma Compounds the Consequences of Clinician Burnout During COVID-19" drew national attention to the sometimes deadly hazards of burnout (Feist et al., 2020).

You may have worked during this outbreak, or like many others marveled at those who did. Perhaps nurses' grit and grace during this crisis inspired you to go to nursing school.

Given the stressors of working as a nurse, it helps to remember that your own body plays an important role. Remember that the body's stress response throws your sympathetic nervous system into high gear before you can even name what is happening. Your primal brain becomes flooded with neurotransmitters as your blood rushes adrenaline throughout your body to fight, flee, or freeze. You may understand intellectually that while this primitive survival response is natural and adaptive, your role as a nurse demands that you don't give into it completely. Instead, you need as much of your prefrontal cortex and executive function as you can get, plus muscle memory and physical dexterity to move into compassionate action (Bergland, 2013; Haglund et al., 2007; Singer & Klimecki, 2014).

When you need to perform with great skill, an unregulated survival response or "prefrontal takeover" could harm your ability to perform (Bergland, 2013; Hougaard & Carter, 2018). So, it stands to reason that freaking out won't serve you, your team, or your patients particularly well. What may be less apparent, however, is that while you perform, you are also leading, because others are consciously and unconsciously picking up on your cues. Whether or not you and others are aware of it, how you show up in the moment leads others through the power of *your* example.

Knowing all this helps to make some sense of why fight, flee, and freeze feel like such involuntary responses. However, managing your stress response in the moment is not an *intellectual* problem to be solved. It's an *experiential* one to be managed.

Self-Care During the COVID-19 Crisis

What does leading under pressure look like? A new nurse manager working during the COVID-19 crisis described how she used self-care to regulate the way she showed up:

> Each day as I enter the hospital, I take a deep breath, not knowing what I'm going to encounter during that workday. It's a feeling that brings initial trepidation, but through mindfulness I've channeled that energy into grit and determination. It's easy to get caught up in the frenzy and become unfocused in the chaos, but one thing I've learned is to take the day [one] hour at a time. When I feel overwhelmed, I remind myself why I went into the profession. I wanted to make a difference, help others, and provide purpose (Cathcart, 2020, p. 20).

Notice that she makes a series of inner moves. She feels and recognizes her initial physiological response. As a ritual, she takes a deep breath to calm her nervous system. But she doesn't stop there. She uses *mindfulness*—that is, paying attention with an attitude of open curiosity and goodwill—to channel her energy into grit and determination so she can act skillfully when she goes into work. She also manages her own attention, shifting from awareness of the frenzy and chaos to one hour at a time. This perceptual shift makes her experience more manageable. She stays attentive to her feelings of overwhelm as they arise but remembers her values and purpose to steady herself so she can move forward effectively with grace, or grounded compassion, for herself, her team, and their patients.

This nurse manager understands a paradoxical truth: Caring for herself in this pressure-filled moment simultaneously serves others and the mission to alleviate suffering. In her example, we see that self-care is not an escape from stress, but rather is a means to move through stress skillfully and respond more effectively. Her wisdom rests on a foundation that recognizes the essential interdependent and dynamic relationship between inner experience and outer behavior.

Leading Mindfully: A Model for Showing Up

Would-be and newer leaders often focus on acting the part, but that is only half of the showing up equation. Think about how you read your own leaders. Like most, you watch their behavior for deeper clues (and often reassurances) of what they really know, believe, or feel. In other words, you want to gauge the leader's *ethos*, or your perception of their trustworthiness (Aristotle, 1926). When a leader's inner experience and outer behavior appear to be in sync, we think of them as "credible" or "authentic" and open ourselves to their influence (Halpern & Lubar, 2004). So the work of showing up needs to be understood as more than skin deep.

For example, issues arise when inner experience and outer behavior appear out of sync. From the leader's point of view, suppose you had to give a big speech. You may fear public speaking. Or you may not believe in the message you have to give. Either way, think how hard you would have to work to appear confident or believable on the outside. And even if you managed to mask your real feelings, you might feel like (and risk looking like) a big phony. From the audience's point of view, suppose you were watching a leader give that speech and detect that something doesn't seem quite right. Perhaps the anxious delivery does not match the speaker's words. Or the leader's past actions don't seem consistent with what he or she is saying now. As a result, you doubt the leader's credibility or authenticity.

In these ways and more, the interplay between the inner and outer dimensions of showing up represents a learning priority for bringing the two into harmony. To visualize the dynamic connection between a leader's inner experience and outer behavior, Figure 23.1 depicts an infinity loop that links the two.

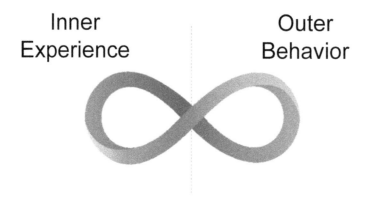

FIGURE 23.1   Foundation of leading mindfully.
Note: Inner experience and outer behavior are mutually connected and dynamic throughout a given moment.

This diagram forms a basis for what my colleague, Jeremy Hunter, and I call "Leading Mindfully" (Powell & Hunter, 2020). We use the active verb "leading" to highlight leadership as an active practice. We use "mindfully" to refer to the qualities of mind and action developed through traditional mindfulness, as well as other contemplative and active practices. (To learn more about the variety of contemplative practices, see the Center for Contemplative Mind in Society: http://www.contemplativemind.org/.)

As we explain in our article for "Leader to Leader":

> With this approach, leaders learn to improve their ability to inquire into themselves and manage their inner experience so that they can act and interact more effectively in the world. They can move from a simple awareness of inner experience and outer behavior while leading to practicing "inner moves" and "outer moves" that result in better choices and better results. . . . Skillful action then becomes a basis for skillful interaction and coordinated action [with a team] toward a common goal, which of course is what leadership is really all about. (Powell & Hunter, 2020, p. 54, 57)

In sum, your ability to lead mindfully begins with adopting mindful practices first for yourself. With experience, qualities that mindful practices encourage—improved awareness, focus, open curiosity, goodwill, and compassion—begin to translate into better choices, words, and actions that reflect these qualities. Through your example, these qualities can influence the work culture of your team. In time, you may also improve your team's collective attention and shared ability to work together with such mindful qualities. For the long term, the intention is to inspire your team to apply awareness, focus, open curiosity, and compassion to pursue worthy goals at work and in the world (Hougaard & Carter, 2018, Powell & Hunter, 2020; Sutcliffe et al., 2016).

Manny's Leading Mindfully Story

One day during an interprofessional course I teach called "Leading with Presence in Healthcare," a student's comment brought the issues of performing well under pressure and leading mindfully alive. Though he was able to learn eventually how to manage the inner and outer experience of leading mindfully, he needed first to understand how to deal with his work stress. The student, who for confidentiality I'll call "Manny," was a graduate nursing student who also worked fulltime in a critical care unit. When I asked students what caused their own work stress, Manny said in a monotone, "My every day is my patient's worst-ever day."

When I asked Manny what he meant, he explained that for his patients and their families, the experience of staying in an ICU was among the worst-ever days of their lifetimes. But for Manny, helping people in their situation was his everyday reality. In many ways, the pressures of his job were taking a toll on him. Unfortunately, Manny felt so burnt out after only two years on the job that he was considering whether he wanted to leave nursing altogether.

If anyone needed to learn how to manage his stress so he could perform well under pressure, it was Manny. In a sense, he was applying too much grit without enough grace. Part of the trouble was that he expected himself to perform every day like a sports car that never runs out of gas. And yet, of course, that's not humanly possible. Manny knew this *intellectually*, but he did not yet believe it *emotionally*.

So he kept up this belief and the work and life habits that went with it, in spite of evidence to the contrary.

No matter their profession, most people have a story they live by that shapes their attitude and behavior toward work (Scott, 2019). In Manny's case, this story ran deep. As the son of immigrants from Guatemala to the United States, his parents and he had bought heavily into the American Dream. He also gained deep personal fulfillment from being a nurse. With a tendency toward perfectionism, encouragement from his upbringing, and, as it turns out, norms in his workplace, Manny believed "the harder you work, the better you will perform." This work ethic bled over into his attitude about nursing: "The more I care and sacrifice for others, the better nurse I will be." Taken to an extreme, Manny was treating his body, emotions, mind, and spirit like a perpetually running machine.

But the human body is not a perpetual machine. Even a person who wants to train for a marathon learns this. The standard advice for marathon training goes something like this: Work up to running a few miles three to four times a week. Every seven to 10 days, go for a long run. Increase your distance slowly over time. Mix in speed work, intervals, and tempo runs to increase cardio capacity. Work in adequate rest and recovery to prevent physical injury and mental burnout (Winn, 2018). Contrary to the way many professionals actually work, elite athletes understand that alternating exertion and recovery are essential to their ability to perform at high levels over time (Groppel, 1999). Otherwise, they run the risk of sidelining themselves due to injury.

Minding the Illusion-Reality Gap

To illustrate the gap between popular belief and physiological reality, look at Figure 23.2. This graph shows how levels of performance quality vary with levels of arousal, psychologists' term for energy or stress (Gino, 2016). Manny's belief or *perpetual machine mindset* is represented by the straight line—"The harder I work, the better I'll perform." But the actual relationship between performance and arousal is represented by the bell-shaped line. This line, known as the

Yerkes-Dodson curve, means that performance is optimal at moderate levels of arousal. Not enough arousal, and performance suffers. Too much arousal, and performance suffers. The goal then is to experience some stress to improve performance, but not too much (Gino, 2016). People who understand this relationship tend to have a mindset that is reminiscent of Stoic philosophy's adage, "All things in moderation."

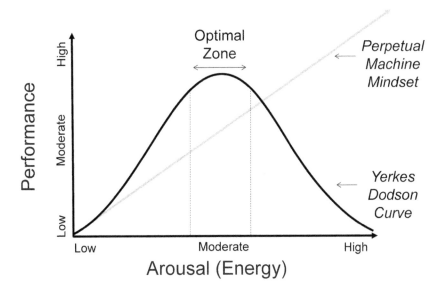

FIGURE 23.2   Perpetual machine mindset vs. Yerkes-Dodson curve.
Note: Optimal performance is actually produced at moderate levels of arousal or energy.

Take a moment to internalize Figure 23.2 by interpreting it in terms of a kind of pressured performance familiar to students—taking a test. If you go into a test with a perpetual machine mindset (straight line), you may think you can work nonstop overnight for your morning test under the belief that you will perform very well.

Reading the bell curve from left to right tells a different story. If you go into a test with low energy because you feel apathetic or fatigued (or worse, burnt out), you probably won't perform so well. Most likely, you'd be in a mental fog and have a hard time concentrating, making a decision, or moving into action. But when you go into a test feeling rested, prepared, and at a moderate level of arousal (optimal zone between dotted lines), you tend to perform better because your mind, body, and abilities are more in sync. The moderate arousal helps you feel more focused and able to respond decisively in the moment.

That said, you don't want to be so wound up that you tip over into anxiety and overwhelm (or worse, panic). In this case, you feel too scattered, everything seems equally important so it's hard to make a decision, you move into hyper-multitasking, or start to freeze and draw a blank. As this happens, your performance also suffers.

Now here's the kicker:

If you bought into the perpetual machine mindset and what you get is overwhelm and indecision, now there's a huge gap between your expectations and your actual ability to perform. With this realization, your energy plummets as you feel disappointed, angry, guilty, or ashamed. This is the situation that Manny found himself in. His unrealistic expectations of himself—fed by his deep-seated hard-work beliefs, his identity as a compassionate caregiver, and his workplace's culture—set him up for great disappointment.

Mapping Energy and Resilience

Now remember that Manny said *every day* was his patient's worst day.

It is one thing to have a bad day. It's another when there are only bad days, day in and day out. So, Manny's challenge is not about how to take a single test or deal with a bad day. Instead, he needs to learn how to manage his energy, work performance, and work environment on an ongoing basis (Schwartz & McCarthy, 2007). In other words, he needs to learn about resilience.

To help Manny begin to envision a new plan, I asked him to do an exercise I call "Resilience Mapping." The exercise begins with "neuroeducation," meaning a brief tutorial in how the body's autonomic nervous system (ANS) works and how fluctuations between sympathetic and parasympathetic responses are ideally balanced within a "resilient zone" (Leitch, 2017). (You can read more about resilience in Chapter 4.) Figure 23.3 depicts an "all things in moderation approach" in which an ideal sine wave fluctuates between an upper range of hyper-arousal and a lower range of hypo-arousal.

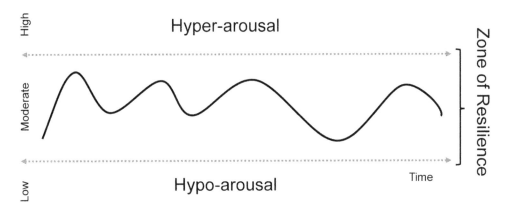

FIGURE 23.3   Resilient zone.
Note: Moderate effort and recovery over time leads to resilience.

In this diagram, when the line goes up, it represents the "charge" of sympathetic nervous system activating the ANS. When the line goes down, it represents the "release" of the parasympathetic nervous system calming the ANS. Above a healthy range of charging, hyper-arousal becomes less healthy, ranging from hyperactivity and hypervigilance to anxiety, rage, and pain. Below a healthy range of calming, hypo-arousal ranges from fatigue or depression to numbness and exhaustion (Leitch, 2017). Suffice it to say that the farther off of the middle level of arousal one travels, especially for extended periods of time without adequate recovery, the greater the risk for stress injury and illness such as clinical anxiety or depression (Kueter, 2020).

Resilience Mapping begins with the resilient zone chart like the one in Figure 23.3, except without a wavy line. I ask students to draw a line that maps their energy levels on the blank chart. The period of time can range from a work shift, a day, a week, a month, or a year. Figure 23.4 depicts the Resilience Map that Manny drew to represent his energy levels as they fluctuated throughout a typical workday.

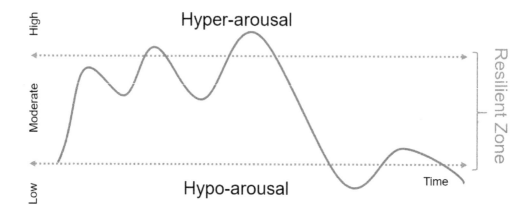

FIGURE 23.4   Manny's initial Resilience Map.
Note: Manny wakes up tired, goes through waves of hyper-arousal at work, and then crashes into hypo-arousal when he gets home.

Then I asked Manny to narrate his experience for me. He explained:

> I usually wake up still feeling exhausted. I drag myself out of bed, make a big thermos of coffee, and go straight to work. I get there just in time to start my 7:00 a.m. shift. As the night shift gives me the rundown on each patient, I'm getting anxious. I start picturing all the things that could go wrong that day. After she leaves, I go in and assess each patient for myself. I clean up the small supply cart in each room. I get so irritated by all the empty wrappers! Arranging everything makes me feel a little better though. Then I put on my roller skates and zoom in and out of rooms all day. Nobody takes lunch. Nobody pees. We just keep motoring through. I start

to drag late morning but have more coffee to keep me going. Then a patient might get in trouble early afternoon. My heart wants to jump out of my throat. It is all hands on deck. People on the unit pull together when something bad happens, but we are so short-staffed that I'm usually on my own. Except for our manager, who's always ready to chew us out for doing something wrong. She's old-school and always tells us to "suck it up." After we get things under control, I start to crash. I start feeling like I'm going through the motions. I'm watching the clock, just waiting for the next hand-off. I don't clean up the carts. They're never straight for me! I just want to get the hell out of there. When I get home, I eat some leftovers while I watch the news. I live by myself, so I binge-watch some TV, drink a few beers, until about 12:30 a.m. I get up at 6:00 a.m. and do it all over again for the next two to three days depending on my schedule that week. I swear I'm doing the best I can, but life feels pretty empty and I feel like I'm slipping. Something's gotta give, or I'm just going to quit.

Manny's narrative shows signs of being caught in a classic fight-flight-freeze survival mode, which in modern times might take these forms:

- **Fight**—Suppressing resentment; getting caught in a blame game directed at the situation, other people, or oneself; exploding in anger

- **Flight**—Avoiding conflict; numbing out in the evening with beer and TV; quitting a relationship or job

- **Freezing**—Feeling paralyzed; plunging into despair and burnout; hoping for a miracle

It was clear that Manny's unmanaged stress response and an unhealthy work environment had begun to take a toll on his quality of life. Without a change in this situation, his risk levels were bound to rise. The risks could range from Manny's health and well-being, to the quality and effectiveness of his team, to costs for his manager and the hospital if he makes a mistake or leaves, and regrettably to the safety of patients. (See Chapter 17 for a discussion of healthy work environments.)

Manny could have waited for outside forces to initiate change at work. Change could be triggered by poor patient outcomes or family complaints, changes in hospital policy and staff, or his manager or team members noticing his distress and taking steps to alleviate it. But after talking it over in class, Manny decided he didn't want to wait for these things. He wanted to take positive actions himself. He decided to lead from where he was today with two resilience practices in his pocket—grit and grace. As Manny discovered, grit and grace would not only help him improve his own resilience, but prepare him to use graceful grit to lead a change in his unit.

Starting With Small, Strong Steps for Self-Care

The Resilience Map exercise was itself a kind of mindful or contemplative practice. It helped Manny reflect, put things in perspective, and come to a decision. Though unsettling, accepting the challenges as real was essential to his decision to make a change.

Beginning to care for himself differently was a good place to start. Manny's self-care would require self-leadership because it involved motivating himself and making intentional choices about the things that were important to him. By starting with self-care, he not only gained the direct benefits of the care, he also exercised grit and grace at a beginning level. Once he felt more confident in his ability to call on grit and grace, he could apply them to the resilience challenges on his unit.

I encouraged Manny to start small. For starters, Manny thought he could improve his personal resilience by changing his sleep habits. So he chose to work toward getting eight hours of uninterrupted sleep a night.

Manny quickly realized, however, that this goal was going to be like going on a diet to lose a few pounds. He would need to make a number of small, strong changes over time to make a difference. Taking lessons from formal grit and grace practices that he'd learned in class (see the sidebar "Arrive-Breathe-Connect" later in the chapter), Manny applied them to small choices throughout the day that would affect his sleep.

It was summer and Manny lived close to the hospital, so he decided he would start walking to work, mainly to get some sunlight so he would sleep better at night. Manny used his walks to and from work as a kind of mindful practice. Some days he didn't feel like walking, but then calling on grit with its focus and determination, he remembered his intention to improve his resilience and walked anyway. While he walked, he intentionally noticed pleasant things and how they made him feel. This See-Hear-Feel exercise practiced on the go served as a way of growing grace with its qualities of calm and care. The trees, the fresh air, kids playing, and flowers blooming were a pleasant counterpoint to the cold technical environment of his critical care unit.

Gradually, Manny also made other changes to improve his sleep. After he ate, he skipped TV and beer and either called a friend or took a hot shower. After that, he didn't do any screens. Instead, he got in bed with a novel, followed by lights out around 10:00 p.m. With each of these changes, he did the inner work. With grit, he encouraged himself to stick to his plan, and with grace, he fell into the pleasant and more wholesome way he was beginning to feel.

Importantly, Manny had to learn to value progress and avoid striving for perfection. Manny wrestled with a loud inner critic, which he learned to counter with a more trustworthy inner coach. Some days, especially rainy ones, he'd "give in" and take the bus home. But instead of criticizing himself, he offered himself grace, also known as self-compassion. Allowing himself more give and take was an important part of his self-care too.

Taking on these self-care practices, Manny started to feel like he was better able to regulate his energy throughout the day. But he also was strengthening his abilities to call on grit and grace when making a change. In this way, self-care was teaching him inner work skills that would help him to show up and lead mindfully on his unit.

Practicing Grit and Grace

Recall that being in hyper- or hypo-arousal feels very much like being off balance. It's important to honor what you feel ready for as you attempt to move back into the resilient zone. If you are struggling with high degrees of hyper- or hypo-arousal, work initially to feel more grounded or centered. (See Chapter 4 for a discussion and specific practices.) When you feel steady enough to begin moving into mindful action, then you'll be ready to work more effectively with grit and grace.

As a yoga practitioner and teacher, I've experienced and taught that yoga trains you for embodying mindfulness in action. Drawing on traditional principles of hatha yoga, you can use yoga to train your attention on physical sensations, emotions, mind states, and spirit while you are moving. For many, this produces a more balanced and purposeful state of mind, not only while practicing yoga, but also off the mat. Learning to make inner and outer moves that adjust your steadiness and manage your energy in the moment can then be transferred to a host of everyday activities, including nursing and leading. In the yoga tradition, life force, *prana*, is a kind of inner work that can be subdivided into five energies or "winds"—*prana, apana, samana, udana,* and *vyana* (Anderson, 2013). *Drishti,* or yogic gaze, is used for focusing attention on a spot, but also refers to "a vision, a point of view, or intelligence and wisdom" (Life, 2017, para. 6). Here, I'm suggesting that working with grit and grace is analogous to working with the *prana vayus* and *drishti.*

A cousin of mindful leadership, *embodied leadership* is emerging as another mind-body approach to leading (Palmer & Crawford, 2013). Embodiment practitioners develop ways of holding their own bodies to generate a particular attitude, belief, or intention in themselves that shines into the way they lead. Grit and grace practices develop the inner poise and outer stance to lead mindfully. You can also develop skills for channeling these qualities into your verbal and nonverbal communication, helping you interact and respond more mindfully. Diverse leadership practitioners emphasize the embodied power of posture to shape mental attitude to convey a commanding presence. For example, the Army imparts the value of military bearing, physical training, confidence, and resilience as part of the presence and image of a professional (Department of the Army, 2012). Amy Cuddy's work on leadership presence emphasizes "power poses" for shaping inner attitudes and conveying confidence (Cuddy, 2012, 2015; Cuddy et al., 2013). Monica Sharma's work on transformational leadership emphasizes "standing in your full power" and embodying values (Sharma, 2017). Joan Halifax encourages combining strength and compassion with a "strong back, soft front" (Halifax, 2018).

In the beginning, practice grit and grace solo or with an experienced teacher. As you gain confidence, you can incorporate these inner moves into everyday situations. Starting with low-stakes situations is best. Then you can graduate to higher stakes situations, such as having a difficult conversation or acting decisively yet compassionately during a defining moment (Powell, 2016, 2020a-c; Powell & Hunter, 2020).

It's in this spirit that I designed a very portable practice that I call "Arrive-Breathe-Connect." Here's a brief introduction to the essential inner moves that you can practice on your own.

Arrive-Breathe-Connect

- **Arrive:** Take a moment to fully arrive in the present moment. Arrange your body in an alert yet relaxed position. Physically and mentally turn away from distraction. Turn off any sense of being on autopilot. Temporarily, disconnect from what you were just doing and from whatever's coming up next. Let go of your remembering mind and your planning mind. Simply bring your full awareness to the unfolding of the present moment. Right here, right now.

- **Breathe:** Now shift your attention to your breath. Rest in the awareness of your body breathing. Notice the quality and sensations of breathing. Watch the breath as the body inhales and exhales. If desired, breathe more deeply and fully on each inhalation and exhalation. You may count to four as you inhale and then four again as you exhale. You may also count each successive round of breath, especially if this helps to steady your mind. If distracting thoughts come up as you do this, simply let them go, like a cloud passing in the sky.

continues

continued

- **Connect:** If continuing to focus simply on your breathing feels right, stay connected to the sensations of breathing. If you are ready to move on to feeling more grounded, connect to the sensations of the body with solid surfaces—your feet on the floor, your bum in your seat, or your hands on your legs or on a table. From this grounded place, you may move on to connect to grit and grace.
  - *To feel into Grit*—Connect to the part of your body that you associate with feeling focused, powerful, and determined. Perhaps it's the sensation of your feet, standing your ground. Perhaps it's the sensation of length and strength in your back. Perhaps it's the sensation of your head and jaw, sitting with dignity at the top of your spine.
  - *To feel into Grace*—Connect to the part of your body that you associate with feeling calm, human, and caring. Perhaps it's the sensation of your breastbone, keeping an open heart. Perhaps it's your palms facing upward, as if to offer a hand in need. Perhaps it's your arms, ready to embrace and comfort.

Akin to learning to ride a bike, at first it may take a good deal of dedicated attention to learn Arrive-Breathe-Connect. Eventually with practice, it begins to feel more like second nature. In time, you'll imprint the moves into your mind and body's muscle memory, so you can call on them at a moment's notice. You may also begin to associate the sensations you feel with deeply held beliefs, such as your values or sense of purpose.

Be open to nuance and trust your experience. For example, it's enough initially to focus on just feeling grounded, especially if you have been feeling overwhelmed. Or you may find that practicing grit motivates and energizes you more than grace, or vice versa. All this is okay. It may be worth comparing notes with a friend, or talking with someone you trust about the small and large things you are observing and experiencing. The objective is to keep practicing and remain open to what you learn along the way.

Beyond this formal practice, you may start noticing grit and grace coming up in other respects. Grit may come from showing up to do your practice, even when you feel distracted or unmotivated. Grace may come by shifting your attention away from your judging mind and toward a sense of open curiosity, acceptance, goodwill, or compassion, whether directed toward yourself, other people, or a challenging situation. In time, you may be able to channel grit and grace simultaneously and blend them dynamically as a situation unfolds.

Shifting From Self-Care Into Leading Mindfully

After making self-care changes in his personal life, Manny started importing his grit and grace practices into his work life. At first, he watched to notice when and how grit and grace ebbed and flowed naturally throughout the workday. He noticed that he spent most of his day putting forward grit, so much so that his ability to call on grace was suffering.

As a small, intentional grace practice, he focused on his annoyance and resentment about the wrappers on the cart. Instead of rehearsing mental recriminations toward his colleagues, he reframed his actions as a way of caring for overstretched caregivers on the previous shift. When he saw things that way, cleaning up the wrappers transformed from a daily gripe to a daily kindness that made him feel good. He was surprised when the same outer behaviors (cleaning up the wrappers) started to feel differently on the inside just by changing his mindset about them. He realized his judging mind had created most of his suffering. Now he felt freer to focus on what mattered more.

Manny's inner work helped him understand that he was not the only one on his unit who overworked the grit side of resilience and under-exercised the grace side. To him, the perfect example of this was the team's habit of skipping lunch.

When he revisited his initial Resilience Map, Manny recognized that loading up on coffee and skipping lunch put him at a real deficit in the afternoons. (And all that afternoon coffee was probably also affecting his sleep.) He guessed the same was probably true for his coworkers.

The issue on Manny's unit wasn't a policy one. Manny's hospital allowed lunch breaks, but everyone worked right through them anyway. Manny read some articles about this. One cited "abundant evidence that correlates shift work, overtime, and long hours with errors, emotional disturbances, and occupational injury" (Witkoski & Dickson, 2010, p. 490). Skipping breaks was so commonplace in healthcare that the state of Washington had even passed a law referred to as the "breaks bill" or "nursing staffing" legislation that led to new requirements for uninterrupted meal and rest breaks for nurses, technicians, and technologists (McDonald, 2019).

Applying Grit and Grace to the Real Issue

Manny realized that the real issue on his unit was a collective habit that had become an unconscious and unspoken norm. No one took lunch because no one took lunch. People on the unit seemed to be buying into a perpetual machine mindset—"the more I sacrifice, the better nurse I am." But in actuality, this practice, fueled by an over-abundance of grit, was not only causing harm for themselves, but possibly their patients. To question their habit of skipping lunch felt taboo and an affront to their shared beliefs, so no one dared.

As before, Manny quickly realized that taking lunch would require many small, strong steps. But unlike before, he could not just take these steps independently. If Manny wanted to take lunch, he would need to interact mindfully by negotiating and collaborating with his coworkers, including his nurse manager.

As a very junior nurse, Manny's work culture sent the message that he was supposed to "stay in his lane," meaning he needed to know his place and just do his job. He didn't have a title or any kind of formal authority. While this was true, he wasn't powerless. He could still lead from where he was.

First, Manny had to acknowledge the power he did have, which was credibility and the power to lead by example. Manny was a very skilled nurse, proving early on that he had the clinical chops to do the job. And for all the misgivings that he had had about work and colleagues, he'd been careful not to act out on them at work.

So, he had a good base of trust and credibility to build from.

Manny started summoning grit and grace in conversations with his coworkers. He used grit to get up the nerve to ask a more experienced nurse who had worked elsewhere whether she had ever worked in a critical care unit that took breaks. Instead of getting all up in arms on the issues, Manny listened with grace to her descriptions of how nurses on her previous unit covered for each other. After a few conversations like this, Manny started wondering aloud whether the nurses on their unit might start doing the same thing.

One day Manny went out on a limb. With grit, he made a gracious offer to the experienced nurse when she was having a really tough day. "What if I cover you, so you can take lunch?" he said. She hesitated at first. Manny said it was really okay, they could just try it as a quiet experiment first. Though this felt awkward for both of them, they tried it. His colleague was so appreciative. Then one day the experienced nurse offered to cover for Manny so he could take a break. He used it to eat his lunch outside and get more sunlight.

In time, Manny and the experienced nurse felt more confident about talking about their experiment with others on the unit. The biggest concern was with the old-school nurse manager. By sharing their story with a few trusted colleagues, Manny and the experienced nurse gained a few allies. Together they started building their case to take to their nurse manager.

Influencing With Grit and Grace

How they made their case would be important for gaining the nurse manager's acceptance. Going in with a list of angry demands was sure to fall flat. Instead, they had to put aside their resentment and imagine the challenges she faced. With empathy and compassion, they realized she was acting so hard-core because her boss was holding her to high standards to ensure patient safety and reduce staff turnover. Realizing this made them feel more forgiving. But it also helped them understand how they could influence her.

To make a long story short, Manny, the experienced nurse, and a few others approached the nurse manager. They told her they had come up with an idea they thought would improve patient safety and staff turnover, which got her attention immediately. For grit, they presented research they had gathered on how occupational health and patient safety correlated with taking uninterrupted breaks during 12-hour shifts. They shared a method of staggering lunch breaks with coverage that they thought they could manage on a pilot basis. They bolstered their pitch by referencing the AACN standards for creating a healthy work environment, which included "skilled communication" and "true collaboration," explaining that they felt this project was helping them to gain these skills among them (American Association of Critical-Care Nurses, 2005). For grace, they said they recognized the nurse manager's own pressures and offered to include covering her lunch breaks in their plans too. Lastly, they invited her to raise her concerns so they could work through them as a team.

It took a few conversations to discuss their discomforts and worries about the pilot and to debug the plan. Eventually, they gave it a try for a month. Although there were a few hiccups, they learned from them and kept improving. In the end, they decided together to make the new norm stick.

In Real Practice

The Young-Brice and Dreifuerst study (2020) explores the concept of grit to examine one way that Black students "succeed in predominantly White pre-licensure nursing programs" (p. 46). In this secondary analysis of qualitative interview data, the authors identified persistence, the unwillingness to give up on goals, and persevering through challenges as factors critical in predicting academic success in nursing school. Grit factors included a commitment and determination to help others and to succeed in the face of adversity. Students also recognized that nursing programs are challenging for everyone, and that short-term failures do not determine long-term success. Faculty can foster grit in students by creating challenging but supportive environments and by helping students develop a "growth mindset."

Closing Thoughts

As long-time leader Ken Chenault is fond of saying, "The role of a leader is to define reality and give hope" (Wharton, 2013, para. 18). The ability to do these things, however, cannot spring from a distracted mind or a dry reservoir of energy. They require the focus and determination of grit to see things as they really are and the care and calm of grace to inspire optimism. And they require doing all this under pressure. Just as Manny did, trust that taking time for self-care in the form of practicing grit and grace will not only benefit you, but also people around you, whether patients and colleagues, or perhaps loved ones and your community too. May the ideas in this chapter help you grow your own grit and grace so you can do worthy things in your world.

Key Points

- No matter exactly where you are in your nursing education and career, now is a great time to grow your capacity for grit and grace.

- Grit helps you focus and take decisive action. Grace helps you care and act with grounded compassion. Blended, grit and grace are a powerful combination for living, learning, nursing, and leading.

- Leading mindfully means managing your inner experience and your outer behavior, which mindful practices can help you do.

- Taking care of your own resilience first offers lessons in grit and grace that you can leverage to lead mindfully.

- You can grow grit and grace through formal practices and in everyday life. Start today to improve conditions for you, other caregivers, and your patients.

References

American Association of Critical-Care Nurses. (2005). *AACN standards for establishing and sustaining healthy work environments: A journey to excellence* (2nd ed.). [Executive Summary]. https://www.aacn.org/~/media/aacn-website/nursing-excellence/healthy-work-environment/execsum.pdf?la=en

Anderson, S. (2013). The five prana vayus chart. *Yoga International*. https://yogainternational.com/article/view/the-5-prana-vayus-chart

Aristotle. (1926). *The art of rhetoric* (J. H. Freese, Trans.). Harvard University Press. (Original work published ca. 350 BCE)

Bergland, C. (2013, Feb. 2). The neurobiology of grace under pressure. *Psychology Today*. https://www.psychologytoday.com/us/blog/the-athletes-way/201302/the-neurobiology-grace-under-pressure

Cathcart, E. B. (2020). The new nurse manager survival guide, part II. *Nursing Management, 51*(6), 17–20. https://doi.org/10.1097/01.NUMA.0000662704.97080.df

Clear, J. (2018). *Atomic habits: An easy and proven way to break bad habits and build new ones.* Random House.

Coats, C. H. (2019, August 12). Grit and grace: A power combination for women leaders. *Forbes*. https://www.forbes.com/sites/forbescoachescouncil/2019/08/12/grit-and-grace-a-power-combination-for-women-leaders/?sh=2a9e2920404a

Cuddy, A. (2012, June). *Your body language may shape who you are* [Video]. TED Conferences. https://www.ted.com/talks/amy_cuddy_your_body_language_may_shape_who_you_are?language=en

Cuddy, A. (2015). *Presence: Bringing your boldest self to your biggest challenges.* Little, Brown and Company.

Cuddy, A., Kohut, M., & Neffinger, J. (2013). *Connect, then lead*. Harvard Business Review. https://hbr.org/2013/07/connect-then-lead

Department of the Army. (2012). *Army leadership*. Army Doctrine Reference Publication (ADRP) No. 6–22. https://www.benning.army.mil/mssp/PDF/adrp6_22_new.pdf

Duckworth, A. (2016). *Grit: The power of passion and perseverance.* Scribner.

Feist, J., Feist, C., & Cipriano, P. (2020, August 6). Stigma compounds the consequences of clinician burnout during COVID-19: A call to action to break the culture of silence. *NAM Perspectives*. Commentary, National Academy of Medicine. https://doi.org/10.31478/202008b

Fontaine, D., Haizlip, J., & Lavandero, R. (2018). No time to be nice in the intensive care unit. *American Journal of Critical Care, 27*(2), 153–156. https://doi.org/10.4037/ajcc2018401

Gino, F. (2016, April 14). Are you too stressed to be productive? Or not stressed enough? *Harvard Business Review*. https://hbr.org/2016/04/are-you-too-stressed-to-be-productive-or-not-stressed-enough

Groppel, J. (1999). *The corporate athlete: How to achieve maximal performance in business and life.* Wiley.

Haglund, M., Nestadt, P., Cooper, N., Southwick, S., & Charney, D. (2007). Psychobiological mechanisms of resilience: Relevance to prevention and treatment of stress-related psychopathology. *Development and Psychopathology, 19*(3), 889–920. https://doi:10.1017/S0954579407000430

Halifax, J. (2018). *Standing at the edge: Finding freedom where fear and courage meet.* Flatiron Books.

Halpern, B. L., & Lubar, K. (2004). *Leadership presence: Dramatic techniques to reach out, motivate and inspire.* Gotham.

Hanson, R. (2018). *Resilient: Find your inner strength.* Rider.

Hapangama, S., Gelabert, L., & Norris, S. (2020, August 10). The wounds are still fresh. *The New York Times.* https://www.nytimes.com/2020/08/10/opinion/coronavirus-doctors-nurses-healthcare.html

Hougaard, R., & Carter, J. (2018). *The mind of the leader: How to lead yourself, your people, and your organization for extraordinary results.* Harvard Business Review Press.

Kueter, C. (2020). *4 tips to prevent stress injuries for healthcare workers on the frontline.* School of Nursing, University of Virginia. https://www.nursing.virginia.edu/news/stress-first-aid/

Leitch, L. (2017). Action steps using ACEs and trauma-informed care: A resilience model. *Health and Justice.* 5, 5 https://doi.org/10.1186/s40352-017-0050-5

Life, D. (2017). See more clearly by practicing drishti. *Yoga Journal.* https://www.yogajournal.com/yoga-101/the-eye-of-the-beholder

McDonald, L. (2019, June 3). *New requirements for uninterrupted meal and rest break and hospital staffing policies for nurses, technicians, and technologists.* Washington State Hospital Association. https://www.wsha.org/articles/new-requirements-for-uninterrupted-meal-and-rest-breaks-and-hospital-staffing-policies-for-nurses-technicians-and-technologists/

Palmer, W., & Crawford, J. (2013). *Leadership embodiment: How the way we sit and stand can change the way we think and speak.* CreateSpace Independent Publishing.

Powell, L. (2016). Three important lessons in mindful communication. *Mindful.* https://www.mindful.org/can-we-talk/

Powell, L. (2020a). *Leading mindfully: COVID-19 and the Big Human Pivot, part 1.* Ideas to Action. Darden School of Business, University of Virginia. https://ideas.darden.virginia.edu/leading-mindfully-COVID19-and-the-big-human-pivot-part-1

Powell, L. (2020b). *Leading mindfully: COVID-19 and the Big Human Pivot, part 2.* Ideas to Action. Darden School of Business, University of Virginia. https://ideas.darden.virginia.edu/leading-mindfully-COVID19-and-the-big-human-pivot-part-2

Powell, L. (2020c). *Leading mindfully: COVID-19 and the Big Human Pivot, part 3.* Ideas to Action. Darden School of Business, University of Virginia. https://ideas.darden.virginia.edu/leading-mindfully-COVID19-and-the-big-human-pivot-part-3

Powell, L., & Hunter, J. (2020, June 26). How to recapture leadership's lost moment. *Leader to Leader.* https://doi.org/10.1002/ltl.20519

Schwartz, T., & McCarthy, C. (2007, October). Manage your energy, not your time. *Harvard Business Review.* https://hbr.org/2007/10/manage-your-energy-not-your-time

Scott, K. (2019). Making sense of work: Finding meaning in work narratives. *Journal of Management & Organization,* 1–21. https://doi.org/10.1017/jmo.2019.43

Sharma, M. (2017). *Radical transformational leadership: Strategic action for change agents.* North Atlantic Books.

Singer, T., & Klimecki, O. (2014). Empathy and compassion. *Current Biology, 24*(18), R875-R878. https://doi.org/10.1016/j.cub.2014.06.054

Sutcliffe, K., Vogus, T., & Dane, E. (2016). Mindfulness in organizations: A cross-level review. *Annual Review of Organizational Psychology and Organizational Behavior, 3*, 55–81. https://doi.org/10.1146/annurev-orgpsych-041015-062531

Watson, J. (2006). Caring theory as an ethical guide to administrative and clinical practices. *Nursing Administration Quarterly, 30*(1), 48–55. https://doi.org/10.1097/00006216-200601000-00008

Wharton. (2013). *American Express CEO Kenneth Chenault: Valuing EQ over IQ.* Knowledge@Wharton. Wharton Business School, University of Pennsylvania. https://knowledge.wharton.upenn.edu/article/american-express-ceo-kenneth-chenault-valuing-eq-iq/

Winn, Y. (2018). *How to train for a marathon.* REI Co-op Expert Advice. https://www.rei.com/learn/expert-advice/training-for-your-first-marathon.html

Witkoski, A., & Dickson, V. V. (2010). Hospital staff nurses' work hours, meal periods, and rest breaks: A review from an occupational health nurse perspective. *American Association of Occupational Health Nurses (AAOHN) Journal, 58*(11). https://doi.org/10.1177/216507991005801106

Worline, M., & Dutton, J. (2017). *Awakening compassion at work: The quiet power that elevates people and organizations.* Berrett-Koehler.

Young-Brice, A., & Dreifuerst, K. T. (2020). Exploring grit among Black prelicensure nursing students. *Nursing Education Perspectives, 41*(1), 46–48. doi:10.1097/01.NEP.0000000000000473

Index

NOTE: Page references noted with a *t* are tables; page references noted with an *f* are figures.

N

S

CPSIA information can be obtained
at www.ICGtesting.com
Printed in the USA
LVHW060934210723
753014LV00006B/201

9 781646 480807